DR. PAUL SLY AND
DR. NATHALIE BEAUCHAMP

SmartCuts

Biohack Your Healthspan: Cutting-Edge Protocols For Greater Energy And Performance

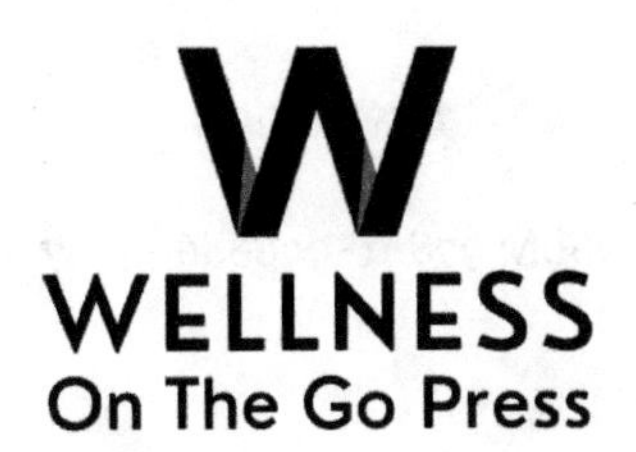

First published by Wellness On The Go Press 2023

The material in this book is not intended to be a substitute for the medical advice of a licensed physician. All material is provided for your information only and may not be construed as medical advice or instruction. No action or inaction should be taken based solely on the contents of this information; instead, readers should consult appropriate health professionals on any matter relating to their health and well-being.

The information and opinions expressed in this book are believed to be accurate, to the latest date, based on the best judgment available to the author, and readers who fail to consult with appropriate health practitioners assume the risk of any injuries or consequences.

Suggestions and recommendations of supplements and vitamins made in this book have not been evaluated by the Food and Drug Administration or Health Canada and should not be construed as claims to diagnose, treat, cure or prevent disease, as they are NOT intended to act as drugs nor to replace any drugs and/or treatments prescribed by a licensed physician. Lifestyle, dietary and supplement recommendations should be always be used in a supportive role.

Please be advised that the book is formatted to fit Canadian standards, thus the spelling of certain words will differ from American standards.

First edition

ISBN: 978-1-998886-06-7

Contents

Acknowledgements

To my patient and beautiful wife, Janet, and my sons, Coleman and William, you are the driving force behind everything I do. This book represents love and joy for life, and it also reflects the deep love I have for each of you. While it's true that writing this book took time that I couldn't spend with you, I believe it will prove meaningful and worthwhile. Thank you for being my greatest motivation and the foundation of my happiness.

With All my Love,
Paul (Dad)

* * *

To my most patient husband, for the countless times you've seen me coming with a new supplement, gadget, or strange concoction and thought, "here we go again," yet never fled—thank you. Your resilience in humorously weathering my ceaseless biohacking experiments, always game to try the next big idea, and steadfast in your belief that I've not completely lost my marbles, has been a source of relief and wonder.

With laughter and love,
Nathalie

Introduction

So much has been written about health. Why then are people more confused than ever about where to start when they decide to work on their health and wellness? It comes down to being inundated and overwhelmed with too much information that is disjointed and pieced together throughout time.

The aim of this book is to break down and simplify health information that encompasses all areas of your life, and to encourage you to feel your best by making simple lifestyle changes backed by science–essentially the "why" behind our suggestions. Only you can decide what you'll take from this information. That's why we encourage you to be your own health advocate–to customize your approach to the tools we give you.

There is no one-size-fits-all as we look across variables; men and women, age and stage of life, metabolic health and activity level, shift working and sleep, the variables are endless. This makes it impossible for anyone to give you an exact prescription for what to do, what to take, and how to live. Even in the situation where we work one-on-one with an individual, they still need to pay close attention to how they respond to different protocols. This is where you get to be your own health advocate or scientist if you will.

Now let's take a look briefly at human evolution and see why we've arrived where we are now.

The human body today does not function the way it did in the past. The last common ancestor of chimps and humans lived about 6 to 7 million years ago, representing the length of our evolution. Our current body first appeared as "early modern humans" about 40,000 years ago.

About a quarter of those 40,000 years, roughly 12,000 years, represents the agricultural revolution where our bodies looked like they do now. Additionally, only the last several hundred years have defined the industrial revolution or what we might call the modern lifestyle:

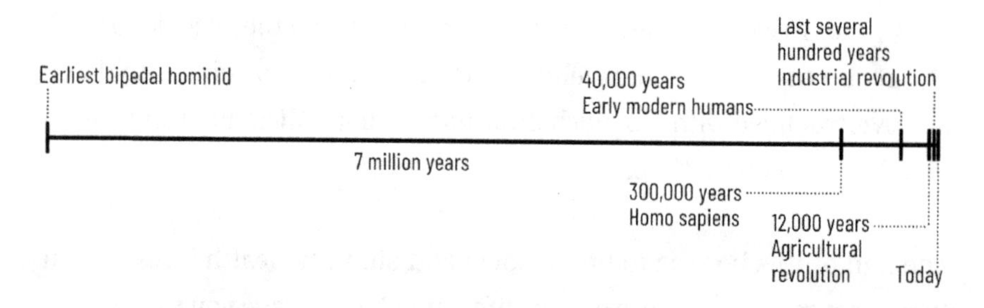

We are, in fact, animals, and for the overwhelming amount of time we have been on this earth we have been hunter-gatherers, working hard for our food, moving to where it was available, getting up with the sun and going to bed when it got dark. We moved and worked hard with our bodies in nature under the sun, with our feet on the ground. We were exposed to extremes of temperature. We could use glucose for fuel or fast and use ketones. We could store fat when food was abundant and use the fat when food was not available. In other words, we were metabolically flexible.

During the tiny fleck of time that represents our modern lifestyle, we have engineered out of our lives virtually all of the things that our bodies evolved and adapted to do.

According to Statistics Canada, the average Canadian adult spends almost 10 waking hours each day being sedentary. (1) Additionally, 84% of Canadians don't get the recommended minimum of 150 minutes per week of moderate to vigorous physical activity, and this is a ridiculously low minimum. (2) In the United States, the average adult sits 6.5 hours per day and teenagers 12-19 years of age sit 8 hours per day. (3)

Is it any wonder that approximately 65% of adults are overweight or obese and that 10% of the population has Type 2 diabetes? (4) As a result, we see waves of preventable diseases including diabetes, osteoporosis, heart disease, stroke, kidney disease, some allergies, dementia, depression, anxiety, insomnia, sleep apnea, and others.

Those waves have created a disease care system. Our overworked and overwhelmed medical professionals do an excellent job dealing with acute injuries and disease processes but have neither the incentive, interest, time or knowledge to help us look after our bodies and prevent disease processes from taking root in the first place.

If you visited your primary care physician and proclaimed: "I feel great, no complaints. I want to decrease my chances of getting atherosclerotic cardio-vascular disease (heart attack or stroke), diabetes, dementia/Alzheimer's, and cancer. What do you have for me?" If you are not met with a blank stare, you might be told to not smoke, drink less alcohol, stay out of the sun and wear sunscreen, and eat less red meat. Not exactly cutting-edge information, and in fact the latter two suggestions may well contribute more harm than good.

What has been termed by the popular press and culture as "biohacking" is simply health optimization. "Hacking", borrowed from web terminology, implies some level of dishonesty or cheating. That is not what you will find in this book.

Current science informs us how to optimally eat, sleep, rest, work, and spend our leisure time. While cutting-edge science often takes years or decades to filter into everyday medical practice, if at all, the keen and knowledgeable observer can extract relevant and timely information from these studies and apply them. Our goal is to present this cutting-edge information to you within a framework of protocols that you can apply to your everyday life and scale according to your level of commitment.

We must learn to take care of our bodies and lower our risk of preventable diseases ourselves, not only for our health but for developing the maximum potential we have for physical and mental performance. Our hope for you is that you become your best, most resilient self. Why? Developing resilience in both our mental and physical well-being is crucial. Mental resilience equips us to cope with adversity, maintain a positive outlook, and persevere toward our goals. Physiological resilience involves nurturing a strong body that can adapt and recover efficiently. Resilience is vital for personal growth, optimal performance, and navigating life's challenges.

What dictates not only your health but your ability to perform at your best is the way you sleep and rest, breathe, move and exercise, eat and metabolize food and use and maintain the integrity of your brain and nervous system. We will help you develop ways of optimizing all of these with protocols and tools that are often low or no cost, and introduce you to proven interventions that you may choose to invest in for yourself and your family. Some may be new variations on things you are already aware of. A lot will undoubtedly be things you have never heard of or did not even know were available.

We are all busy, but very few people who honestly assess the amount of time per day spent watching Netflix or mindlessly scrolling social media cannot find at least an hour per day to spend on themselves. In many cases, the tools we present may be incorporated into things you are already doing, taking no additional time or even saving you time. Some tools may require you to add something to your routine, but others will be a deletion. This is why we refer to them as SmartCuts. We want you to work smarter, not harder. The bottom line is you can influence your health in a positive way without spending any additional money or time. When you choose to invest, we will help you do so wisely.

This book is divided into the 5 following sections:

1. Sleep, Rest & Recovery
2. Hydration, Fuel & Foundationals
3. Movement, Exercise & Detoxification
4. Neurotransmitters, Hormones & Brain Wiring
5. Epigenetics, Ageing & Healthspan

The first three sections of the book discuss protocols critical to the most important basic care of your body. In plain terms, how to provide it with the rest it needs, how to feed and water it, and how to exercise and move it. If you get those correct and dialed into your routines, you will have improved your healthspan, lifespan and vitality immensely.

Once this foundation has been solidly laid, these concepts are further reinforced in Sections 4 and 5, as numerous protocols that enhance your physiological resilience also contribute to a happier, healthier mind, improved learning abilities, and increased resistance against the effects of time and ageing. These protocols often overlap with or resemble those outlined in the initial three sections, with additional justifications for their implementation. Furthermore, these sections will delve further into optimizing brain function and provide more advanced techniques to elevate your overall health.

Each section will provide you with multiple smart protocols, considerations, tools, upgrades, and resources to choose from to improve and optimize not only your lifespan but your healthspan.

Some of the protocols are basic, fundamental requirements that are frankly, non-negotiable for human health. Sleep is a great example of this. While many people are able to sleep 6, 5 or even 4 hours and still function in their day to day lives, sleep is one of the most crucial aspects vital to our health. You will learn that research has taught us that this amount of sleep hinders learning, negatively affects motor coordination, impacts hormones, and does not allow your brain enough time to pump out toxins—a factor in the development of dementia and Alzheimer's disease. Really, the list goes on. Gaining a solid foundation in such fundamental health practices will allow you to add in other protocols to enhance your personal health. Some may become part of your daily routine. Others may be things you do weekly, monthly, quarterly, or even yearly.

There is no substitute for the "N=1 experiment". You are the 1. We are all different, and we will change over the course of our own lives in terms of requirements and needs. Good stressors, known as hormetic stressors, like hot, cold, fasting periods, exercise etc., are amazing tools for finessing adaptations in your body. But during times of high stress, these should be used sparingly, or not at all.

There are practices your body needs and craves, but the details and nuances of how they are applied will vary. For instance, time is necessary for your digestive system to do its job and recover to prepare for the next day. This is the fasting period, hence the term "breakfast." We will provide ranges and even an average ideal place to start, but what works best for you? Only you will be able to tell.

You are on a discovery journey about yourself. Pay attention to what your body tells you and adopt those tools and practices that, when given a fair attempt, help you feel and function better.

Furthermore, it's important to note that the protocols we suggest are often low-cost or free lifestyle modifications, and can be readily incorporated into your routine. Our objective is to minimize reliance on external factors whenever possible and promote a sense of adaptability and self-sufficiency. This ensures that you can maintain well-being even in challenging circumstances. Consider the scenario of being dropped on an island without access to your belongings. Can you thrive without them?

It is also important to implement changes to your routine slowly. One protocol per week or two is what most people can manage. Effort and consistency are the keys to building habits. One of Dr. Paul's favourite quotes, which sits above his cold plunge at home, is very appropriate here:

"The comfort zone is where dreams go to die."

Get comfortable with some discomfort—where you start to get uncomfortable is where growth begins. Be consistent and have fun. Becoming stronger, healthier, and more resilient is just a few Smartcuts away, so let's get started!

How To Use This Book

Part 1—Embark on your Smartcuts journey by visiting our website and downloading the complimentary PDF that comprises all the suggested protocols in the book. Just go to smartcuts.life/summary-protocols or scan the following QR code:

As you read the book you can jot down your thoughts directly into the PDF for each of the protocols. Each protocol is delineated by its name and is accompanied by an approximate cost indicator, ranging from no cost to low ('$'), medium ('$$'), or high ('$$$') expense. After checking out each protocol, decide whether it's something you're already doing, something you want to start doing, or something you're not ready to tackle just yet.

Here is an example:

PROTOCOL—Mouth Taping - $

☐ *Currently doing* ☐ *Want to integrate* ☐ *Not for now*

Part 2—At the end of your SmartCuts reading journey in the book's conclusion, we will provide thorough guidance on how to help you incorporate the book's protocols into your daily life. We recognize that valuable information alone is insufficient without practical implementation. Therefore, our aim is to empower you with the tools and support needed to effectively apply these protocols and make a meaningful impact on your everyday well-being.

To Your Health,
Dr. Paul & Dr. Nathalie

Section 1—Sleep, Rest & Recovery

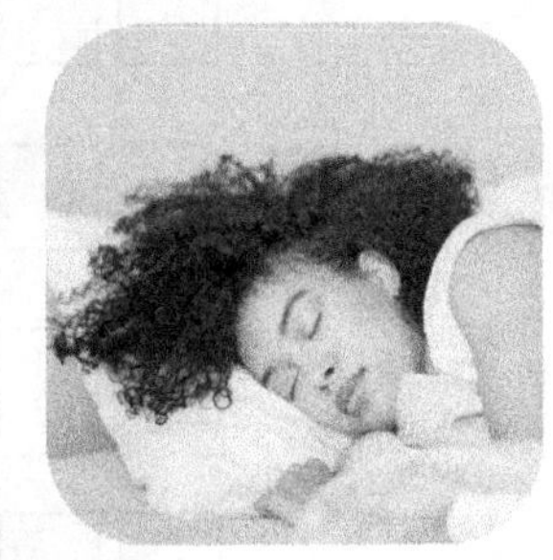

"Sleep is an investment in the energy you need to be effective tomorrow."

— Tom Roth

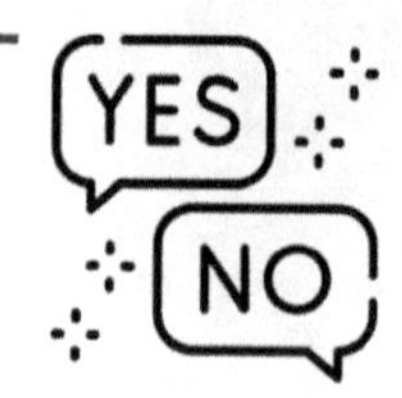

SELF EVALUATION-DISCOVERY QUESTIONS

Question		
Do you sleep 7-9 hours per night?	Y	N
Do you feel refreshed upon awakening?	Y	N
Do you go to sleep and wake up within a 1-hour window most nights?	Y	N
Do you feel your regular sleep position is comfortable?	Y	N
Do you breathe through your nose when you sleep?	Y	N
Is your mouth dry when you wake up?	Y	N
Have you been told that you snore?	Y	N
Do you have a routine to wind down before sleeping?	Y	N
Do you spend time outside exposed to sunlight first thing in the morning and at times throughout the day?	Y	N
Do you limit bright light exposure after sundown?	Y	N

Do you use white light therapy to supplement sunlight when you don't have access to natural sunlight?	Y	N
Do you have digital devices in your bedroom?	Y	N
Do you use hot exposure on a regular basis?	Y	N
Do you use cold exposure on a regular basis?	Y	N
Do you sleep in a dark room?	Y	N
Do you use sleep support supplements?	Y	N
Do you eliminate caffeine use in the afternoon?	Y	N
Do you pay attention to your body signals to figure out if you are not fully recovered?	Y	N
Do you have a way to track your sleep and recovery?	Y	N

Sleep and recovery are crucial to human health and performance. Many healthy practices can be sabotaged by failing to give your body the rest and chance to recover that it needs. Here are some fabulous protocols to help you do just that!

How Long Should We Sleep?

While sleep needs can vary between individuals, it doesn't vary as much as you might think. The consensus in the literature today is that adults require 7-9 hours of sleep per night for optimal function. Notice we said "optimal function" not "getting by". While you can subsist on less, and that has become the common thing to do, adequate sleep is absolutely necessary for immune function, consolidation of memory and learning, addition and preservation of lean muscle mass, and clearing the brain of toxic metabolic by-products via the glymphatic system.

Among the studied consequences of poor sleep:

- Weight gain
- Muscle loss (higher catabolic rate)
- Diminish your willpower
- Negatively affect your mood
- Decrease immune system function
- Lower anabolic hormones (muscles building) such as testosterone and IGF-1.(1)

To quote many of the scientists in the field of health...

Best nootropic (brain performance enhancer): SLEEP
Best stress-relief: SLEEP
Best trauma release: SLEEP
Best immune booster: SLEEP
Best hormone augmentation: SLEEP
Best emotional stabilizer: SLEEP

And the list goes on. We can't escape our biology. Find a way to spend enough time in bed to give yourself a minimum of 7 hours of sleep.

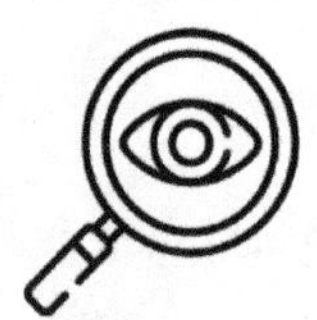

SMART CONSIDERATION

Stay On Schedule

One of the biggest disruptors of sleep, otherwise known as circadian rhythm, discussed below is inconsistent sleep and wake times, especially on our cherished weekends. A best practice is definitely to keep to a 1-hour window of sleep and wake times. Consistency is key. You are going to have nights when you stay up later than usual and we are not proposing that you never do. After all, social interaction is critical to health as well. As painful as it may be though, it is best to wake up no later than an hour past your usual time, and then use yoga Nidra or NSDR (more on this later) which was coined by Dr. Andrew Huberman, and stands for non-sleep deep rest. Your overall sleep rhythm will thank you for it. (2)

SMART CONSIDERATION

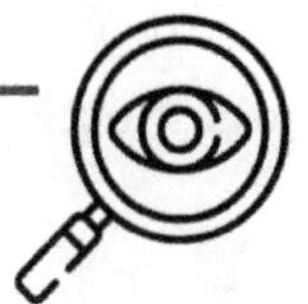

Sleep Position Pointers

There continues to be much debate regarding ideal sleep posture. Here are some suggestions regarding posture depending on your preferred position.

If you are a back sleeper, make sure your pillow is not too high; you want to avoid having your pillow push your neck forward. Additionally, remember to put a pillow under your knees to allow your lumbar spine to maintain its natural curve. Thankfully, for most people, this adds another level of comfort.

If you're a side sleeper, make sure your pillow is thick enough to fill the space between your shoulder and neck to keep your spine straight. Using a pillow that is too thin, and brings your head too close to your shoulder, can trigger pain and inflammation in the shoulder, potentially causing tendonitis or bursitis. You may also find it comfortable to cuddle a pillow to your chest to put your arm around. Finally, if sleeping on your side, draw your legs up slightly towards your chest and sleep with a pillow (a body pillow can be comfortable for some people) in between your legs/knees.

If you are a stomach sleeper, this can be tricky as sleeping on the stomach can be good for a select few who have breathing issues and also to help keep the cervical spine curvature and flexibility. However, many find that sleeping on their stomach makes their neck and lower back stiff when they get up, so this one is not black and white. If you don't need to sleep on your stomach, our recommendation would be to focus on the first two sleeping positions mentioned above. If you are going to sleep on your stomach, you may also consider placing a pillow underneath your abdomen/pelvis area to ease back strain and mitigate stiffness.

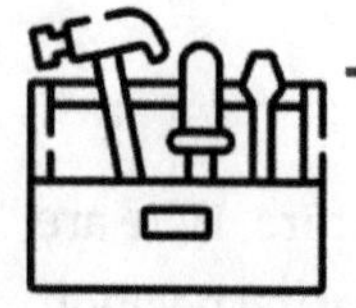

SMART TOOLS

Sleep Tracker

Tracking your sleep has become increasingly popular in recent years and for good reason. Sleep trackers are devices or applications that monitor and analyze your sleep patterns. These insights include sleep efficiency (the percentage of time spent asleep while in bed), sleep latency (the time it takes to fall asleep), and sleep quality (based on factors like sleep interruptions and time spent in different sleep stages). Some trackers also provide recommendations and suggestions for improving sleep habits based on the gathered data. If you own a smart device, chances are there is a sleep monitoring application installed, or you can choose a wearable device like Oura or Whoop.

SMART CONSIDERATION

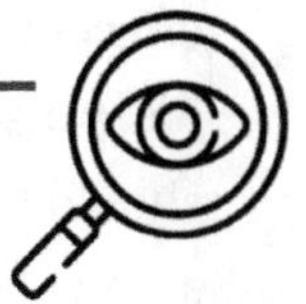

Key Biomarkers To Track To Optimize Sleep

Understanding the importance of, and optimizing sleep is crucial for your overall health and well-being. These biomarkers can be used to monitor both the quality and quantity of your sleep, allowing you to identify areas that may require improvement. With this knowledge, you can make the necessary adjustments to your sleep routine in order to achieve optimal recovery and reap the benefits of restorative rest.

Here are a few markers to consider:

- **Total Sleep**—7 to 9 hours
- **Sleep Efficiency**—Reflect the % of time spent asleep compared to time spent awake while in bed. For adults, a sleep efficiency of 85% is a sign of peaceful and uninterrupted sleep.
- **% of Deep Sleep**—Deep sleep is the most restorative and rejuvenating sleep stage. Makes up from 0 to 35% of total sleep. On average adults spend 1 to 1.5 hours in deep sleep but this slightly decreases with age.
- **% of REM Sleep**—REM sleep is associated with dreaming, memory consolidation, and creativity, and makes up anywhere between 5 to 50% of total sleep time. For healthy adults, an optimal amount of REM sleep starts at around 1.5 hours on average, although this duration may slightly decrease as individuals age. Research findings indicate a direct correlation between reduced REM sleep and elevated all-cause mortality rates. (3)
- **Restfulness**—Tracks the wake-ups, excessive movement, and getting up from bed during sleep. Too much tossing and turning can have an effect on overall sleep quality.
- **Sleep Latency**—The amount of time it takes to fall asleep. Ideally should be within 15 to 20 minutes. If less than 5 minutes could be a sign of over tiredness.

Sleep Position And The Glymphatic System

What does the way we sleep have to do with the glymphatic system? First, let's go over what the lymphatic system is. The lymphatic system consists of vessels and nodes that carry a fluid called lymph from tissues and organs to the bloodstream. Lymph is meant to help the body filter and clean toxins, debris, and pathogens that accumulate in our circulatory system as a result of toxic environments, medications, and an unhealthy diet. Lymph fluid passes through lymph nodes in our organ tissues. The nodes act as filtration stations that move the lymph fluid to the surface of our skin near the neck, abdomen, armpits, and groin.

Think of the lymphatic system as a city waste-removal service; garbage is removed regularly, and if not, the garbage will build up and eventually overwhelm a household. Our lymphatic system can become blocked and congested, causing stagnation in circulation and, therefore, having adverse effects on the body.

Now, what about the glymphatic system? It turns out that the brain has its own lymphatic system called the glymphatic system (a.k.a. brain drain) which is responsible for waste clearance for the central nervous system (CNS). Research is showing that when the glymphatic system is not working optimally it can lead to a higher incidence of diseases of the CNS such as Alzheimer's disease. Glymphatic system impairment may also play a role in traumatic brain injury, cortical spreading depression (slow, propagating waves of altered brain activity), and stroke. (4) The glymphatic system is most active during sleep. During sleep, the brain's interstitial space volume expands compared to its size during wakefulness or arousal. Increased interstitial space with sleep results in faster waste removal. (5)

Researchers confirmed that glymphatic transport and clearance were superior in the lateral and supine sleeping positions. The researchers proposed that sleeping on your side has evolved to optimize waste removal during sleep and that posture is considered ideal for glymphatic transport. Sleeping on the left side can help facilitate lymphatic drainage since the left side of the body is dominant in lymph nodes. This position allows the body to efficiently filter and eliminate waste materials. (6) Raising your bed height a few inches, with your head above the feet, can also help promote better lymphatic drainage. This can be easily achieved by using bed risers, adjustable bed frames, or placing sturdy blocks under the bed legs. This position also benefits heart health by reducing strain on the heart, improving blood flow, and enhancing circulation. It can help prevent acid reflux by keeping the stomach positioned below the esophagus, and it supports optimal breathing by allowing the lungs to expand more freely. In certain situations, sleeping with your feet elevated is recommended to promote circulation and reduce fluid retention.

Who would have thought that there was so much to consider when deciding on your best body position? Now, you may have your own limitations when it comes to positions as you may have a sore left shoulder or hip, so you have to take all of these factors into consideration before deciding on your most favourable sleeping position.

The Importance Of Restoring Nose Breathing At Night

As the old saying goes, noses are for breathing, mouths are for eating, drinking, and speaking. Nasal breathing almost all the time, most especially at night, is the optimum. Mouth breathing during sleep dries the airways, making any breathing difficulties worse. It makes it easier for your tongue to fall back against the airway, causing snoring and even sleep apnea. You lose 42% more water by mouth breathing. (7) In contrast, nasal breathing regulates your breath rate, making it easier to relax. Your nose cleans the air you take in, exposing it to your immune system and preparing it for your lungs, so you are not taking raw air into your lungs all night long.(8)

SMART PROTOCOL

Mouth Taping - $

There's really only one way to train yourself to do this. Take a small piece of 1" paper or micropore tape, and tape your lips in a lightly closed position, either vertical or horizontal. No need to press your lips together or pucker, just close your lips and tape.

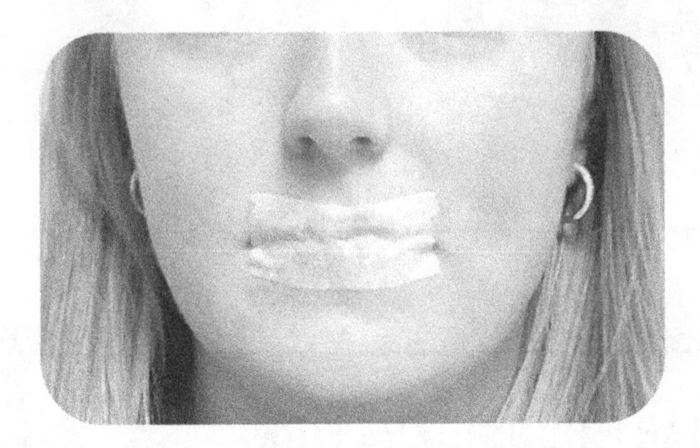

You may wake up without the tape. You may pull it off in your sleep during the night. Most people will adapt to it over a few weeks. It takes about 3 months to train yourself to breathe through your nose at night. After that, you may choose to discard the mouth taping, use it intermittently, or you may like the feeling and decide to use it nightly or periodically—your choice.

If you cannot stand the idea or feeling of having your lips sealed shut, or you want to have your child's mouth taped (nose breathing is critical for the development of the airways, teeth, and craniofacial structure). (9) Consider MyoTape which gently presses the lips together without sealing them.

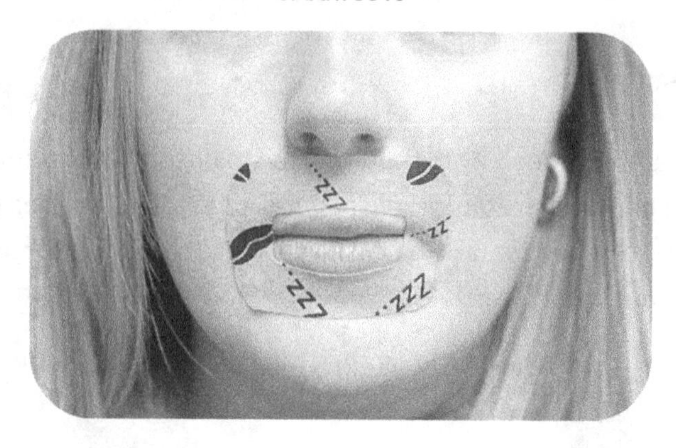

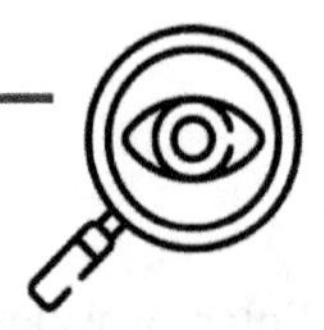

SMART CONSIDERATION

Reduce EMF Exposure

Cell phones are low-power devices that work on electromagnetic fields and they emit radiation in the radio frequency region of the electromagnetic spectrum. There continues to be considerable debate about human health risks with regard to cancer and other disorders and diseases. (10)

Why take the chance? You don't need your phone at your bedside close to your head, and for that matter, you don't need your home Wi-Fi turned on while you and your family are asleep. Leave the phone out of the bedroom, and put your Wi-Fi on a simple timer to turn it off at night.

Natural Light Exposure

The primary determinant of our sleep/wake cycle is exposure to light. Circadian rhythms follow a 24-hour cycle and can affect us both physically and mentally. If you find you are staying up too late at night, and are looking to shift to an earlier bedtime, make sure you are viewing bright light as soon as you wake in the morning. The low solar angle of the morning sun (less than 30 degrees to the horizon) has been shown to help stimulate the retinal ganglion cells in our eyes called melanopsin cells, which help trigger the production of melatonin, which helps you fall and stay asleep at the end of your day.

Sunlight also triggers your body to produce optimal levels of daytime hormones and neurotransmitters. The melanopsin cells are activated most efficiently by the wavelengths of natural sunlight, even on a cloudy or overcast day. The timing of exposure to light is what informs our bodies that it is time to go to sleep and time to wake up.

Everyone has experienced the different colours we see during sunrise, daytime, and sunset. Our bodies get information from these different wavelengths of light that inform us of what time of day it is. It is important to allow our bodies to access these light cues throughout the day.

SMART PROTOCOL

Morning Light Exposure - $0

This is one of those situations where the mechanism of action is complex, but the protocol is dead simple—get outside in the sun. Get exposure to 5-30 minutes of sunlight as early in the day as possible, preferably within two hours of sunrise. More on dull days. Less if bright.

- 5 minutes on clear bright days
- 10-20 minutes on overcast days
- 30 minutes on very dull days

No sunglasses. No windows. Prescription glasses or contacts are said to be fine but some companies are now stepping it up a notch and have designed prescription glasses that allow 55-60% of beneficial UV lights to enter the eyes. They claim that the issue with regular prescription lenses is that they are designed to block 100% of UVA and UVB rays, therefore not allowing the full spectrum of the sun and its benefits. There is a growing number of companies offering prescription glasses as well as clip-on artificial light protection. VivaRay® is among these companies, providing both prescription glasses and Clip'N'Go, a 3-in-1 solution which effectively reclaims nature's dark/light cycles in just one pair of glasses.

When outside, there is no need to stare at the sun, just "bathe" in the sunlight and let your eyes do their job. Never look at light that is painful and can be uncomfortably bright. You don't need to stare at the sun. Just let the sunlight all around you get to your eyes.

Do this again late in the afternoon, if possible within an hour of sunset. Any opportunity to get out in the sun throughout the day is good. This is how our bodies get information from the environment.

Don't worry if you live in a part of the world where sunlight in the winter months is limited. As soon as practical, get exposure to bright light—an inexpensive selfie ring light will do. There is no need to buy a pricey sunrise simulator. Keep that on for as long as practical. It takes up to 10 times longer to activate the relevant brain circuits with artificial light. Then get out and get some sun as soon as it rises.

SMART CONSIDERATION

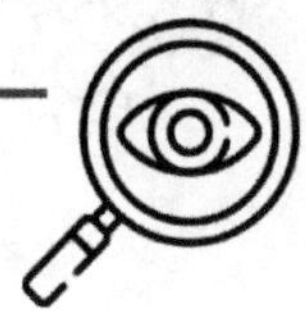

Follow The Sun

There are free Apps that will tell you the exact angle of the sun to the horizon. However, keep in mind that the sun moves through the sky about 15 degrees per hour, so you can use this information to calculate the approximate angle of the sun at different times of the day. If you want to be outside for the health benefits of sunrises and sunsets, note that the sun is below 30 degrees to the horizon in the east for the first two hours after sunrise and in the west for two hours before sunset.

Limit Light Exposure Later In The Day

Equally as important as getting light in your eyes at certain times, is NOT getting light in your eyes at others. While your circadian rhythm depends on the light at the above-mentioned times, it also depends on the absence of light, especially between 11 pm and 4 am. Every effort should be made to minimize bright light and eliminate blue light after sundown. In one of those cruel peculiarities of our nervous system, it takes less light during those hours to disrupt circadian rhythm than it takes to activate it early in the day.(11)

SMART PROTOCOL

Limiting Pre-sleep Light Exposure - $0

Limit computer and screen time after sundown. Wear blue-blocking glasses, and turn the blue light off on your screen in settings if you must use devices. Try to keep the light low, and consider red light bulbs in rooms you use after sundown. Keep your bedroom ultra-dark. Consider using an eye mask for complete darkness. It is a common mistake to wear blue-blocking glasses during the day. We want light, preferably natural and of all wavelengths, into our eyes during the day. Blue blocking glasses are for after sundown if you are going to be exposed to bright lights and screens.

SMART CONSIDERATION

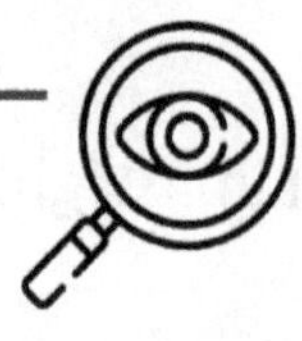

Choose Better Bulbs

Red light has very little effect on the circadian clock, so it is better to use an incandescent dim red light at night. LEDs (light-emitting diodes) & CFLs (compact fluorescent lights) do save money, but, unfortunately, they produce flickering blue light and dirty electricity which may have a negative impact on overall health. To avoid the harmful flickering of LED and fluorescent bulbs opt for incandescent lights (maximum 150W) or halogen (halogen light is a type of incandescent light) instead. (12)

Sleep Temperature

Our body temperature also follows the 24-hour circadian rhythm. It is lowest about 2 hours before our average awakening time, and peaks in the late afternoon or early evening, roughly 12 hours later. (13) The drop in body temperature that follows the peak helps us access sleep and is important for REM sleep and restful slow-wave phases of sleep. Either extreme of temperature is detrimental to sleep, but it appears that being too hot is more disruptive than being too cold. (14) Body temperature drops a degree or two as we initiate sleep, and this helps us to get and stay asleep. Taking a warm bath or shower, or for some people even a sauna an hour or so before bed causes the body to reflexively cool, helping this process of lowering body temperature.

SMART PROTOCOL

Sleep Temperature - $0 to $$$

Do your best to keep the temperature in the room where you sleep between 60 and 67 F. Try to start in the mid to upper range, and adjust down if you are able. Below 60 F is likely too cold and will actually trigger your body's warming mechanisms, which is obviously not desirable.

SMART UPGRADES

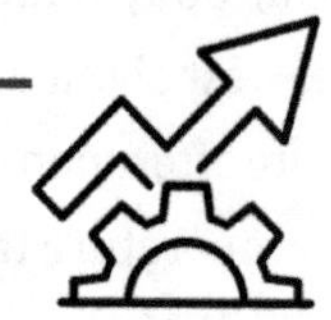

Temperature Regulator

Depending on where in the world you live, cracking open windows in your room even in winter can aid in keeping room temperature down, and the fresh air won't hurt! If temperature control is difficult, you may consider investing in a sleep temperature system for your bed, such as a Chilipad or an Eight Sleep System.

Recovery And Stress Management

Managing short, medium, and long-term stress is critical to health and wellness. Stress is an adaptive response that turns on systems that we need to deal with a particular situation and turns off systems we don't need. Stress is a combination of psychological and physical factors. It is inevitable, and while we cannot control the external world, we can and should learn to control how we respond to it. It is extremely difficult to control the mind with the mind, but we have the ability to use our body, our physiology, to control the mind.

Our autonomic nervous system controls the stress response by turning on the sympathetic branch. Heartbeat and breathing increase in speed, pupils constrict, and digestion and sexual responses are suppressed, all to prime our body for action, the so-called "fight or flight." The opposite response, the parasympathetic branch, is known as "rest and digest." These responses all happen without conscious thought, however, the one that we also have the ability to control is breathing. This makes breathing the remote control for our autonomic nervous system, and we can control our breath to modulate our stress response.

Our diaphragm is a large umbrella-shaped skeletal muscle that sits between our lungs and our abdominal organs, and it both receives messages from our brain and sends messages to our brain. When we breathe fast, the diaphragm sends a message to the brain saying, "Pay attention and become alert. I'm moving quickly." When we breathe slowly, it sends a message to the brain saying, "Relax. I'm moving slowly."

It should be obvious that we want to spend the vast majority of our time in rest and digest mode. The fight or flight response was intended to help us escape from the lion that we came across while foraging for food. Our problem is that the modern-day lion is our cell phone, job, traffic, financial strain, and relationship stress—all things that keep our sympathetic system on overload. This means our blood sugar stays high, we gain weight, we don't sleep well, and we begin spiralling into ill health.

It is this combination of autonomic and conscious control of our breath and diaphragm that makes it the ideal tool to manage the stress response in the short, medium, and long term.

Using Breathwork To Help Manage Stress

Did you know that breathing is one of the most impactful ways we can regulate our nervous system? Breathwork is often referred to as the remote control of the nervous system and it can change your physical and emotional state in seconds, helping you become calmer or more alert.

Light, Slow And Deep Breathing—To Be Calmer

According to Patrick McKeown, author of the books, *The Oxygen Advantage* and *The Breathing Cure*, the goal of Light, Slow, and Deep (LSD) breathing, is to help us be more calm, efficient, and resilient. (15) There are 3 components of functional breathing: biochemistry, biomechanics, and psychophysiology. Let's dig deeper into how to optimize these 3 components and what their benefits are.

Because it is a smaller opening, our nose regulates the amount of air we take in and out. The increased resistance to the air helps to activate our diaphragm. The nose is a major part of our immune system, filtering the air and exposing it to immunoglobulins and nitric oxide which help to sterilize the air. Nitric oxide is also a vasodilator that helps with gas exchange in the lungs. The nose warms and moisturizes the air, and recaptures moisture on the exhale. These are all things our mouths do not do for us with regard to breathing. Mouth breathing should be used only in times of extreme effort, or as a backup in the case of the nose being blocked.

Breathing **light** for biochemistry—the goal is to develop a decreased sensitivity to CO_2/increased tolerance to CO_2. Why? Here are the benefits:

- Increased blood flow circulation
- Decreased breathlessness
- Decreased respiratory rate
- Increased sleep quality
- Increased focus and concentration
- Calmer mind
- Increased oxygen delivery to the cells

To access light breathing, try to take very quiet breaths, breathing in and out slightly less volume than you normally would. You know when you have achieved this if you feel a slight air hunger, but tolerable enough that you don't have to take a big breath to make up for it. Try to anchor your concentration on where you feel the breath. That may be feeling slightly cooler air when it enters your nostrils and slightly warmer air when it exits. Or it may be the sense of air moving across the back of your throat, or the rise and fall of your abdomen. As your mind wanders, just gently take it back to where you feel the breath.

Breathing **slow** for cadence (and, as mentioned in the bedtime breathing section)—the goal is to breathe slowly at 4.5 to 6.5 breaths per minute to optimize autonomic nervous system function. Why? Here are the benefits:

- optimized sympathetic and parasympathetic balance
- stimulated vagus nerves
- increased gas exchange in the lungs
- increased resilience
- increased focus and concentration
- calmer mind

Try using a metronome (there are free apps available) or just watch a clock and breathe in for 4 seconds and out for 6 seconds, taking you to 6 breaths per minute. You can toggle the time up or down to experiment and see what feels best for you. You can try equal inhales and exhales, but a slightly longer exhale tends to be more relaxing.

Breathing **deep** for biomechanics—the goal is to use the diaphragm as the primary breathing muscle with proper recruitment. Why? Here are the benefits:

- increased lung volume
- increased oxygen uptake in the blood
- increased spinal stabilization
- increased lymphatic drainage
- calmer mind
- increased focus and concentration

To feel your diaphragm move, sit up nice and straight in a chair. Put your hands against your lower ribs, the web between your thumb and index finger against the rib, your thumb towards your spine, and your fingers towards your abdomen. Breathe in and out through your nose, and try to limit or eliminate vertical (up and down) movement of your shoulders and chest. You should feel your hands moving out slightly as you breathe in, and moving in as you breathe out, signifying the motion of the diaphragm. Your breath should cause this horizontal expansion of your ribs and abdomen, not a vertical (taller) expansion of your chest.

Now that you understand the power of breathwork, and before you start integrating the 3 components of breath together to leverage your physiology, let's figure out what your Control Pause number is so you can measure your progress in your breathwork practice.

Take The Control Pause (CP) Breath Test

McKeown also has popularized the Control Pause Test which is a self-assessment measure to accurately gauge one's level of functional breathing. It is an indirect measure of the body's sensitivity to CO_2. There are some other similar tests, such as the Carbon Dioxide Tolerance Test (CO_2 TT) or the Maximum Breathlessness Test, however, we prefer the Control Pause as it is the only one that does not involve the confounding factor of willpower when done correctly.

A CP of less than 25 seconds is indicative of a breathing pattern disorder, with a lot of room for improving functional breathing. The ideal CP for maximizing mental and physical performance is at least 40 seconds.

In order to test your CP, all you need is a device to measure in seconds, which could be your phone, stopwatch, or a clock with a second hand.

To take your CP:

- Sit comfortably and relax for 3 to 5 minutes.
- When ready, take a normal breath in through your nose, a normal breath out through your nose, pinch your nose, and start the timer.
- Hold your breath only until you feel the first definite physiological urge to breathe. This will usually be a contraction of your diaphragm in your belly or the muscles around your throat.
- Resume breathing and note the time in seconds. That is your control pause.
- This is NOT a maximum breath hold, and it is done on the exhale. If you resume breathing at the first definite urge, your next breath back in will be as soft and relaxed as your last breath before the hold.

Evaluating your CP:

- 40-60 seconds indicates normal healthy breathing and excellent physical condition.
- 20-40 seconds indicates a mild breathing impairment and some decrease in exercise tolerance.
- Less than 25 seconds is indicative of a breathing pattern disorder.
- 10-20 seconds indicates significant breathing impairment and poor tolerance to exercise.
- Less than 10 seconds indicates a severe breathing impairment, very low exercise tolerance, and often chronic health conditions.

In Section 3—Movement, Exercise & Detoxification, you will learn protocols aimed at increasing your control pause (CP). These protocols will enhance your respiratory control and optimize your breathing patterns. Monitoring your CP regularly is essential as it serves as a vital indicator of your progress along the way. In the meantime, begin by prioritizing nasal breathing, particularly during the night, to help improve your overall respiratory function.

SMART PROTOCOL

Know Your Control Pause - $0

For a period of at least 2 weeks, test your CP daily. It is best to do it at the same time every day as it will vary somewhat at different times of day. First thing in the morning is the best time to do it. Once you know this baseline over a couple of weeks, your CP can be used as a measure of readiness. If you are properly rested and you are healthy, your CP should be within a few seconds of your baseline. Significant decreases can mean you need more rest and/or your body may be fighting illness.

Oxygen Advantage Breathwork—Putting It All Together

To optimize your breathing and maximize your benefits, start by performing the LSD functional breathing exercise for 3 to 5 minutes per session, and aim to do about 20 minutes total per day. You can do it while in line at the grocery store, in your car driving, before going to bed, or anytime you want to calm yourself down. As we bring attention back to our breath by keeping it LIGHT, SLOW AND DEEP, not only are we going to be able to improve our CP score in the long run and experience the long-term benefits of keeping our nervous system in a more parasympathetic state, but we will also find ourselves calmer during stressful situations.

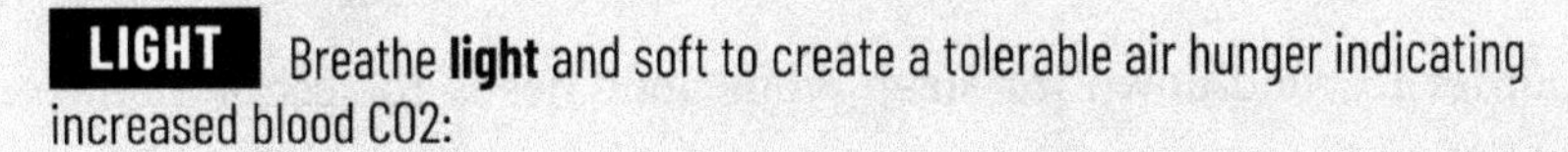

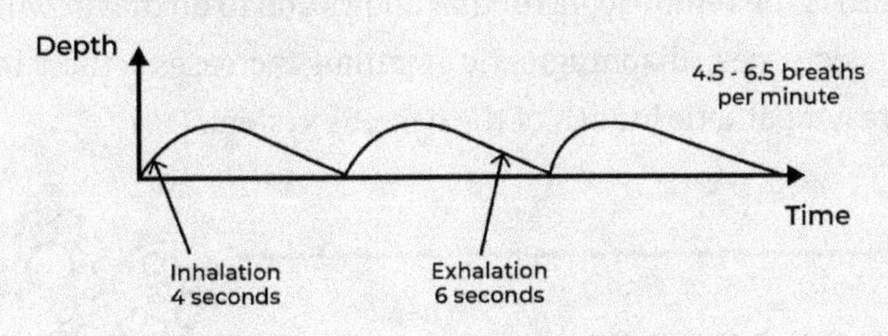

SLOW Breathe **slow**, 4.5 to 6.5 breaths per minute to optimize autonomic nervous system function:

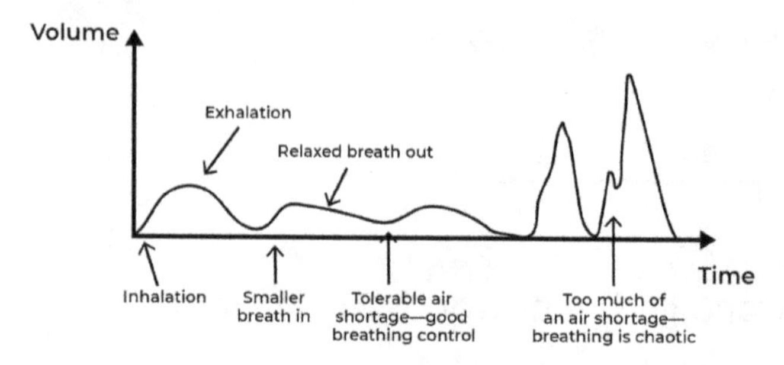

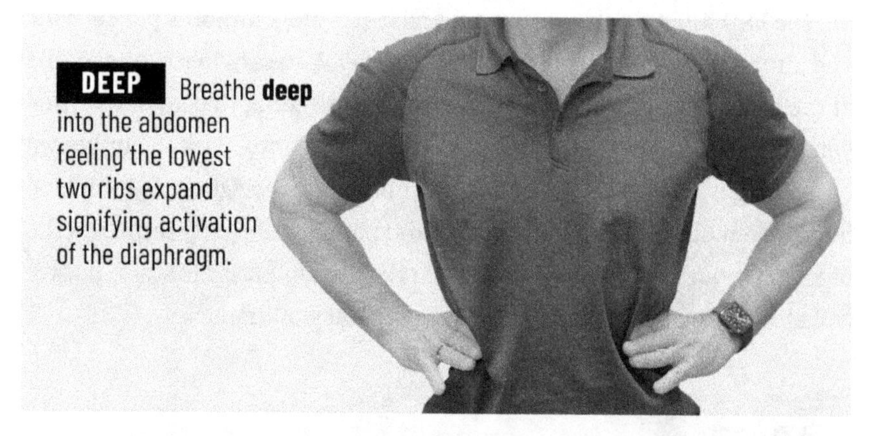

In order to wind down for sleep, your body needs to access a relaxed state. Your breath is the remote control that allows you to do that at will. Controlled light, slow, deep diaphragmatic breathing increases activity in the calming parasympathetic branch of the nervous system. (16)

SMART PROTOCOL

Breathe Yourself To Sleep - $0

Performing LSD breathing for 5-20 minutes prior to sleeping can transform your ability to fall asleep as well as access deep sleep. Lie on your back, get comfortable and give it a try.

Managing Short-Term Stress In Real-Time

In as little as one breath, you can calm the nervous system down. To make something extremely complex quite simple, we have a mechanism called respiratory sinus arrhythmia. What that means is that when you inhale, your heart speeds up, and when you exhale, your heart slows down. You can think of your exhalation as putting the breaks on the sympathetic response. If you consider a common stressful situation as a confrontation with a co-worker or family member, it is helpful to think of creating "space" between the stimulus that triggers you, and your response to it. In that space is an opportunity to calm your nervous system down. Take 1-3 breaths, more if you have time, in and out through your nose, and prolong the exhale. As a rough guide, make the exhale 1.5 times as long as the inhale. No need to count, or perform the breathing in a way that anyone would know what you were doing.

SMART PROTOCOL

Managing Short-Term Stress - $0

If you need more time to calm yourself down, do the following. Sit down in a comfortable position. Take a breath in and out through your nose, pinch your nose, and hold your breath for a count of 5 seconds. Take one or two breaths in and out through your nose, and repeat. The breath hold time can be up to ½ of your BOLT score time.

Managing Medium And Long-Term Stress

"Doing breathing exercises to calm the body is one thing. Having a daily breathing practice that creates a calm body is another." -Anon

Among the myriad of ways to relieve stress and create a calm body, regular focused breathing practice is among the most efficient. This can be done in as little as 5 minutes a day, up to several sessions of 20 minutes, depending on your level of stress and anxiety and what works for you.

SMART PROTOCOL

Managing Medium To Long-Term Stress - $0

Sit down or lie down in a quiet space. Set a timer for 5-20 minutes and practice light, slow, and deep breathing as described above.

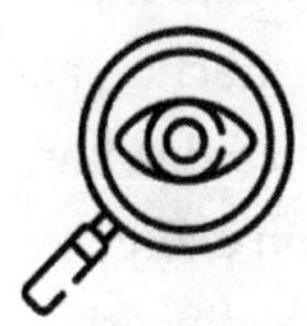

SMART CONSIDERATION

Breathe The Box

An alternative breathing practice to relax is called Box Breathing, sometimes referred to as Tactical Breathing due to its popularity with Special Forces personnel. It is simple. The length of the inhale, a hold, the exhale, and another hold, are of equal time. A good place to start, for instance, would be to inhale for a count of 3 seconds, hold for a count of 3 seconds, exhale for a count of 3 seconds, and hold for a count of 3 seconds. Repeat. You can play with the length of time (for example 4-4-4-4 or 5-5-5-5 etc.), finding what feels good for you. Remember to keep the breathing nasal.

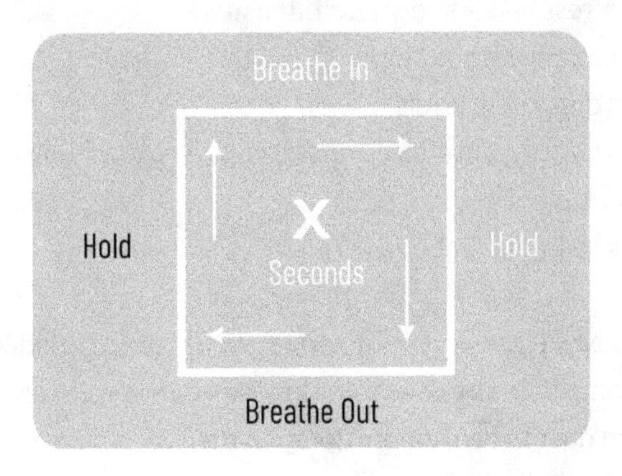

There are numerous breathing techniques and exercises designed for different purposes and outcomes, far too many to list in this book. If you are looking to dive deeper, or simply enhance your breathwork practice, an excellent tool is the BreathSource App. This App connects you to leading breathwork experts and provides comprehensive guidance on exercises and methods, helping you harness the profound benefits of breathwork.

Yoga Nidra

Another option is to practice Yoga Nidra, or Non-Sleep Deep Rest (NSDR). You simply relax and follow the directions from an audio script that prompts your brain to drift between a state of sleep and consciousness. You focus on different parts of the body systematically while concentrating on breathing. It allows your brain to get into a state very similar to REM sleep.

Some of the positive effects of Yoga Nidra are:

- Lowers cortisol levels
- Reduces stress levels and stress intensity
- Reduces anxiety symptoms
- Increases dopamine levels
- Improves sleep quality, sleep onset, and sleep duration
- Can help with insomnia
- Enhances immune function (17)

Yoga Nidra or NSDR can be done anytime you are feeling anxious, stressed, fatigued, having difficulty concentrating, or when you are trying to access sleep. You can do it in bed, on the floor, on the couch, or even lying on the ground outside - anywhere you can get horizontal and comfortable.

SMART PROTOCOL

Yoga Nidra/NSDR - $0

To begin a Yoga Nidra session, start by picking an audio track from the Smart Resources at the end of this Section, or by searching for Yoga Nidra and NSDR online. Choose a 10-Minute, 20-Minute, or 40-Minute practice, depending on your available time and needs. If you wish to incorporate breathwork, consider using Patrick McKewon's 20-Minute session from the Oxygen Advantage Method. Find a comfortable spot, lie down, and use a pillow, blanket (weighted if possible), or sleep mask for added comfort. Finally, follow the audio script as you practice Yoga Nidra.

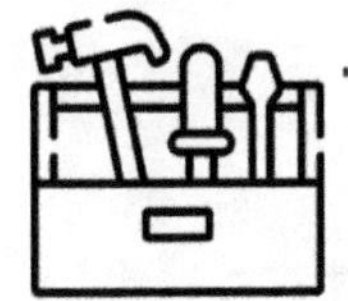

SMART TOOLS

Weighted Blankets

Weighted blankets have gained popularity in recent years. Potential benefits of a weighted blanket may include improvement in anxiety, depression, insomnia, chronic pain, and restless leg syndrome. A weighted blanket has a filling that makes it heavier than traditional blankets and provides pressure to the person's body, not so different from an oxytocin-releasing hug.

According to one of the many studies on it—more are needed—the Deep Touch Pressure Stimulation (DTPS) offered by the blanket gives the feeling of safety, relaxation, and comfort, helping to improve anxiety. (18)(19) DTPS has been shown to help reduce cortisol levels in our system as well as help decrease sympathetic arousal—our fight or flight system while increasing parasympathetic arousal—our rest and digest system to help us feel calmer. Two or more hormones come into play here, too: serotonin and melatonin. Serotonin is also known as our 'happy' hormone, and melatonin is our sleep hormone. Both of these hormones are released into our system when we experience DTPS.

Weighted blankets can be filled with different materials. Look for organic cotton shells and non-conductive materials like glass pellets or even flaxseeds. One should look for about 10 percent of their body weight, so if you weigh 150 pounds, a 15-pound blanket would likely be best.

Use a smaller weighted blanket for your meditation or Yoga-Nidra practice or on your bed as a full blanket.

Hot And Cold Therapy

The use of hot and cold in various forms dates back to ancient times. The science behind these practices is now becoming clear. The use of hot and cold is the intersection between recovery and mental and physical well-being.

The concept of hormetic stress or eustress embodies the old saying "What doesn't kill you makes you stronger!" Subjecting yourself to deliberate stress in the form of uncomfortable heat (i.e., sauna) or cold (i.e., cold shower or plunge) forces your body to adapt in a variety of ways at the cellular level that is good for overall health and promotes longevity. Hormetic stress can help repair cellular damage, repair DNA, work against oxidative stress, produce new mitochondria (energy packs of cells), reduce inflammation, help eliminate toxins, and help blood sugar regulation. (20)

Hormetic stress is also an excellent form of stress inoculation. If you can lean into the discomfort and control your body when your mind is telling you to get out of the situation, you learn to control your response to stress. You are learning to control your physiology and psychology.

Examples of hormetic stressors include hot and cold exposure which are the present subject, but also other practices found in this book such as time-restricted eating, intense exercise, and intermittent hypoxia breathwork.

Deliberate Heat Exposure

When we expose ourselves to short-term stressors like heat, our body undergoes a series of reactions, one of which involves activating the dynorphin system. This system acts as a regulator, influencing the release of different neurotransmitters, including endorphins. Endorphins are well-known for their ability to promote positive emotions and reduce the perception of pain.

The dynorphin system interacts with other neurochemicals in our brain, such as dopamine and serotonin, which further contribute to the overall improvement of mood. It also stimulates the production of endogenous opioids, which are natural substances in our body that relieve pain. These opioids not only alleviate physical discomfort but also induce a sense of euphoria and general well-being.

Heat stress also induces a cardiovascular response similar to that of moderate cardiovascular exercise. This similarity presents an excellent opportunity for individuals who may be unable to engage in conventional exercise due to disability or other reasons. Moreover, when individuals combine sauna sessions with regular exercise, their cardiorespiratory system experiences even greater improvements compared to doing either activity alone.

A Finnish sauna cohort study of more than 2000 sauna users found that 3-7 saunas a week were associated with a 40% lower all-cause mortality, compared with one sauna per week or no sauna. (21) One of the main effects is the increase in heat shock proteins. As our cells function, they create by-products that damage proteins and cause them to "clump." These protein clumps are a common feature of cardiovascular disease as well as nerve-damaging diseases such as Alzheimer's, Parkinson's, and Huntington's. Heat shock proteins repair the damaged proteins and may protect against these diseases. According to Søberg et al (2021), 57 minutes per week of sauna exposure over 2-3 sessions is adequate for optimizing the benefits. (22) Deliberate heat exposure should be approached gradually to allow the body to adapt and acclimatize to the heat. It is important to listen to your body and pay attention to any signs of distress.

SMART PROTOCOL

Deliberate Heat Exposure - $0 to $$$

Three sessions of 20 minutes each per week is a great goal for sauna use. How hot? "This is hot. I want to get out, but I can safely stay in."

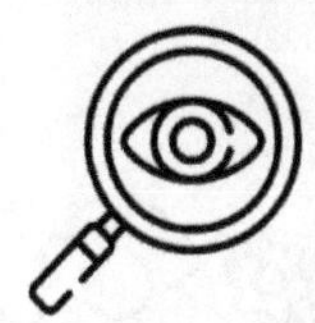

SMART CONSIDERATION

Feel The Heat

A hot tub or hot bath in the absence of access to a sauna is an option, though difficult to get warm enough for positive effects and still be able to tolerate. Remember—uncomfortably warm but safe.

Deliberate Cold Exposure

Cold exposure of sufficient intensity likewise has many beneficial effects. It increases noradrenaline, used in many antidepressants, to improve your mood. It boosts neurotransmitters like dopamine that increase motivation and focus. In about one minute, glucose consumption increases along with a metabolic rate increase of 350%. Cold shock proteins are activated, which help with cellular repair processes. Cold exposure and the adrenaline release that goes with it shift white fat to beige and activate brown fat—which is thermogenic—thus increasing fat burning. (23) Cold exposure can reduce systemic inflammation and inflammation in the brain. According to Søberg et al, 11 minutes total per week is optimum. Note that immersion to the neck is better than a cold shower, which is better than cold air. (24) When doing a cold plunge, it is best to get into the water quickly. Your body heat will warm the layer of water surrounding you creating a protective thermal layer. Movement disrupts this layer, diminishing its insulating effect so if you want an extra challenge move your arms and legs a little.

SMART PROTOCOL

Deliberate Cold Exposure - $0 to $$$

The ideal cold exposure time frame is to spend 11 minutes total per week, divided into 2-4 sessions. Immersing yourself to the level of your neck will benefit you more than taking a cold shower. Most people would find the most accessible way to do this is to start by ending your shower with 30 seconds of full cold, and work your way up from here.

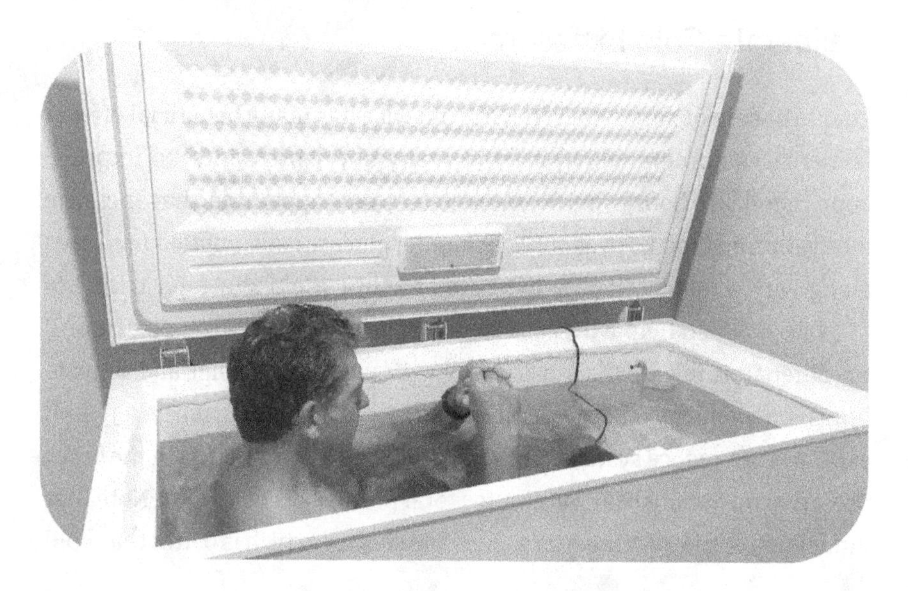

How cold? "This is cold. I want to get out, but I can safely stay in." Remember, always do this exercise with a buddy. As a reference, at 0 degrees Celsius, it takes more than 15 minutes of exposure to cause hypothermia.

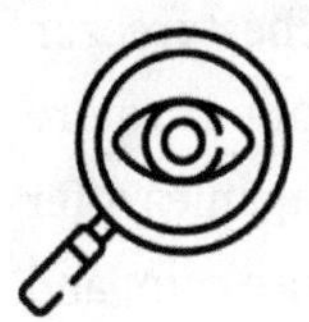

SMART CONSIDERATION

Get Chilly

In the absence of access to a cold plunge, the next best thing is to fill your tub with cold water and use ice as necessary. A good safe starting point would be 60 deg F or 16 deg C. Inexpensive thermometers like those used for a pool can be purchased in a variety of places. The next best option is cold showers. People have a visceral reaction to cold - they can't fathom themselves doing this. You may start by splashing cold water on your face and holding your hands in cold water for 15 seconds. Build up to a minute, then end your showers with 10-15 seconds cold, and gradually increase to a few minutes. Build your way up gradually and tolerably.

SMART UPGRADES

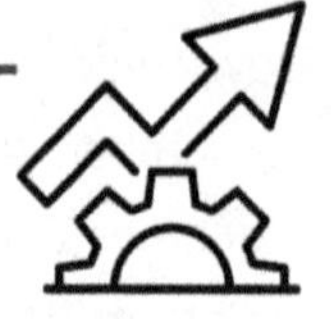

Cold Plunge

If you're interested in building your own cold plunge using a chest freezer, a valuable resource can be found at chestfreezercoldplunge.com. If you're leaning towards a pre-made cold plunge, many reputable companies offer great products. Check out sites like morozkoforge.com, coldture.com, and icebarrel.com for a diverse selection. While some options might be on the pricier side, you should be able to find a unit that aligns with your budget and requirements.

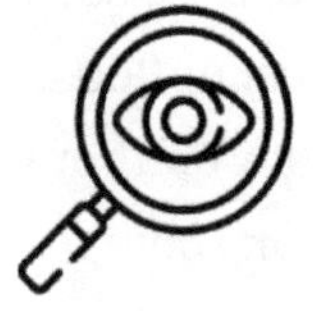

SMART CONSIDERATION

Hot Or Cold?

A note on using both heat and cold. You may choose to go back and forth from cold to hot, and this can be a great practice. According to Søberg et al, to preserve the benefits of cold exposure you should end these cycles with cold and let your body re-warm naturally. (25)

SMART CONSIDERATION

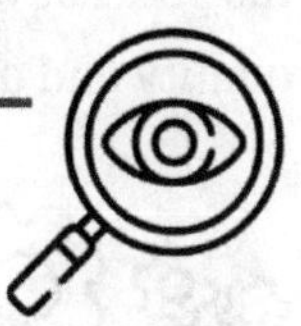

Timing Is Key

In the realm of bodybuilding and athletics, it's often advised to refrain from cold exposure post-workout. This is due to the anti-inflammatory properties of the cold, which can potentially dampen the body's muscle-building abilities. For those focusing on muscle growth through resistance training, it's preferable to avoid cold exposure on training days or, if unavoidable, to create a minimum 4-hour buffer between the two activities. However, for the average individual pursuing general fitness goals, a short period of cold exposure following a workout can convey the advantages typically associated with such a practice. As always, it is essential to make individualized decisions based on your specific needs and goals.

Sleep Supplements

When you have all the lifestyle elements nailed down—your relationship to and use of light, temperature, the comfort of the bed, breath control and/or Yoga Nidra and NSDR, enough time to sleep 7-9 hours—and you are still having trouble accessing good quality and quantity sleep, there are some supplements that can help.

The following recommendations come from Dr. Andrew Huberman from his podcast when he shared researched supplement use for enhancing the quality and quantity of sleep. (26)

SMART PROTOCOL

Difficulty FALLING Asleep - $

If you have trouble falling asleep, try:

- Magnesium Threonate or Glycinate, 145mg, 30-60 minutes before sleep
- Apigenin: 50mg daily, 30-60 minutes before sleep
- L-theanine at a dosage range of 100-400mg, 30-60 minutes before sleep

These supplements can be taken individually or all together. You need to find what works for you. They all have a wide safety margin, but you should check with your physician and/or pharmacist before adding anything to your supplement regime.

In roughly 5% of people, magnesium threonate can cause gastrointestinal irritation, in which case it should not be used. L-theanine has a wider potential dose, so start on the low end and increase if needed. For some people, L-theanine can cause vivid dreams to the point that it is uncomfortable, in which case it also should not be used. As always you need to experiment to find what works for you.

Difficulty Staying Asleep

If you have a hard time staying asleep, especially waking up between 2 and 4 am, some different considerations may be necessary.

A blood sugar dip in the middle of the night is a common cause of awakening. A continuous glucose monitor, in this case, can be helpful to see if a drop in blood sugar is the problem (see Section 2—Hydration, Fuel, & Foundationals). Yes, this goes against the idea of time-restricted eating, but again this is a case where what works for most may not work for you. Consider a trial of eating a judicious amount of quality protein and fat closer to bedtime.

During times of greater stress, your cortisol response may be prolonged or early, causing you to awaken. Cortisol is a hormone produced by the adrenal glands. It regulates a wide range of processes throughout the body, including regulating metabolism and helping to control blood sugar levels, memory formation, blood pressure, and affecting immune responses such as inflammation. It also plays an important role in helping the body respond to stress. Cortisol peaks in the first hour or so of your day, and is important in helping your body wake up.

Try using an adaptogen like Ashwagandha to modulate your cortisol response. It is suggested to take two doses of Ashwagandha daily, one in the afternoon and one in the evening closer to bed. This dose schedule allows cortisol to peak normally in the morning as it should, but not later in the day. It is recommended to take it only during times of stress, or for a maximum of one month and then 2-4 weeks off.

Myo-inositol can be helpful in improving sleep quality. A study published in the Journal of Clinical Psychiatry found that taking 12 grams of inositol before bedtime significantly improved sleep quality in participants with depression. (27) Other research has also reported improvements in sleep quality in individuals taking inositol, including increased deep sleep and reduced sleep onset latency (the time it takes to fall asleep). According to Dr. James DiNicolantonio in his book, *Win*, inositol can have a mild laxative effect on some people, which may necessitate dividing the dosage over the course of the day to as little as 500 mg 4 times per day, or a single dose before bedtime. As with anything it is wise to start at the low end of the recommended dose range and increase as necessary. (28)

A number of studies have been conducted on the use of glycine as a sleep aid, with generally positive results. For example, a study published in the Journal of Clinical Biochemistry and Nutrition found that taking 3 grams of glycine before bedtime significantly improved sleep quality in participants with sleep disturbances. Other studies have also reported improvements in sleep quality, including increased deep sleep and reduced sleep onset latency in individuals taking glycine. (29)

There is some research suggesting that supplements containing GABA may be effective in improving sleep quality and duration. For example, a study published in the Journal of Clinical Psychopharmacology found that taking a GABA supplement before bedtime significantly reduced the time it took for participants to fall asleep and increased the amount of time they spent in deep sleep. (30)

These supplements are generally safe to experiment with to see if they help you, after checking with your health professionals as suggested above. For instance, Dr. Huberman suggests alternating their use, taking glycine and GABA together one night and inositol the next, not taking either more than a few times per week.

Again, you as an individual may benefit from some, all, or none of the above suggestions.

The use of melatonin is widespread, however, melatonin is a hormone and is the only one that can be taken without a prescription. The doses taken are extremely high compared to what is made in your body. Hormones typically have multiple effects, for instance, melatonin delays puberty in youngsters and adolescents. The supplements mentioned are likely a safer alternative.

SMART PROTOCOL

Difficulty STAYING Asleep Or Accessing Better Sleep Quality And Duration - $

- Consider a trial of eating a judicious amount of quality protein and fat closer to bedtime to prevent a blood sugar dip.
- Take two doses of 250-300 mg of Ashwagandha, one in the afternoon and one in the evening closer to bed.
- Take myo-inositol at a dosage range of 900 mg-4 g an hour before bed. If you find it has a laxative effect at higher doses, divide the doses and take 4 times per day.
- Take glycine at a dosage range of 2-3 g before bed.
- Take 100 mg of gamma-aminobutyric acid (GABA) an hour before bed.

SMART CONSIDERATION

Delay Caffeine Consumption

Sometimes what you don't take is as important as what you do take. These authors both use caffeine in the form of coffee and are proponents of its benefits. Even if you are the type who can drink coffee or other forms of caffeine and fall asleep, however, it is most probably disrupting the quality of your sleep in the form of disrupting your natural sleep rhythms. Coffee works by blocking the receptors for adenosine.

Adenosine is a neurotransmitter made in the brain, and it binds to adenosine receptors, causing drowsiness by slowing down nerve cell activity, promoting sleep, and suppressing arousal.

Adenosine builds up in your system over the course of the day. Caffeine is an adenosine receptor antagonist, which means it blocks the receptors but does not mimic its actions. In this way, caffeine acts as a stimulant, and recent research has even shown that adenosine receptor antagonists can modify brain dysfunctions and diseases like Alzheimer's disease, Parkinson's disease, Huntington's disease, epilepsy, pain/migraine, depression, and schizophrenia. Researchers are using caffeine and other adenosine receptor antagonists and agonists as therapeutic tools against neurodegenerative diseases. (31)

Along with the many effects discussed, caffeine also increases cortisol production. When you wake up in the morning after a night of adequate sleep, your adenosine is at a low baseline level and cortisol rises. Because of this delicate balance of the body awakening, adenosine clearing, and cortisol rising, and the fact that caffeine modulates these factors, many doctors and scientists believe it is best to delay caffeine intake for 90-120 minutes after waking.

There are two considerations. The first is that because cortisol is already peaking, you are wasting the stimulating effect of the caffeine, which would be more helpful once cortisol has started to drop. (32) The second is the theory that this interference of caffeine with the normal clearing of adenosine and rise in cortisol contributes to the early to mid-afternoon crash in energy many people experience. (33)

As painful as the prospect may seem to some, the optimum use of caffeine may be to delay its use for 90-120 minutes after waking to allow the adenosine receptors to clear properly, and eliminate its use in the afternoon, certainly beyond 3 or 4 pm, depending on your usual sleep time, and maybe earlier. Caffeine has a half-life of approximately six hours, which means that half of the caffeine consumed will still be present in the body after this time. This can lead to difficulty falling asleep, shorter sleep duration, and reduced sleep quality, ultimately leading to fatigue and reduced productivity the following day. It is wise, therefore, to limit caffeine consumption to the early part of the day. Certain individuals may have a reduced ability to eliminate or process caffeine effectively, resulting in its lingering effects. Despite consuming caffeine late in the day, these individuals might still manage to fall asleep, but the consequences of this can be more subtle and impactful. Specifically, the quality of their sleep architecture may be altered, leading to shallower and less restorative sleep. This disruption can impact various aspects of sleep, including the time spent in deep sleep and rapid eye movement (REM) sleep, which are crucial for physical restoration, memory consolidation, and overall cognitive functioning.

SMART CONSIDERATION

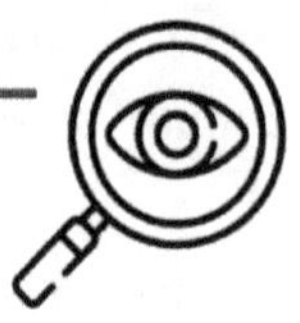

Transmission Timeout

We are big fans of tracking and quantifying certain metrics for monitoring health, however, we are not as enthusiastic about constantly transmitting data through these various wearable devices.

As mentioned previously, Electromagnetic Fields (EMFs) are invisible areas of energy that are produced by electrical and wireless devices. Some people have raised concerns about the potential health effects of EMFs, particularly in relation to wearable devices such as smartwatches and fitness trackers. Switch your devices to airplane mode whenever possible, you do not need to be constantly switched on to still be able to track your health data.

While there is currently no strong evidence to suggest that the low levels of EMFs emitted by wearable devices pose a significant risk to human health, most studies on the health effects of EMFs have focused on higher levels of exposure, such as those encountered near power lines or cell phone towers. It is also important to note that the long-term health effects of low-level EMF exposure from wearable devices are not fully understood and more research is needed to determine their safety.

How To Know If You Are Adequately Recovered?

Recovery is a complex and multifaceted concept, both in practice and in measurement and assessment. Make no mistake, the number one and the most underutilized recovery tool is optimizing your sleep. If you are a lover of technology, and/or you have time and money to spend, there are some advanced tools that can help you measure and enhance your recovery.

Assessing And Measuring Recovery

By recovery we are talking about physiological recovery, meaning that the body's systems are working well at producing and utilizing energy and repairing tissues for optimal performance. Elite athletes are paying more and more attention to recovery and its measurement because they understand that rest is crucial for muscles to repair, rebuild and strengthen.

The first step is to learn to listen to what your body is telling you. If you feel stressed, agitated, moody, overtired, have a hard time sleeping, or have a poor appetite, this may be a rest day instead of a workout day.

There are an increasing number of technologies now to help you track your body's state of recovery. A simple tool widely available to measure grip strength can be used every morning and is a very good proxy for how well you are recovered. More advanced tools measure temperature, heart rate, heart rate variability, sleep quality and quantity, and more. These varied tools are not an exact science just yet but they help you to track some numbers, identify patterns, and become more in tune with how your body is responding to changes and the integration of new health protocols.

SMART PROTOCOL

Assess Your Recovery - $

As you integrate many of the protocols outlined in this book, you will periodically want to assess how well your body is responding to these changes and how well you are recovering. The metrics in this 3 step protocol are invaluable tools to help assess both readiness and recovery.

1. **Control Pause Test**—Utilize the CP test and evaluation explained earlier on in this Section to measure your functional breathing level. Once you establish your baseline, use the Control Pause (CP) as a readiness indicator. A slight deviation from your baseline may suggest the need for additional rest on that particular day.
2. **Grip Strength**—Evaluating grip strength goes beyond merely measuring hand strength; it serves as an excellent indicator of overall muscular strength and function. A robust grip is often associated with better physical performance and can reflect your body's ability to recover effectively. Tracking changes in grip strength over time can help identify possible fluctuations in your physical readiness and alert you to potential signs of fatigue or overtraining. We will discuss grip strength more in depth in Section 3—Movement, Exercise & Detoxification.
3. **HRV (Heart Rate Variability)**—HRV is a key metric that assesses the variations in time intervals between successive heartbeats. It's a powerful tool for monitoring the balance between your sympathetic (fight-or-flight) and parasympathetic (rest-and-digest) nervous systems. Higher HRV generally indicates a well-regulated and adaptable autonomic nervous system, reflecting better stress management and

recovery. On the other hand, lower HRV can be an early sign of physical or mental strain, suggesting the need for additional rest and recovery strategies. In Section 4—Neurotransmitters, Hormones, & Brain Wiring, we will go more in detail on how regularly assessing HRV can help you make informed decisions about your training intensity and lifestyle choices to optimize overall health and performance.

Advanced Recovery Tools

We can't say often enough how important the basics are when it comes to sleep and recovery. You need to be sleeping a minimum of 7, and preferably 8, quality hours per night. If you have the basics down, here are some tools that have a good track record that you may want to integrate into your daily or weekly routine.

SMART UPGRADES

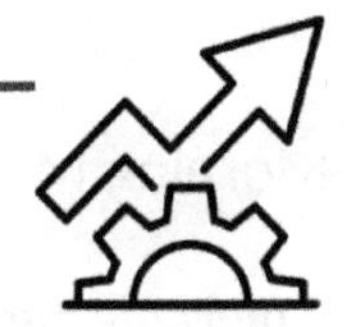

Photobiomodulation Or Red Light Therapy

Red Light Therapy—also known as photobiomodulation (PBM)—is a non-invasive therapy that delivers beneficial wavelengths of light to the skin and cells. Full-spectrum light encompasses many colours, including wavelengths we can't see, but only a select range of red and near-infrared light has therapeutic value for the purposes of photobiomodulation.

The photons of red and near-infrared react with the mitochondria in your cells, where they stimulate the electrons during cellular respiration. That is the process responsible for adenosine triphosphate (ATP) production, which is our cellular energy fuel.

Most red light therapy devices will provide red light delivered at 660 nm and invisible near-infrared light delivered at 850 nm. Red light is readily absorbed by surface tissues and cells, leading to enhanced skin health and healing. Near-infrared light penetrates into deeper tissues, leading to enhanced recovery and inflammation support.

SMART UPGRADES

Morning Movement Routine

A morning movement routine doesn't have to be long or complex. In fact, the more complex, the more likely we are to push certain tasks off. The truth is, you don't need to devote hours to your routine to set yourself up properly for the day.

Taking just 5 to 10 minutes every morning to leverage movement can go a long way to start your day right. A good option for a movement sequence is the Five Tibetan Rites which are an ancient yoga practice that consists of a sequence of 5 exercises to help increase energy, mobility, flexibility, calmness and mental clarity. (34) Each movement is performed 10 to 21 times (the sequence takes about 5 to 15 minutes) and has a mantra attached to it to help build concentration and focus.

SMART UPGRADES

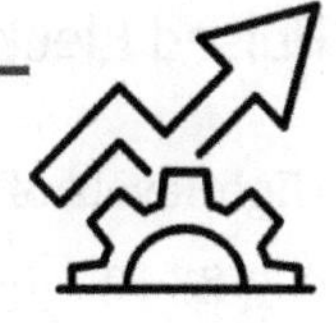

Heart Rate Variability Monitor

Heart rate variability (HRV) is a powerful indicator of overall health and recovery. It measures the variation in time intervals between consecutive heartbeats, reflecting the balance between the sympathetic and parasympathetic nervous systems. High HRV is generally associated with good physical and mental health, while low HRV may indicate an increased risk for health problems, such as heart disease or depression. We will go more in-depth on HRV in Section 4—Neurotransmitters, Hormones & Brain Wiring, however, tracking your heart rate variability is an indispensable tool for monitoring your sleep and recovery.

Numerous smart devices exist for sleep and HRV tracking, one standout being Hanu. This wearable technology, coupled with a mobile app, delivers precise capture and analysis of HRV patterns. It equips you with insights into your body's reactions to various activities and stressors, aiding in identifying prime recovery strategies and refining your training protocols.

SMART UPGRADES

Pulsed Electromagnetic Field (PEMF)

High levels of activity and daily stressors slowly drain your body of its energy to function optimally. By the end of the day, you're mentally, physically, and emotionally depleted. Think of PEMF as a battery charger for our cells. Electromagnetic pulses at low frequencies pass through the skin and penetrate deep into muscles, bones, tendons, and even organs to activate the cell's energy and encourage its natural repair mechanisms.

Although PEMF therapy may seem like a novel technology, it has been safely and effectively used across America and Europe for over five decades and is backed by many studies and clinical trials. (35) The benefits of PEMF therapy include improved circulation, reduction of pain, muscle relaxation and enhancement of physical performance, reduction of swelling and inflammation, improved oxygenation in the tissues, improved quality of sleep, and enhanced cellular repair and recovery.

SMART UPGRADES

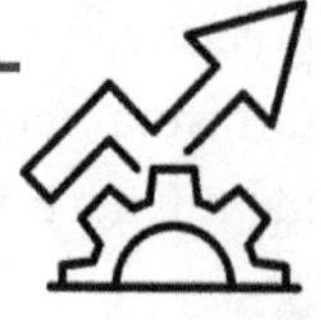

Percussion/Vibration Therapy

Handheld percussion/vibration devices have exploded in popularity in the last few years, from professional athletes to weekend warriors looking for help loosening tight and stiff muscles.

The physiological effects of vibration include increased metabolism, increased ROM, improved vascularization, the release of trigger points, and reduction of fascia densification, scar tissue, and calcifications. (36)

Other benefits may include reduced pain, faster rehabilitation, increased lymphatic flow, reduced lactic acid build-up, and stimulation of proprioceptive (body awareness) functions. They can be a great tool to add to your recovery arsenal.

Another benefit of these percussion and vibration therapies is their impact on sleep. Research showed that Therabody and Biostrap's findings concluded that Theragun's percussive therapy was able to help 87% of participants fall asleep almost 5 minutes faster than they usually do on a "normal night." In addition, 70% of participants slept longer throughout the night, with an average of 7% fewer awakenings per participant. Finally, the results indicated that 56% of participants enjoyed a higher overall sleep score, which takes into account factors such as sleep duration, deep sleep, efficiency, wakening, and movement. (37)

Section Wrap-Up

Sleep, rest, and recovery are not indulgences or time wasted; they are the foundations upon which our overall health and performance are built.

Neglecting these fundamental aspects of self-care can hinder our potential, both in our personal and professional lives. By giving yourself permission to rest, prioritize your sleep and recovery, you are investing in your long-term well-being and setting yourself up for success.

Just as sleep provides the necessary rejuvenation for our bodies and minds, the food we consume acts as the fuel that powers our daily activities and sustains our physiological functions. In Section 2—Hydration, Fuel, & Foundationals, we will explore the role of nutrition in enhancing our health and performance, protocols to optimize hydration, and highlight the importance of how proper nourishment lays the groundwork for a vibrant life.

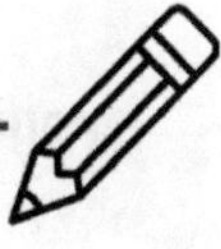

PROTOCOLS QUICK REFERENCE CHECKLIST:

PROTOCOL—Mouth Taping - $

☐ *Currently doing* ☐ *Want to integrate* ☐ *Not for now*

PROTOCOL—Morning Light Exposure - $0

☐ *Currently doing* ☐ *Want to integrate* ☐ *Not for now*

PROTOCOL—Limiting Pre-sleep Light Exposure - $0

☐ *Currently doing* ☐ *Want to integrate* ☐ *Not for now*

PROTOCOL—Sleep Temperature - $0 to $$$

☐ *Currently doing* ☐ *Want to integrate* ☐ *Not for now*

PROTOCOL—Know Your Control Pause - $0

☐ *Currently doing* ☐ *Want to integrate* ☐ *Not for now*

PROTOCOL—Breathe Yourself To Sleep - $0

☐ *Currently doing* ☐ *Want to integrate* ☐ *Not for now*

PROTOCOL—Managing Short-Term Stress - $0

☐ *Currently doing* ☐ *Want to integrate* ☐ *Not for now*

PROTOCOL—Managing Medium To long Term Stress - $0

☐ *Currently doing* ☐ *Want to integrate* ☐ *Not for now*

PROTOCOL—Yoga Nidra/ NSDR - $0

☐ *Currently doing* ☐ *Want to integrate* ☐ *Not for now*

PROTOCOL—Deliberate Heat Exposure - $0 to $$$

☐ *Currently doing* ☐ *Want to integrate* ☐ *Not for now*

PROTOCOL—Deliberate Cold Exposure - $0 to $$$

☐ *Currently doing* ☐ *Want to integrate* ☐ *Not for now*

PROTOCOL—Sleep Nutraceuticals Falling Asleep - $

☐ *Currently doing* ☐ *Want to integrate* ☐ *Not for now*

PROTOCOL—Sleep Nutraceuticals Staying Asleep - $

☐ *Currently doing* ☐ *Want to integrate* ☐ *Not for now*

PROTOCOL—PROTOCOL—Assess Your Recovery - $

☐ *Currently doing* ☐ *Want to integrate* ☐ *Not for now*

SMART RESOURCES

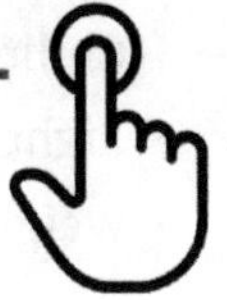

- Mouth Tape—oxygenadvantage.com/product/myotape/
- Blue blocking glasses—vivarays.com
- Breathwork App—thebreathsource.app
- Oxygen Advantage App for Apple—apps.apple.com/us/app/oxygen-advantage/id1589260950 and Playstore—play.google.com/store/apps/details?id=com.oxygen.advantage
- 10-Minute Yoga Nidra Practice
- 20-Minute Yoga Nidra Practice
- 40-Minute Yoga Nidra Practice
- Cold plunge—chestfreezercoldplunge.com or if you want to purchase one already made, many companies are now producing great products like: morozkoforge.com or icebarrel.com or coldture.com
- Percussion Therapy Device—therabody.com

SMART TOOLS AT A GLANCE

- Oura ring—ouraring.com
- Hanu—hanuhealth.com or Whoop straps—whoop.com
- Chilipad—chilisleep.com
- Eight Sleep System—eightsleep.com
- Weighted blankets

Section 2—Hydration, Fuel & Foundationals

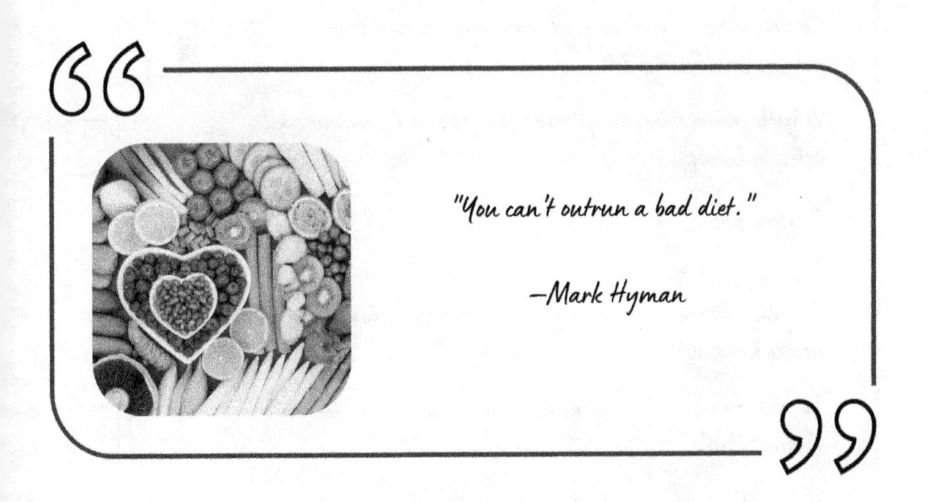

"You can't outrun a bad diet."

—Mark Hyman

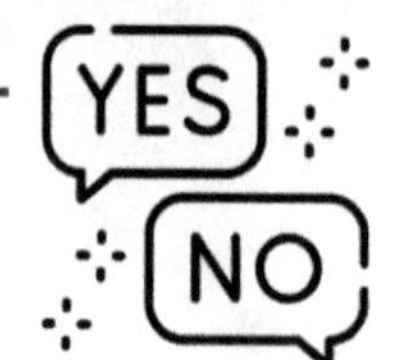

SELF EVALUATION-DISCOVERY QUESTIONS

Question		
Do you know what your optimal daily water intake is?	Y	N
Do you know how to adapt your water intake to your exercise output?	Y	N
Do you eat 80% of your food from scratch and from whole/unrefined foods?	Y	N
Is your protein intake optimal for your body weight and activity level?	Y	N
Do you spend time in natural sunlight daily?	Y	N
Do you consume your daily caloric intake within an 8 to 10 hours window?	Y	N
Do you spend at least 15 minutes with your bare feet on the ground daily?	Y	N
Do you know if your daily diet covers your basic vitamins and mineral needs? If not, do you supplement?	Y	N
Are you taking any key foundational supplements to optimize what you might be lacking in your diet?	Y	N
Do you ever experience symptoms of blood sugar imbalance-feeling lightheaded or 'hangry'?	Y	N

Do you regularly consume probiotic-rich foods? Y N

Does your oral care routine support your oral microbiome? Y N

Does your diet support your ideal healthy weight? Y N

Do you periodically track your macronutrient intake? Y N

The way we hydrate and fuel ourselves plays an immense role in how we think, feel, and perform in our day-to-day lives. As simple as it may sound, knowing what to eat and drink is arguably one of the most complex and contentious subjects. Different perspectives from a myriad of scientific research, cultural norms, and religious doctrines create a plethora of confusing and often contradictory advice.

Your unique bodily system—your metabolism, physiology, personal beliefs, and values are essential elements that guide your nutritional needs. A universally accepted 'best diet' simply does not exist. What nourishes and fuels one person might not work the same for another. That said, there are several principles with strong scientific backing that anyone can consider when evaluating their hydration and nutrition strategies.

Here's what there is a good scientific basis for—hydrate adequately with clean water and electrolytes, eliminate refined and processed foods including seed oils, practice time-restricted eating–commonly referred to as intermittent fasting, consume adequate quality protein for the preservation of muscle, and use the sun and the earth as the energy sources they are.

We have to remember that food is there to fuel us and give us energy, so what is cellular energy and how does it work? Cells in the human body obtain energy through a process called cellular respiration, which converts glucose (a type of sugar) into ATP (adenosine triphosphate). ATP is the primary source of energy for the body's cells and is used to power a variety of cellular processes, including muscle contractions, nerve impulses, and chemical reactions.

Overall, cellular respiration is a complex process that is essential for the production of energy in the human body. It enables cells to perform the functions that are necessary for maintaining life and good health.

So let's get started on the journey of hydration, fuel, and optimal energy production.

Hydration

The human body is amazing. We can survive between one and two months or even longer without food, depending on fat stores, body composition, and activity. However, you would be hard-pressed to last more than 3 days without water. According to Dr. Andy Galpin, a 2% dehydration (for our purposes a 2% decrease in body weight excluding other inputs and outputs) causes a significant increase in perception of difficulty in exercise, and a decrease in endurance performance, speed, power, and accuracy. (1) A 2% dehydration has also been shown to impair cognitive performance. (2)

Exercising in a hot environment can cause the loss of 1-2 litres of water per hour, equivalent to 1-2 kg or 2.2-4.4 lbs. (3) This means a 150-lb individual could be as much as 3% dehydrated in 1 hour.

Where does our water intake come from? Typically 50% comes from water, 30% from fluids such as coffee, tea, etc., and 20% comes from food. This is assuming a good, whole-food diet that is low in processed food. Processed food is water sparse and heavy in salt.

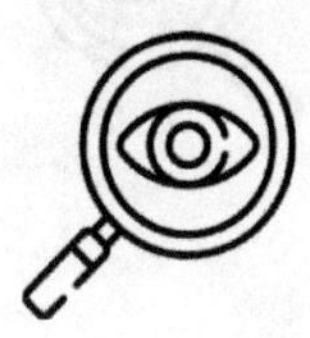

SMART CONSIDERATION

Eat Your Water

The water content of food:
Vegetables 90-96%
Fruit 80-90%
Eggs 75%
Meat 65%

How Much Water?

Dietitians of Canada recommend 2.2 L (9 cups) for females and 3.0 L (12 cups) for males. (4) The U.S. National Academies of Science, Engineering, and Medicine recommends a slightly higher 2.7 L (11.5 cups) for females and 3.7 L (15.5 cups) for males. (5) These recommendations, of course, do not take into account individual variations in weight, diet, activity, etc. A more customized approach, recommended by Dr. Andy Galpin and others, is to consume one-half daily of your body weight in pounds, in ounces of water. As with all general recommendations, this is an excellent place to start, and pay attention to what your body is telling you. If you eat a highly processed diet, you will likely need more water. If you consume a pure whole-food diet, you very likely need to consume less water.

SMART CONSIDERATION

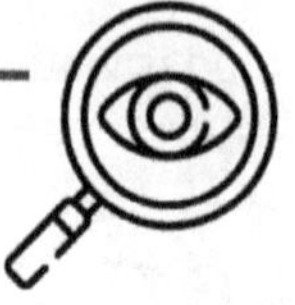

Daily Water Intake - $0 to $

Consume in water Body Weight (lbs)/2 in ounces per day

For example, if you weigh 150 lbs, 150/2=75, consume 75 ounces of water per day.

SMART CONSIDERATION

Quick Conversions

1 litre = 1 kg = 2.2 lbs = 35.3 oz
16 oz = 2 cups = 1 lb
1 oz = 30 ml
1000 ml = 1 litre

Using the table of conversions, it would be wise to assess your sweat rate with different workouts. Try to urinate prior to working out, and then weigh yourself before and after your workout, and account for fluid intake.

For example, if you weigh 68 kg (150 lbs) prior to working out, and 67 kg after (147.8 lbs), and you consumed 500 ml (.5 kg) of water during the workout, you have lost 1.5 kg or 1.5 litres of water during the workout (68 kg-67 kg + .5 kg). Note: if you urinate (or defecate) during the workout the math gets a little complicated—do it a few times until you have a complete workout during which you don't urinate. You don't need to do this calculation every time you workout, but if you do it occasionally you will get a pretty good average. Again, Dr. Andy Galpin has a formula for peri-hydrating around an exercise bout. He recommends consuming body weight in pounds divided by 30, in ounces of water per 15 minutes of exercise.

SMART PROTOCOL

Exercise Hydration - $0 to $

During exercise, consume in water Body Weight/30 in ounces per 15 minutes

For example, if you weigh 150 lbs, 150/30=5 ounces of water per 15 minutes.

Now let's make it a little more complicated. When you sweat you don't just lose water but also electrolytes, especially sodium (Na+), chloride (Cl-), potassium (K+), Magnesium (Mg+), Calcium (Ca+), and also some glucose.

SMART CONSIDERATION

Evaluate Electrolyte Loss

There are various methods of testing hydration and electrolyte loss in sweat (see Smart Upgrades) but on average in 1 litre of sweat, we lose:

Na^+ 500-2000 mg (average 1200 mg)
Cl^- 500-3000 mg
K^+ 100-500 mg
Mg^+/Ca^+ 0-100 mg

Where does our salt come from? Typically, 10% of intake is from food, 15% is added at the table, and 75% is processed food. Note the whopping amount from processed food, and it is hard to keep track of and calculate.

Before adding salt to your hydration protocol, you must honestly assess your health status and the purity of your diet. If you are not pre-hypertensive or hypertensive (high blood pressure), and if you do not have kidney disease, you probably should not be afraid of adding salt. That is provided that you eat a whole-food diet with minimal to no processed food. According to Dr. James DiNicolantonio, author of *The Salt Fix*, it may even be optimum for humans to consume 3.2-4.8 g of sodium per day, which is 1.5 to 2 times the current medical recommendations. (6) According to Dr. Andrew Huberman, studies show that beyond 6 g of sodium per day is definitely hazardous to health. (7) Therefore, if you are adding salt to a highly processed diet you could easily exceed that amount of 6 g per day.

SMART PROTOCOL

Electrolyte Replenishment For Heavy Sweating - $

To hydrate with electrolytes for heavy sweating (exercise, sauna, work in intense heat, etc.):

In 1-1.5 L of water, add
1/4 teaspoon salt (Redmond Real salt, Celtic sea salt)
1/4 teaspoon Morton Lite salt (potassium chloride salt)
1/4 teaspoon Sodium Bicarbonate (baking soda)

This provides just over 1100 mg sodium, just over 1600 mg chloride, 350 mg potassium, 7 mg calcium and 2 mg magnesium.

Or

1/2 teaspoon of Boulder Salt (brand name).

This provides 992 mg sodium, 1500 mg chloride, 300 mg potassium, 75 mg calcium and 140 mg magnesium.

To either of these, you could add a teaspoon of honey for a shot of glucose and fructose, and potentially a squeeze of lemon juice for flavour, and you have an excellent electrolyte replacement water for a fraction of the cost of a commercial electrolyte blend.

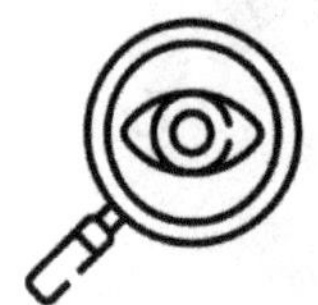

SMART CONSIDERATION

Shut Your Mouth

Mouth breathing results in 42% greater water loss than nasal breathing.(8) So breathing through the mouth, especially at night during sleep, results in a much greater water loss and needs to be considered in hydration. See mouth taping in Section 1—Sleep, Rest & Recovery.

Exploring The Concept Of Structured Water

The scientific community is engaged in ongoing debate and discussion regarding the validity and merits of water structuring, which contributes to the uncertainty surrounding this concept. Structured water, also known as the gel phase or Exclusion Zone (EZ) water, is believed to be crucial for proper hydration. While we are familiar with the water existing as liquid, ice, and vapour, the gel phase introduces a distinct state of water. It is present within the cells of our bodies, as well as in plants and natural surroundings.

Moreover, water in the gel phase possesses energy akin to a battery, holding extra electrons, and is denoted as H302 by Dr. Gerald Pollack, author of the book, *The Fourth Phase of Water: Beyond Solid, Liquid, and Vapor.* In his book, Dr. Pollack explores this unique phase of water and its significance in various contexts, shedding light on its remarkable properties and potential applications. (9)

EZ water is formed when water is exposed to infrared light, specifically at a wavelength of 1200 nanometres (nm). Exposing our bare skin to sunlight, which includes near-infrared and ultraviolet (UV) radiation, can help structure the water already present in our bodies. When water molecules absorb this infrared light, they vibrate, and the energy from the vibrations is transmitted from one molecule to another, similar to ripples in a pond. As a result, the water molecules become denser and more viscous, moving closer together to stabilize themselves. This structured water stores energy in the form of a negative charge, akin to a charged battery, ready to be delivered. Having more EZ water in the body means storing up more energy that can be sent to cells that require it.

The concept of water structuring is a topic of ongoing debate among experts. While some people believe that certain substances and methods can structure water, scientific evidence supporting these claims is currently limited. Various products, such as wands, devices, and filters, claim to assist in water structuring by utilizing mechanisms like magnetic fields, vortexing, or specific materials.

Understand Our Body's Energy Systems

As mentioned earlier, we could not talk about energy without talking about our cells and, more specifically, our mitochondria. Inside each of the trillions of cells that make up all the tissues of our body are tiny organelles called mitochondria. They are our cellular power generating stations, producing about 90% of our energy.

Our mitochondria are constantly renewed to fulfill the vast energy demands of muscle and other tissues in our bodies. As we get older, mitochondrial renewal declines and dysfunctional mitochondria accumulate in the cells. This age-associated mitochondrial decline can lead to a progressive decrease in our metabolism, energy levels, and resilience.

The food we eat is transferred and used by our bodies to produce energy from our mitochondria. We are not going to give you a biochemistry lesson here as the process of producing energy is complex, but the gist is that we eat food that contains macronutrients: protein, carbohydrates, and fats, and micronutrients: vitamins and minerals. As we digest our food, our body breaks down proteins into amino acids, carbohydrates into glucose, and fats into glycerol and essential fatty acids. These are then further broken down into energy units that the cell mitochondria use to produce energy. In consideration of macronutrients, it is helpful to think of protein as the building blocks of your body, and fat and carbohydrates are the energy supply.

When you think about it, you truly are what you eat.

Proteins—The Building Blocks

Protein is a valuable source of energy and renewal. It is found in muscle, bone, hair, and virtually every other tissue in the body.

Proteins are essential for cell growth, tissue and cartilage repair, transporting oxygen and nutrients to cells, the production of immune cells that fight off bacteria and viruses, and much more. Amongst the most important functions of adequate protein intake is the preservation of lean body mass, which is primarily muscle.

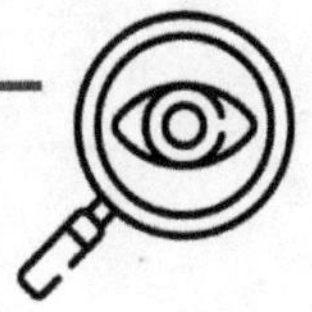

SMART CONSIDERATION

Prioritize Protein

Humans lose muscle mass and strength as we age, and we die overwhelmingly from frailty and fragility. Adequate exercise (see Section 3—Movement, Exercise & Detoxification) and protein intake are the remedies for this at any age. Strive to build and maintain as much muscle mass as possible, especially if you are still young, as this is absolutely a prerequisite to ensure stability and gracefulness well into your golden years.

Proteins can be acquired from both animal and plant sources. It is important to note that animal sources of protein are complete, meaning they have all the amino acids our body needs. Simply put, the best way to build muscle is to eat animal muscles. Plant protein sources are incomplete, meaning we need to carefully combine plant protein sources in order to get all the amino acids we need.

For our purposes here we are going to focus on the amount of protein in the diet. Where you get your protein depends on your beliefs and values, but understand if you choose to not eat meat, you need to be very careful about getting both adequate amounts and quality of protein.

The RDA (recommended daily allowance) for protein, like other nutrients, has been focused on preventing deficiency as opposed to optimizing health. The RDA of 0.8 g/kg of body weight or 0.36 g/lb is woefully inadequate, especially in the case of an active person, let alone one who is exercising at a level that is healthy. Recent studies point to at least 1.2-1.6 g/kg (0.5-0.7g/lb) as healthy levels of protein intake. (10) (11)

SMART CONSIDERATION

Add Amino Acids

For individuals who do not consume sufficient dietary protein (less than 1.6 g/kg ideal weight per day), essential amino acid (EAA) supplementation can provide an effective means of increasing their intake. EAAs are amino acids that the body cannot produce on its own and must be obtained through diet or supplements. These amino acids are crucial for supporting various biological functions, including muscle growth and repair, immune function, and hormone synthesis.

Of all the EAA, leucine stands out as a key amino acid crucial for muscle protein synthesis. For this reason, most EAA supplements contain a higher ratio of leucine to others. Supplementing with essential amino acids in general, ensures that our muscles receive the necessary building blocks to stay strong and resilient, ultimately supporting muscle health and overall physical performance.

SMART PROTOCOL

Daily Protein Intake - $

Aim to ingest 1 g of protein for every 1 pound of ideal body weight, or 2.2 g of protein per kg of body weight. 1.2–1.6 g/kg (0.5–0.7 g/lb) is the minimum goal.

Fats—The Energy Reserve

Fats are no longer the villain, nor should they have ever been. Our bodies *need* saturated and unsaturated fats from animal or plant sources.

Healthy fats are necessary to help our bodies:

- Absorb fat-soluble vitamins (vitamins A, D, E, and K)
- Insulate and protect our organs
- Balance hormones
- Improve insulin function
- Provide satiety and flavour to food

A quick primer on fats or triglycerides. They can broadly be divided into saturated and unsaturated fats.

Saturated fats are solid at room temperature and have a high melting point. They include fat in pork, beef, cheese, whole milk, eggs, coconut oil, and butter. There are many studies linking saturated fat with heart disease, and there are many studies refuting that link. If you are exercising and as active as you should be (refer to Section 3—Movement, Exercise & Detoxification) and if you do not suffer from heart disease, diabetes or any other chronic condition, these fats from clean sources are acceptable additions to a healthy diet. This is contrary to the official narrative. The American Heart Association recommends saturated fat makes up, at most, 5-6% of total daily caloric consumption. (12) According to these guidelines, this would mean that a person consuming 2000 calories a day could have at most 120 calories from saturated fat. This equates to about 13 grams or 2 slices of cheddar cheese.

Unsaturated fats can be subdivided into trans fats, monounsaturated and polyunsaturated fats. Trans fats are solid at room temperature and have a high melting point. Trans fats can be in the form of natural or ruminant fats or artificial trans fats.

Natural or ruminant (as in ruminant animals) fats make up 2-5% of the fat in dairy products and 3-9% of the fat in beef and lamb. These are healthier sources of trans fats.

Artificial trans fats are manufactured by taking vegetable oils and adding hydrogen to them in a process known as hydrogenation. This increases the shelf life and flavour stability. These are found in fast foods, some baked foods, fried foods, artificial coffee creamers, margarine, frozen pizza, etc. These types of fats should be avoided at all costs. In 2013, the United States Food and Drug Administration made a provisional recommendation that partially hydrogenated oil was not safe in food. (13) Enough said.

Monounsaturated fats are liquid at room temperature and have a low melting point. They include olive oil, canola oil, peanut oil, avocados, and most nuts and seeds. These are generally considered healthy fats.

Polyunsaturated fats are liquids at room temperature and start to turn solid when chilled. There are four types, known as omega-3, -6, -7, or -9. Omega-3 and -6 are essential fats meaning they have to come from the diet as our bodies can not manufacture them.

Omega-6 oils come mostly from things like salad dressings, fried foods, and grain-fed beef and they are mostly pro-inflammatory. Omega-3 oils come from flax seeds, walnuts, grass-fed beef, and fatty fish such as tuna and salmon. Omega-3 oils possess anti-inflammatory properties, which means they can help reduce inflammation in the body. Both omega-6 and omega-3 oils are necessary for the optimal functioning of the human body, but they need to be consumed in a balanced ratio. The recommended ratio of omega-6 to omega-3 is 3-4:1, indicating that we should consume three to four times more omega-6 than omega-3 oils. Varying sources put that ratio at 10:1 and as high as 30:1 in a standard American diet. This results in an imbalance of the two types of oils and ultimately leads to increased inflammation. (14)

SMART PROTOCOL

Daily Fat Intake - $

Clean and natural sources of saturated, natural trans, monounsaturated, and polyunsaturated fats in moderation can be part of a healthy diet. Artificial trans fats (which show up on labels as trans, hydrogenated, or partially hydrogenated fat/oil) should be avoided at all costs.

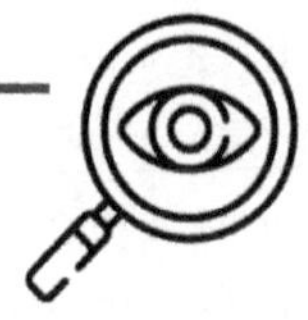

SMART CONSIDERATION

Choose Your Fats Wisely

Many processed oils contain unsaturated fatty acids that are highly susceptible to oxidation. When oils are heated, the increased energy causes chemical bonds to break, leading to the formation of free radicals. Free radicals can cause cellular damage, which contributes to ageing and various health conditions. To prevent oil from becoming rancid, it's important to store it in a cool, dark place and avoid excessive heating during cooking.

As a general guide:

Olive Oil—High heat
Coconut Oil—High heat
Tallow—High heat
Ghee—High heat
Avocado Oil—Medium heat
Butter—Low heat
Nut Oils—Don't cook them
Vegetable Oils—(Grapeseed, canola, sunflower, soybean, corn, safflower). Don't cook them. Its best to avoid them altogether.

Carbohydrates—The Quick Fuel

Carbohydrates are the biggest energy source in most diets and they can be classified as simple, complex, and fibrous. The carbohydrates in fruits and milk are simple, which means they are one sugar molecule or monosaccharide. The carbohydrates in whole grains and vegetables are complex, which means they have long chains of sugars or polysaccharides.

A much simpler and more useful classification of carbohydrates when trying to decide which to include in your diet is fast and slow carbohydrates. Fast carbohydrates raise your blood sugar levels quickly. They are rapidly digested, hunger returns faster, and we eat more. Slow carbohydrates raise your blood sugar levels slowly, keeping you full longer, and because they take longer to digest they raise your metabolism level—they use more energy to digest.

Managing blood glucose levels is essential not only for individuals with diabetes but also for managing cholesterol levels. Elevated blood glucose levels can contribute to the formation of harmful cholesterol particles and increase the risk of cardiovascular disease. When blood glucose levels are too high, the body produces more triglycerides, which are a type of fat that can increase the amount of harmful Low-Density-Lipoprotein (LDL) cholesterol in the bloodstream. Additionally, high blood sugar levels can cause damage to the lining of the blood vessels, leading to the accumulation of cholesterol and other substances that can form plaques and cause blockages.

In general, simple carbohydrates, being composed of only one sugar or monosaccharide, are absorbed relatively quickly and thus these are fast carbohydrates. However, whole fruits have a supply of fibre along with vitamins and minerals, and the fibre slows the absorption of the sugar significantly.

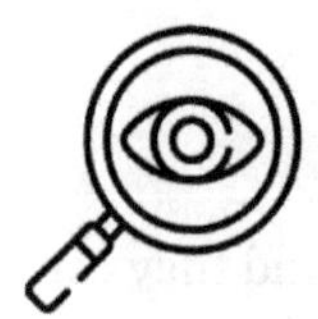

SMART CONSIDERATION

Keep It Complex

Complex carbohydrates, being composed of many sugars strung together or polysaccharides, are slow carbohydrates. Here we are talking about whole grains and vegetables. Just as with simple carbohydrates, complex carbohydrates can be processed as well, stripping them of fibre and causing them to be digested and raising your blood sugar more quickly. These refined or processed carbohydrates include white flour, white bread, white rice, pastries, sodas, snacks, pasta, sweets, breakfast cereals, and added sugars. These are also added to many processed foods.

The processing of fruit juice strips the fibre out, and therefore fruit juice raises blood sugar very quickly. As an example, orange juice contains about 24 grams or 6 teaspoons of sugar in 8 ounces with little or no fibre to slow the absorption. An orange contains about 2 ounces of juice along with its fibre to slow the absorption of the sugar. When including fruit in the diet, choose the whole fruit.

SMART CONSIDERATION

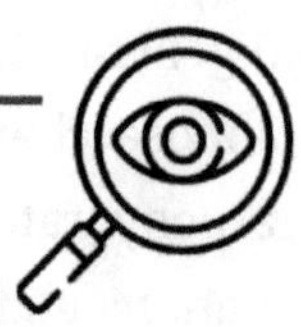

Fibre Facts

Stick to carbohydrates in their whole, unprocessed, or minimally processed forms. If it has an ingredient list, it is not a whole food.

Fibre is a type of carbohydrate that our digestive system cannot break down. It can be classified as soluble, which dissolves in water and forms a gel, and insoluble which does not dissolve in water and keeps its form. Fibre helps to lower cholesterol, control weight, prevent constipation, bind and remove toxins, and control blood sugar levels.

While fibre does not provide us with energy, it does provide energy to our microbiome, the very important "good" bacteria that line our digestive tract. In this way, fibre is a prebiotic, a fertilizer for our microbiome that provides a good environment for it to thrive.

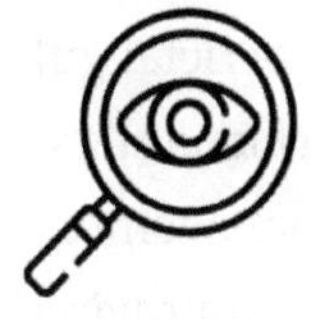

SMART CONSIDERATION

Feast On Fibre

Try to include a variety of the following foods which are high in fibre and also good sources of carbohydrates like lentils, kidney beans, chickpeas, quinoa, avocado, brown rice, berries, apples, bananas, sweet potatoes (eat the skin), beets, broccoli, Brussels sprouts, almonds, and dark chocolate which contains 3 grams of fibre per ounce!

A great way to increase total fibre intake is to add a plain unflavoured soluble fibre to your morning coffee or tea. Stirring in a tablespoon or so of acacia powder, partially hydrolyzed guar gum, or wheat dextrin will start your day off with about 5 grams of fibre and will not change the texture or flavour of your drink at all.

Resistant Starch—Nourishing Gut Bacteria Or Fueling Inflammation?

Resistant starch is a type of dietary fibre that behaves like starch but resists digestion in the small intestine. Instead of being broken down and absorbed, it passes through the digestive system largely intact until it reaches the large intestine. Once there, it undergoes fermentation by the gut bacteria, producing beneficial compounds and by-products. It is found in green bananas, legumes, cooked and then cooled rice and potatoes, green mango, and semi-raw oats. Resistant starch offers potential benefits such as improved digestive health, including nourishing beneficial gut bacteria and reducing the risk of digestive disorders; aiding in blood sugar regulation for diabetes management; supporting weight management by increasing feelings of fullness and enhancing fat burning; improving insulin sensitivity, important for conditions like type 2 diabetes; and promoting enhanced colon health through the production of beneficial compounds.

However, there is one caveat—some emerging research has uncovered that certain types of gut bacteria, specifically those that produce endotoxins, can thrive on a diet rich in resistant starch. (15) These endotoxins, known as lipopolysaccharides (LPS), are molecules found in the outer membrane of some types of bacteria, including some in the gut. High levels of LPS in the bloodstream have been associated with chronic inflammation, which is linked to various health conditions such as obesity, insulin resistance, and cardiovascular diseases. When the balance of gut bacteria is disrupted or certain types of bacteria multiply excessively, it can lead to an overgrowth of LPS-producing bacteria. Under normal circumstances, these endotoxins are contained within the gut and pose no harm. However, when there is increased permeability of the gut lining (leaky gut), LPS can enter the bloodstream, triggering an immune response. So, while resistant starch can absolutely be beneficial, if you have compromised digestive function or inflammatory bowel conditions, you may want to avoid or limit your intake.

Deciphering Energy Dynamics—Glucose And Ketones As Fuels

Our body primarily harnesses energy from two main sources: glucose and ketones. Glucose, which is derived from carbohydrates, is either tapped for immediate energy or stashed away as glycogen. If glycogen reserves overflow, surplus glucose is converted into fat. Relying exclusively on glucose can lead to inconsistent energy levels, resulting in sporadic bouts of fatigue and hunger.

Ketones serve as an alternative energy source when glucose is in short supply, such as during fasting, on a low-carb diet, or after rigorous physical exertion. The liver is responsible for ketone production, and once the body is in a state of ketosis, it leans towards using ketones over glucose. While both these elements transform into ATP – our primary cellular energy – they journey through distinct metabolic pathways. The Randle cycle defines whether cells lean towards glucose or fat as their energy source. (16) For optimal glucose metabolism, it's suggested to limit dietary fat to 30% of total caloric intake. However, if you still struggle with diabetes or obesity, you may need to get your fat level down to 15% to 20% of your total calories. Surpassing these limits pushes the metabolic equilibrium toward fat oxidation.

It's vital to recognize that metabolic processes can differ between individuals. For instance, someone with substantial fat reserves may metabolize differently than someone who boasts both metabolic flexibility and robust muscle mass. Muscle plays an indispensable role in metabolism. Diminished muscle mass can decelerate metabolic rates, compromising calorie burn efficiency. Maintaining muscle is pivotal; it actively burns fat, even during rest, ensuring a consistent energy supply. By comprehending the roles of glucose and ketones, we can craft our dietary and lifestyle choices to align with our unique metabolic needs, activity profiles, and performance goals.

SMART UPGRADES

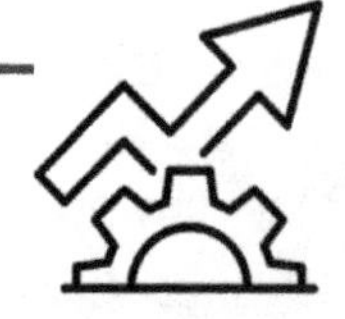

Exogenous Ketones

Exogenous ketones are available in different forms, including powders, capsules, and drinks. These supplements are formulated to increase the levels of ketones in the body, helping individuals achieve the benefits of a ketogenic diet without adhering to a strict low-carbohydrate diet.

Exogenous ketones can be found in two primary forms: ketone salts and ketone esters. Ketone salts are a combination of beta-hydroxybutyrate (BHB) and other minerals such as sodium, calcium, and magnesium. They are often available in powder or capsule form and are more affordable than ketone esters. Ketone salts are known to cause gastrointestinal distress in some people, and they may not increase ketone levels as significantly as ketone esters.

Ketone esters, on the other hand, are pure BHB molecules that are bound to a ketone precursor. They are typically available in liquid form and can be consumed directly or added to drinks. Ketone esters are more expensive than ketone salts, but they can significantly increase ketone levels in the blood, resulting in a more profound effect on the body.

If you're considering exogenous ketones to boost concentration or elevate performance, sifting through the multitude of available options to gauge their quality can be overwhelming. To simplify your search, we've pin-pointed two reputable firms that excel in ketone esters and ketone salts. You'll find their links in the Smart Resources at the end of this Section.

Pre-Pro-Post-Biotics And The Microbiome

The microbiome refers to the trillions of tiny bacteria, fungi, protozoa, and viruses that live in and line our digestive tract. The digestive tract encompasses the entire tube that extends from our mouth to our anus. Scientists now understand that the "gut-brain axis" is a biological circuit in which our gut (digestive tract) is continually communicating with our brain and vice versa. The microbiome changes the way the brain functions by making or facilitating the manufacture of particular neurotransmitters. This in return strongly impacts the way our entire body works. (17)

The microbiome plays an essential role in metabolism by aiding, and in some cases, directly participating in digestion, immune function, and modulating inflammation and brain function. Research has linked the microbiome to mood, psychiatric disorders like ADHD, and even autism.

Discussion of this is beyond the scope of this book, however, it does illustrate the potential power of the microbiome. (18)

Prebiotics, probiotics, and postbiotics are all important components of this ecosystem that can have significant health benefits. Prebiotics are non-digestible fibres that promote the growth of beneficial bacteria in the colon (chicory root, Jerusalem artichoke, garlic, onion, asparagus, bananas, apples, oats, and flaxseed), while probiotics are live microorganisms that directly add to the gut microbiota (yogurt with live and active cultures, kefir, sauerkraut, kimchi, miso, tempeh, kombucha, pickles, buttermilk). Postbiotics, on the other hand, are the by-products of bacterial fermentation and have been shown to have various positive effects on gut health like short-chain fatty acids (e.g. butyrate, propionate, acetate), bacterial enzymes (e.g. lactase, amylase, lipase) and bacterial metabolites (e.g. vitamins, organic acids, antimicrobial peptides).

A recent human study found that four to six, 4-6 ounce servings of low-sugar fermented foods increased microbiome diversity and decreased inflammatory signals in the body. Consistency was the most important factor. Some examples of low-sugar fermented foods are plain yogurt, kimchi, sauerkraut, kefir, and homemade lacto-fermented vegetables. (19)

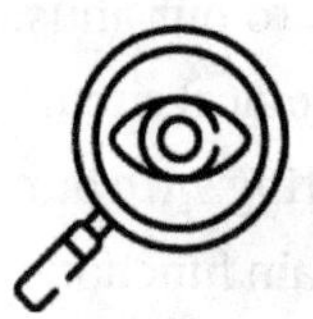

SMART CONSIDERATION

Populate Your Gut With Probiotics

Incorporating a high-quality probiotic into your diet can help maintain an optimal balance of microorganisms in your gut. This is important because our gut bacteria play a key role in digestion and nutrient absorption. Moreover, research has found that probiotics can reduce common biomarkers of inflammation. Interestingly, our gut is also responsible for producing a significant proportion of our immune cells (70%) and serotonin (80%), which is associated with positive mood. (20)(21)

A good daily dose is anywhere from 15 to 50 billion CFU. The dosage depends on a few factors, for example, if you've recently had to take antibiotics (which kill good and bad bacteria), you'd want to supplement with a higher dose. The two most beneficial strains are lactobacillus and acidophilus. It's important to note that it's beneficial to often rotate different good quality brands as they will carry different proprietary bacterial strains. Please note if you follow the recommendations on eating multiple sources of fermented foods every day you should not need a probiotic supplement, except potentially in the (hopefully rare) case of antibiotic use. It's also much cheaper, especially if you make some of your own.

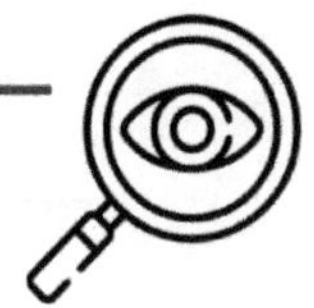

SMART CONSIDERATION

Microbiome Mediators

Adding a short-chain fatty acid supplement, such as a butyrate complex, to your diet can be beneficial for gut health. Unlike fermented foods and probiotic supplements, butyrate complex does not directly replenish gut flora. Instead, it contains a short-chain fatty acid (SCFA) that is produced by friendly gut bacteria during the digestion of fibres and resistant starches found in fruits, vegetables, legumes, and whole grains. These SCFAs promote the production of tight junction proteins in the gut, which strengthens the intestinal lining and reduces permeability. This leads to a stronger and healthier microbiome, which has been shown to provide protective effects against autoimmune and inflammatory diseases and can positively influence gut-brain communication. (22)

Recent research has shown that SCFAs also act as postbiotics, which are metabolic by-products of microbial fermentation that have beneficial effects on human health. SCFAs, such as butyrate, acetate, and propionate, are produced by gut bacteria during the fermentation of dietary fibres, and they play an important role in maintaining gut health and immune system function. Butyrate, in particular, has been found to have anti-inflammatory properties and promote the growth of beneficial gut bacteria. SCFAs also act as an energy source for colonocytes and have been shown to improve insulin sensitivity and reduce the risk of metabolic disorders such as obesity and type 2 diabetes. These findings highlight the importance of maintaining a healthy gut microbiome and consuming a diet rich in fibre to promote the production of SCFAs and other postbiotic metabolites. (23)

SMART CONSIDERATION

Live Cultured Lacto-Ferments

Shelf-stable sauerkraut, pickles, kimchi and the like that are stored on the shelf at the grocery store do not contain live cultures, which are necessary for the probiotic effect. Always look for those products in the refrigerated section instead.

There are also many resources available online for making probiotic-rich foods at home. For example, kefir can be easily made at home by obtaining milk kefir grains. Lacto-fermented vegetables can also be made at home using water, salt, and mason jars, following simple recipes and instructions that can be found online or in books such as *The Art of Fermentation* by Sandor Katz. (24) Sauerkraut can also be made at home using recipes like the one found in Tim Ferriss' book, *The 4-Hour Chef.* (25) Another popular probiotic food, yogurt, can also be made at home using starter cultures, as described in books such as *Super Gut* by Dr. William Davis. (26) It is important to note that lacto-fermented foods are very high in histamines, and may trigger symptoms in those who are sensitive. Histamine intolerance is a condition in which the body has difficulty breaking down histamines and can result in a range of symptoms including headaches, rashes, hives, digestive issues, and more. Diamine Oxidase (DAO) is an enzyme naturally present in the body that helps to break down histamines. To improve histamine intolerance and minimize histamine response, consider taking a (DAO) supplement when ingesting lacto-fermented foods.

SMART PROTOCOL

Daily Fermented Food Intake - $

Add four to six, 4-6 ounce servings of probiotic food per day to your diet. Supplement with DAO if you are histamine intolerant.

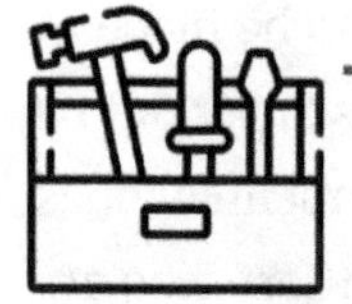

SMART TOOLS

GI Assessment

There are some excellent independent diagnostic labs that can help you assess the health and diversity of your gut microbiome. Utilizing non-invasive stool samples, these tests delve into the equilibrium of gut bacteria, nutrient assimilation, and the presence of inflammation. Such evaluations can pinpoint digestive anomalies and assist in diagnosing conditions like irritable bowel syndrome and inflammatory bowel disease, among others. If you're grappling with digestive concerns or wish to optimize gut and immune health, these tests can be instrumental. The GI Effects® test from Genova Diagnostics and GI MAP® from Diagnostic Solutions Laboratory are two reputable assessment tools.

Oil Pulling—A Natural Approach To Boosting Oral Microbiome Health

Just like the digestive tract, the mouth is home to numerous microorganisms, including both beneficial and harmful bacteria. When the balance of the oral microbiome is disrupted, it can lead to various oral health issues such as tooth decay, gum disease, and bad breath. (27) Oil pulling is an ancient Ayurvedic practice that involves swishing oil in the mouth for several minutes. This traditional technique has gained popularity in recent years as a natural alternative to conventional mouthwashes and oral care products. Research suggests that oil pulling may help promote a balanced oral microbiome by reducing the levels of harmful bacteria while preserving beneficial microbial populations.(28)

The process of oil pulling is quite simple. A tablespoon of oil is taken into the mouth, and then it is swished around for 10 to 20 minutes. The oil is pulled through the teeth and the spaces between them, ensuring that it reaches all areas of the mouth. As the oil is moved around, it adheres to the surface of the teeth and gums, attracting and pulling out harmful bacteria and toxins. Typically, cold-pressed oils like coconut or sesame are used.

Coconut oil is a popular choice due to its pleasant taste and aroma. It contains lauric acid, which has antimicrobial, anti-inflammatory, and antifungal properties making it effective against harmful bacteria in the mouth, and reducing gum inflammation.

Sesame oil has a long history of use in Ayurvedic medicine and is commonly used for oil pulling. It is rich in antioxidants, like sesamol and sesamin, which can help reduce plaque and strengthen teeth. Sesame oil exhibits antimicrobial activity against various bacteria, including those associated with oral health issues such as Streptococcus mutans and Porphyromonas gingivalis.(29) These bacteria are responsible for plaque formation, tooth decay, and gum disease.

Ultimately, the choice between coconut oil and sesame oil for oil pulling comes down to personal preference. Both oils have their own unique properties and benefits. It's important to use high-quality, organic, cold-pressed oils for oil pulling to ensure maximum benefits.

Please note that oil pulling is not a substitute for regular oral hygiene practices such as brushing, flossing, and routine dental check-ups.

SMART PROTOCOL

Oil Pulling - $

Oil pulling is best done first thing in the morning, before brushing your teeth. Put 1 tablespoon of either cold-pressed sesame oil or virgin coconut oil in your mouth. If this amount feels too large to begin with, then start with half the amount as you want to make sure you won't swallow any of the oil unintentionally. Gently swish and swirl it around your mouth. Avoid vigorous movements which can lead to muscle fatigue or an aching jaw. Continue gently swirling the oil for up to 20 minutes. If you are new to the practice, you may need to start with a shorter time frame—aim for 10 minutes to start and gradually increase the time. Spit the oil out into a trash can or napkin. Do not spit it into the sink as it may clog the drain due to the oil's solidifying properties. Rinse your mouth with warm water and then brush your teeth as usual.

Foods To Avoid

Nutrition is so complex and individual, it can be overwhelming when trying to determine what foods are best to eat. However, it's easier to start by knowing what to avoid. Some foods are universally recognized as unhealthy and detrimental to our health when consumed.

Processed, Packaged, And Fried Foods—Refined processed foods are pro-inflammatory, meaning they can cause more inflammation throughout the body. It's best to reduce your consumption of processed foods and especially avoid those containing any hydrogenated or trans fats. Many snacks and junk foods on store shelves contain these harmful fats that are used to preserve freshness and crispness as they sit in stores for long periods. These harmful fats are highly processed oils that can increase the risk of developing inflammatory diseases like heart disease, diabetes, arthritis, and weight gain. Highly processed food has yet another strike against it due to the presence of emulsifiers, which can limit the gut's ability to identify the food and send satiety signals to shut down hunger. This can lead to overeating and increased consumption of unhealthy foods.

Sugars, Artificial Sweeteners, And Simple Carbohydrates—Sugar, in all its various forms, has many harmful effects on health when consumed in large amounts. Processed table sugar, organic cane sugar, corn syrup, honey, soft drinks, juices, and refined and sweet foods such as pastries, bread, and pasta should be avoided as they can trigger inflammatory responses. Overconsumption of sugars can cause chronic low-grade inflammation in the gut and may lead to other long-term effects on health such as obesity, type 2 diabetes, and heart disease. In particular, high fructose corn syrup, which is found in the majority of processed foods contains 50% fructose as compared to fructose in whole, fresh fruit which contains anywhere from 1-10% fructose, with 10% being on the high end.

One of the simple ways to find these processed, refined, and sugary foods is the layout of a modern grocery store. If you walk around the perimeter, you are looking at whole foods. As soon as you start up and down the aisles, you are looking at refined and processed foods. With very few exceptions, if the food has an ingredient list, it is refined and/or processed.

SMART PROTOCOL

Pantry Clean-Up Time - $0

Purge your pantry of garbage, and get rid of sweets, chips, and convenience junk. Shop the periphery of the grocery store. Better yet, go to your local farmers market and get to know the people who produce real food. They are knowledgeable and helpful with cooking suggestions. Ditch the seed oils and try using extra virgin olive oil, ghee, butter, avocado oil, or beef tallow.

Alcohol—Overconsumption of alcohol can cause dehydration and can compromise liver function and increase inflammation in the gut. It's best to eliminate it entirely or minimize intake as the current evidence shows no beneficial levels of alcohol consumption.

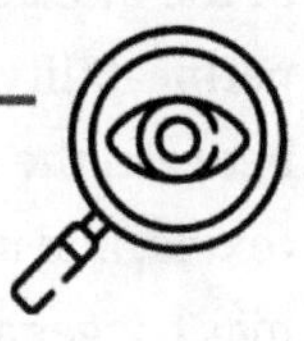

SMART CONSIDERATION

Alcohol Avoidance

The Canadian Centre on Substance Use and Addiction (CCSA) has revised its guidelines and now recommends that individuals should limit their alcohol consumption to no more than two drinks per week. This represents a significant departure from the previous guidelines which categorized 10 drinks per week for women and 15 drinks for men as safe or low-risk. (30) The new guidelines underscore the negative impact of alcohol on health.

Food For Thought—Inflammation Considerations

As previously mentioned, dietary recommendations are highly individualized, making it difficult to provide specific advice. However, if you are experiencing gut issues, inflammation, or any conditions that are resistant to a traditional diagnosis, an elimination diet may be beneficial to get to the root of your issues. This type of diet is considered the gold standard for identifying food sensitivities and promoting gut healing. Typically, an elimination diet involves removing gluten, dairy, corn, and soy from your diet. Lectins and nightshades should also be considered when it comes to inflammation.

Gluten—Gluten, a protein found in wheat, may interfere with the function of the intestinal protein zonulin and trigger what is known as intestinal permeability. This is a condition where the spaces, or tight junctions between the cells of the intestinal lining open up, and allow for bacteria, toxins, and undigested foods to be released into the bloodstream, which may trigger an immune reaction and ultimately cause inflammation.

Dairy—Overly-processed dairy products have also been shown to be pro-inflammatory in some cases, which can lead to digestive issues, allergies, acne, and eczema. These products can also have a harmful effect on bone health. Because dairy is acid-forming and your body likes to maintain a neutral pH balance, it has to compensate for this increased acidity by drawing on its alkaline reserves—the calcium, magnesium, and potassium stored in your bones. This weakens your bones putting them at increased risk for fractures.

Nightshades—For some, inflammation can be aggravated by nightshade vegetables such as eggplants, tomatoes, and bell peppers, as well as black pepper spice. These items contain a chemical compound called solanine which may aggravate inflammation.

Lectins—Lectins are plant proteins that can cause trouble in your digestive system by sticking to your intestinal wall and creating intestinal permeability, another contributing factor to inflammation. The most common sources of lectins include grains, legumes, and nightshades. These plants contain drastically more lectins than other food sources. That said, lectin sensitivity varies widely from person to person. You'll know you have a problem with lectins if you experience inflammation, brain fog, migraines, stomach issues, acne or joint pain after eating a lectin-rich meal. The lectins in nightshades, in particular, are a common autoimmune trigger and can cause sensitivities in many people. To test yourself, fill up on a nightshade-heavy lunch—think tomatoes, peppers, and potatoes—and see how you feel afterward.

Weight Management And Calories

The idea that all calories are not created equally-is based on the concept of nutrient density. The source of the calories you consume can affect your health and weight in different ways, even if the number of calories is the same. Common sense tells even the biggest skeptic that 100 calories from potato chips are not the same as 100 calories from broccoli.

Our eating habits are driven not by the feeling of a full stomach, but rather by the brain's perception of sufficient amino acid intake. This process is rooted in the intricate mechanisms of nutrient and amino acid sensing. Typically, we continue eating until our digestive system signals our brain that we have consumed enough amino acids. These amino acids of course play a crucial role as they serve as the fundamental building blocks for various bodily functions, including muscle growth and tissue repair.

It is possible to eat a diet that is high in calories from processed foods, but low in nutrients, and still, be hungry. On the other hand, you can eat a diet that is lower in calories but higher in nutrients, and feel satisfied and full. Some research suggests that the body processes calories from different sources differently and that the way in which the body uses these calories can have different effects on appetite, metabolism, and body weight.

For example, some studies have found that diets high in protein and fibre can help to reduce appetite and increase weight loss, while diets high in added sugars and refined grains may contribute to weight gain.

A study published in the *International Journal of Obesity* found that when overweight individuals consumed a higher-protein breakfast, they had significantly reduced hunger and desire to eat later in the day compared to those who consumed a lower-protein breakfast. (31)

Another study published in the *British Journal of Nutrition* found that when adults consumed a high-protein, high-fat breakfast, they had significantly lower levels of the hunger hormone ghrelin and higher levels of the satiety hormone peptide YY compared to when they consumed a high-carbohydrate breakfast. (32)

Also, it is important to understand that eating foods that are high in sugar or have a high glycemic index (GI) can cause a rapid spike in blood sugar levels. The glycemic index is a measure of how quickly a food raises blood sugar levels. Foods with a high GI are rapidly absorbed and cause a rapid spike in blood sugar, while those with a low GI are absorbed more slowly and cause a slower, more gradual increase. Consuming high-sugar foods can cause an overproduction of insulin which can cause blood sugar levels to drop too low and lead to hypoglycemia.

A calorie is simply a measure of energy. It is defined as the amount of heat energy required to raise 1 gram of water 1 degree Celsius. We use a certain number of calories as energy a day depending on our activity level, and everything we eat has a certain calorie benefit to provide us with that energy.

If weight loss or gain is your concern, the laws of thermodynamics apply here. If you consume more calories than your body uses, you gain weight. If you consume less, you lose weight. A cheap kitchen scale to weigh your food and an app on your phone (often free in basic form) on which you enter what you eat and the measure of it, and you will know your calorie intake. Track your weight and adjust your calorie intake for the desired outcome. Simple? Maybe not quite.

What Is On Your Plate—Order Does Matter

The order in which we eat our food can have a significant impact on our digestion, nutrient absorption, and overall health. Experts recommend starting meals with foods that are high in fibre, such as fibrous vegetables.

Fibre can help slow down the digestive process, which can help regulate blood sugar levels, promote feelings of fullness, and support healthy gut bacteria. After consuming fibre-rich foods, it is recommended to move on to foods that are high in healthy protein and fats. These foods can help provide sustained energy and support various bodily functions, including hormone regulation and cell repair. Finally, it is recommended to consume carbohydrates, towards the end of the meal. This is because carbohydrates can cause a rapid rise in blood sugar levels, which can be problematic for those with blood sugar imbalances or diabetes. Consuming fibre prior to the carbohydrates blunts the rise in blood sugar. By prioritizing the order in which we consume our food, we can help support healthy digestion and blood sugar regulation.

Furthermore, eating complex carbohydrates during your evening meal can actually have a positive impact on sleep, as carbohydrates help to increase the production of serotonin, a key neurotransmitter that regulates sleep and mood. When serotonin levels are low, it can lead to sleep disturbances and mood disorders such as depression. We will cover neurotransmitters more in-depth in Section 4—Neurotransmitters, Hormones & Brain Wiring.

SMART PROTOCOL

Eat Your Food In This Order - $0

Prioritize fibrous vegetables at the start of your meal, followed by protein and fats, and save carbohydrates for last and complex carbohydrates later in the day.

Sugar—The Forever Trickster

The human body is hardwired to crave sugar, which can make it challenging to resist indulging in sweet treats. This is because sugar molecules can activate the "gut-brain axis," which plays a critical role in driving our preference for sugar. The gut-brain axis is a complex system of neurons and hormones that connect our digestive system and brain, allowing them to communicate and coordinate. Eating sweet foods can trigger a cascade of events in our bodies that can be difficult to resist. When we consume something sweet, the neuropod cells in our gut send signals to our brain, which activate the release of dopamine—the neurotransmitter responsible for feelings of pleasure and reward. This, in turn, can cause us to crave more sweet foods, leading to a vicious cycle of overeating. Interestingly, glucose—the main type of sugar in sweet foods—is the preferred source of fuel for the brain and nervous system. As such, our bodies are hardwired to seek out and consume sweet foods, making it challenging to resist temptation. To combat this, experts recommend consuming sweet foods alongside other foods that are high in fibre, as this can help reduce the glycemic index of the meal and slow down or blunt the release of dopamine. Increasing intake of essential fatty and amino acids may also help to decrease sugar cravings. This can help individuals enjoy their favourite treats without succumbing to cravings and overeating. (33)

What about artificial sweeteners? When it comes to curbing a sweet tooth, some people may turn to artificial sweeteners in hopes of reducing their sugar intake. However, these options may not be as effective as hoped. Artificial sweeteners are designed to activate the tongue's taste receptors, but they do not trigger the sensors in the gut that satisfy the craving for sugar. This means that individuals may still experience cravings and urges to consume sweet foods, even after consuming artificially sweetened options.

One of these sweeteners, sucralose, has been associated with potential disruptions to the composition and function of the microbiome. These disruptions include alterations in microbial diversity, impaired bacterial metabolism, increased gut inflammation, and potential impacts on the gut-brain axis. (34)

As a healthier alternative to artificial sweeteners, many have turned to Stevia. This natural sweetener has gained popularity in recent years because it does not raise blood glucose levels, making it a suitable option for those with diabetes or blood sugar imbalances. Despite its potential health benefits, it's important to note that consuming sweet foods can still lead to increased cravings and appetite. The sweet taste of stevia can stimulate the release of dopamine in the brain, leading to feelings of pleasure and reward that may increase the desire to eat more sweet foods. (35)

SMART CONSIDERATION

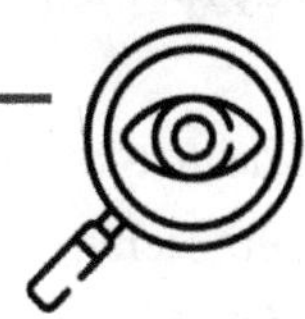

Blood Sugar—A Balancing Act

There are several effective ways to regulate blood sugar levels naturally. Incorporating 1 TBSP of apple cider vinegar (ACV) into your diet before a meal can prevent blood sugar spikes and help maintain stable blood sugar levels. A study published in the *Journal of Functional Foods* found that consuming apple cider vinegar before a meal led to a 20% reduction in postprandial glucose levels in healthy individuals, suggesting that it could be a useful tool in managing blood sugar levels. (36)

Extra virgin olive oil has been shown to have beneficial effects on glucose regulation in the body. (37) The monounsaturated fatty acids (MUFAs) found in olive oil can help improve insulin sensitivity, which is the body's ability to respond to and regulate blood sugar levels. This can be particularly beneficial for people with type 2 diabetes or those at risk of developing the condition.

Studies have also found that olive oil can help reduce postprandial (after-meal) blood glucose levels. (38) This is thought to be due to the high levels of polyphenols and antioxidants found in olive oil, which can help improve glucose uptake in the muscles and liver and reduce the production of glucose by the liver. It's worth noting that while olive oil can have positive effects on glucose regulation, it should be consumed in moderation as it is high in calories. The American Heart Association recommends limiting daily intake of added oils (including olive oil) to no more than 3 tablespoons per day for most adults. (39)

The use of berberine, a compound found in many plants, can also be beneficial. Berberine is known to improve the activity and proliferation of insulin beta cells, which can help balance blood sugar levels. (40) This makes it an effective natural supplement for managing blood sugar in individuals with type 2 diabetes or metabolic syndrome. It is important to use caution when taking berberine, as it has the potential to significantly lower blood sugar levels if not taken properly. There are other over-the-counter supplements that have been shown to lower blood glucose levels, including ginseng, magnesium, yerba mate, chromium, and certain acidic foods. (41)

Lastly, taking a short 10-20 minute walk after a meal can help regulate blood sugar levels, especially in people with type 2 diabetes. It increases insulin sensitivity and glucose uptake in the muscles and aids digestion.

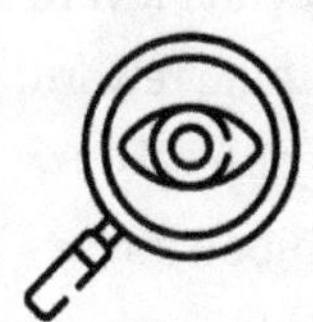

SMART CONSIDERATION

Know Your Numbers

Blood glucose monitors (BGMs) can be a valuable tool for individuals who want to monitor their blood sugar levels as a preventative measure or to determine which foods work best for their bodies. Testing blood sugar before and after meals can provide insights into which foods cause a spike in blood sugar levels, allowing individuals to adjust their diet accordingly. BGMs can also be useful for monitoring the effects of other activities, such as sauna sessions, cold plunges, and exercise, on blood sugar levels. By using a BGM to track their body's response to different activities, individuals can gain a better understanding of how their body uses fuel and make informed decisions about their lifestyle.

SMART CONSIDERATION

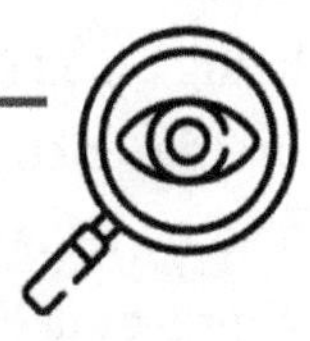

Train Your Brain

To develop healthy food preferences, some experts suggest a conditioning approach that involves pairing healthy foods with those that can elevate blood sugar levels for 7-10 days. The idea is to rewire the dopamine reward system, which can drive our desire for high-calorie, high-sugar foods. By pairing a healthy food, such as a vegetable, with a slightly blood sugar-elevating food, such as a complex carbohydrate, you can create positive associations in your brain between the two. Over time, this can help you to develop a preference for healthy foods and reduce cravings for unhealthy, highly processed options. This approach can be particularly useful for those who are struggling to make healthier food choices and looking for ways to retrain their taste buds and brain to crave more wholesome options. (42)

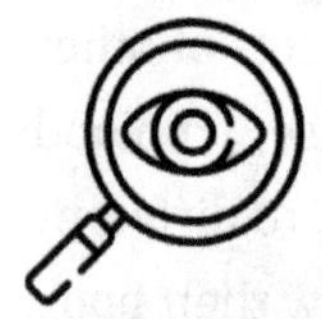

SMART CONSIDERATION

Give Your Gut More Glutamine

Glutamine is an amino acid that can help reduce sugar cravings by stabilizing blood sugar levels and promoting healthy digestion. It is found in protein-rich foods such as meat, fish, dairy, beans, and nuts, and can also be taken in supplement form. Glutamine has also been shown to improve gut health, support immune function, and reduce inflammation. It is particularly effective at healing and strengthening the gut lining, which can become damaged by poor diet, stress, and certain medications. (43)

Time-Restricted Eating

Time-restricted eating has many general benefits for overall health and wellness, including weight management and reducing the risk of various diseases such as obesity, diabetes, cardiovascular disease, neurodegenerative conditions, and cancer, as noted in a meta-analysis of 85 studies published in the *New England Journal of Medicine* in December 2019. (44) Intermittent fasting can lead to metabolic switching from glucose to ketones, making the body more metabolically flexible. This can result in cellular healing benefits such as increased ketone production, mitochondrial stress resistance, antioxidant defence, autophagy, and DNA repair, while decreasing glycogen, insulin, mTOR, and protein synthesis.

Studies have also shown that eating within a condensed window of time can lead to reductions in total body fat percentage, visceral fat, waist circumference, blood pressure, LDL cholesterol, and hemoglobin A1C. (45) Different lengths of fasting can lead to different benefits, including the start of autophagy at about 17 hours and gut reset at about 24 hours, fat-burning at about 36 hours, dopamine reset at about 48 hours, and immune reset after 72 hours or more. (46)

To ensure proper fast-breaking, recommendations for breaking a fast depend on individual goals such as resetting the gut, building muscle, or burning fat. For breaking a fast of 48 hours or more, it is suggested to start with a cup of broth, followed by a probiotic-rich meal with fat, steamed vegetables, and animal protein.

According to Satchin Panda, researcher, and author of the book, *The Circadian Code*, the practice of time-restricted eating has tremendously positive effects on your gastrointestinal tract ("gut"), liver, and brain. It helps balance your blood sugar and hormones, decreases inflammation, and even helps your mood and ability to focus. As an added bonus, it saves time! (47)

Both evidence and time constraints make an 8-hour feeding window optimal. The feeding window could be 6-12 hours. Less is difficult and may actually result in overeating and longer makes the fasting period too short for benefit. As with all aspects of self-care, you will find what works best for you.

The easiest methodology is to extend the natural sleeping fast that we all do. As an example, depending on your personal schedule, you might have your first meal at 11 am, and finish your last meal by 7 pm. While you sleep, your cells are undergoing repair and regeneration processes, and the glymphatic system in your brain is clearing toxins. This is best accomplished without the burden of digestion on your system, so the last meal should be 3 hours prior to bedtime. Social connection is vital, so shifting the feeding window as late as possible without encroaching on that 3-hour period prior to sleep is advantageous to allow for meals shared with family and friends.

What doesn't break your fasting state? During your fasting period, you can and should consume water, as well as unsweetened coffee, tea, or a similar beverage that does not contain calories or cause a significant rise in blood sugar. It's also okay to take supplements during this time. Some people find that adding full-fat cream or MCT oil to their coffee does not break their fast, but it's best to use a blood glucose tester or continuous blood glucose monitor to measure your glucose level and ensure this is the case. As long as your beverages and additives do not contain calories or significantly affect blood sugar levels, they are generally acceptable to consume during a fasting state.

Fasting Considerations For Women

According to author Dr. Mindy Pelz, in her book, *Fast Like A Girl: A Woman's Guide to Using the Healing Power of Fasting to Burn Fat, Boost Energy, and Balance Hormones*, women should fast differently than men due to hormonal differences. Dr. Pelz proposes a hormonal fasting schedule based on a woman's menstrual cycle. During what she calls the power phase (Days 1-10 and Days 16-19), fasting can be done for 13 to 72 hours. During ovulation (Days 11-15), fasting should be limited to 13 to 15 hours. During the nurturing phase (Day 20 to bleeding), no fasting should be done. According to this recommendation, women going through menopause should begin their fasting routine based on the current phase of the moon, with the full moon marking the start of ovulation. (48)

SMART PROTOCOL

Time-Restricted Eating - $0

Choose a time window: Determine the number of hours you want to eat each day, ideally between 8-12 hours. Gradually adjust your eating schedule: Start by pushing back your breakfast by 30 minutes each day until you reach your desired time window. Consume water and electrolytes, and if you wish unsweetened coffee and/or tea, and your usual supplements during the fasting period. Finish your last meal of the day at least 3 hours prior to sleep.

SMART CONSIDERATION

Get Fasting, Faster

You don't really achieve a "fasting" state until you have digested the last meal and your blood sugar has returned to baseline levels. A 10-20 minute walk after eating can help shorten the time to fasted state.

Vitamins

Vitamins are organic compounds vital to the body's basic functions and are found abundantly in whole foods. They help regulate all functions in the body; metabolism, fighting off infection, repair, and growth of body tissues, energy maintenance, fertility, and the onset of numerous enzyme reactions.

Since our bodies can't manufacture vitamins (except for Vitamin D, which can be synthesized by the body from the sun), they need to be ingested.

Vitamins are either water-soluble or fat-soluble. Water-soluble vitamins include the B vitamins and vitamin C, and they can be absorbed easily by the water in our bodies. Fat-soluble vitamins A, D, E, and K, require a source of fat to be efficiently absorbed. This is why it's often recommended to take vitamins along with food.

When vitamins are extracted and taken in supplement form we can help boost nutrient intake and combat deficiencies lacking in the diet.

Minerals

Minerals are inorganic compounds that come from the earth and whose major functions in the body include monitoring water balance, enzyme and hormone production, strengthening bones, and carrying oxygen through the bloodstream.

There are two types of minerals: macrominerals which we need more of, and trace minerals which we need less of, but are just as important. Macrominerals include calcium, phosphorus, magnesium, sodium, potassium, chloride, and sulphur. Trace minerals include iron, manganese, copper, iodine, zinc, cobalt, fluoride, and selenium.

As with vitamins, minerals can be acquired in the diet or in supplement form to help meet nutritional requirements.

To Supplement Or Not?

In an ideal world, it would be best to get all the nutrients we need from high-quality, wholesome foods, but how realistic is that? With our busy lifestyles, we often don't take the time to plan and prepare well-balanced, nutritional meals. Another reason we don't get necessary nutrients from our everyday foods is due to the depletion of nutrients in our earth's soil. Our agriculture is not what it used to be: from genetically modified organisms to herbicides, pesticides, erosion, and increased radiation, the quality of our soil and agriculture has decreased significantly. Nitrogen, phosphorus, and potassium fertilizers have played a big role in depleting our soil of essential nutrients, and when nutrients aren't in our soil, they won't be found in our food. (49) This is why eating organic as much as possible is highly recommended to avoid dealing with chemical side effects.

Not All Vitamins Are Created Equal

When buying supplements, it is important to do your research. Good supplements should be whole-food-based, without chemicals, dyes, binders, or fillers. Find a nutraceutical company that is meticulous with its raw material and nutrient selection, one that aims to maximize the stability, absorption, and metabolism of its formulas. Ensure that they offer nutritional supplements that are free of ingredients commonly associated with negative side effects, that are non-GMO sourced, gluten-free, soy-free, and free of any artificial sweeteners or flavours. They must also be in accordance with the GMP regulations by the NSF international. (50)

Be warned: Taking a poor-quality supplement can be worse than taking no supplement at all. Not only do you get a false sense of security about getting the right amount of nutrients, but depending on the supplement's quality, you could also be ingesting unnecessary fillers or binders.

How Do I Know If I Am Vitamin Deficient?

If you start taking vitamin supplements after suspecting you're deficient, it's important to understand that you shouldn't expect to see instant results. The time it takes for your body to reach a healthy state again can vary depending on the severity of your deficiency. When your body lacks essential vitamins, it can lead to various symptoms and health issues, and simply taking a supplement won't immediately reverse these effects. The process of restoring vitamin levels and addressing deficiencies takes time and patience.

The duration it takes for your body to recover from a deficiency depends on multiple factors—the severity of the deficiency, your overall health, your body's ability to absorb and utilize the supplemented vitamins, and whether there are any underlying conditions affecting your nutrient absorption.

If your deficiency is mild or moderate, and you start taking the appropriate supplements as recommended, you may start noticing improvements in your health in a few weeks. For more severe deficiencies, it may take longer to restore your vitamin levels to a healthy range. In some cases, your healthcare provider may prescribe higher doses of supplements to accelerate the replenishment process. Regular monitoring and follow-ups with your healthcare professional are essential to ensure you're on the right track and to make any necessary adjustments to your supplement regimen.

Combining supplements with a healthy diet and lifestyle is a comprehensive approach to promoting optimal health and addressing deficiencies effectively.

SMART CONSIDERATION

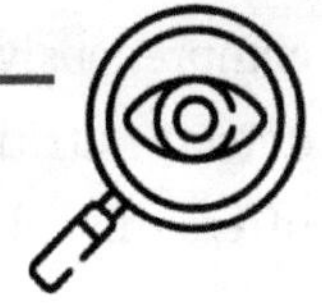

Blood Serum Test

A reliable test to measure some vitamins and minerals in the blood is a blood serum test. This test measures the levels of some vitamins and minerals in the liquid portion of the blood called serum. The most common ones to be measured by routine lab work include vitamin D, vitamin B12, iron, and ferritin, however, your annual regular blood work is most likely not comprehensive enough to test for other specific vitamin and mineral deficiencies. More extensive nutrient panels also exist to measure a combination of vitamins, minerals, and antioxidants that can impact health and can be ordered through a functional health practitioner.

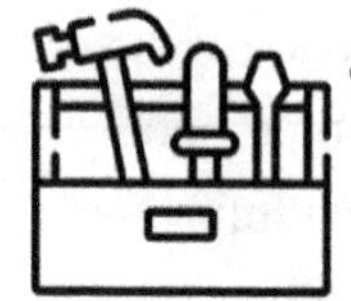

SMART TOOLS

Laboratory Testing For Nutritional Deficiencies

Laboratory tests can precisely measure nutrient deficiencies, helping you understand and address your specific health needs. Companies offer various comprehensive tests to assess these deficiencies. Organic acid testing (OAT) detects nutritional gaps affecting metabolic processes. Mosaic Diagnostics offers this, plus tests for mycotoxins, food sensitivities, and candida.

Genova Diagnostics, a leading clinical lab, offers the NutrEval® assessment, analyzing over 125 biomarkers like vitamins, amino acids, and antioxidants from urine and blood samples. (51) They also provide the Metabolomix + test, a more accessible home test, focusing on metabolic needs and oxidative stress markers. It offers a broader metabolic perspective than OAT by including amino acids and oxidative stress markers, but it isn't as extensive as NutrEval®. Please note that these tests need to be ordered through a licensed health care provider.

While these valuable tests are underutilized and come with a cost, they pave the way for personalized nutrition's future.

Foundational Supplements

Navigating the world of dietary supplements can be overwhelming and complex, with countless options available to choose from. However, there are a few foundational supplements that are essential for maintaining optimal health and well-being, particularly for supporting gut health, reducing inflammation, and improving overall health. While individual supplement needs may vary, we recommend the following supplements as a good starting point for anyone looking to enhance their overall health and well-being.

Vitamin D

Vitamin D works through a variety of mechanisms and has been shown to be beneficial for heart health, immune support, osteoporosis/osteopenia, oral health, mood disorders, and inflammation. It also helps regulate calcium in the body, necessary for the maintenance of strong bones. Unfortunately, only a handful of foods contain significant amounts of Vitamin D. Additionally, exposure to sunlight, our best source for Vitamin D, is not always available, given the long winters that dominate the Northern Hemisphere. Therefore, deficiency of Vitamin D is extremely common and supplementation is recommended.

Vitamin K (K1 and K2) is often included in high-quality formulations because it is needed to work in synergy with vitamin D, as both vitamins D and K are essential for optimal bone and arterial health. Vitamin K helps keep the important bone protein, osteocalcin, carboxylated. Undercarboxylated osteocalcin cannot regulate calcium, causing it to freely circulate in the bloodstream, and potentially be deposited in the soft tissues (calcification) such as arterial walls or kidneys. Although they originate from different sources, the inclusion of K1 along with the highly bioavailable K2 (otherwise known as MK-7), provides a comprehensive scope of vitamin K to complement the vitamin D supplement. (52)

Consider getting your Vitamin D levels tested to find out your ideal intake. The best time to get Vitamin D levels tested is at the end of the summer, especially in areas where winters are long when technically your reserves should be replenished.

Omega-3

Supplementing with high-quality fish oil is also highly beneficial. Omega-3 fatty acids are a precursor to prostaglandins, which help prevent cardio-vascular disease and regulate inflammation in the body. (53)

As mentioned previously, most North Americans are getting a way higher ratio of omega-6 to omega-3 than the recommended 3:1 ratio. (54) This is due in part to the fact that we are consuming more omega-6 from canola oil, soy oil, and corn because we are consuming processed foods made from these substances. Additionally, quality is important here. Be sure to purchase fish oil supplements harvested from smaller fish like sardines and anchovies that carry fewer toxins, such as mercury, in their bodies. Make sure you look for fish oil that also includes an antioxidant like vitamin E to protect the oil from oxidation and rancidity. It is also important to note that fish oils that are offered in a natural triglycerides (TG) form have superior bioavailability compared to fish oils in the ester (EE) form.

You can actually get your fatty acid levels tested to determine whether you have optimal levels of omega-3 fatty acids to effectively reduce your risk of developing diseases. A Fatty Acid Profile typically includes the following: Omega-3 Index, Omega-3 Whole Blood Score, Arachidonic Acid to EPA Ratio, Mono-unsaturated fatty acids, Saturated fatty acids, and Trans fatty acids. Ask your natural health provider as this is not a general annual test that is done, but is well worth the money.

Collagen

Collagen is the most abundant protein in the body, accounting for about one-third of its protein composition. There are 4 main types of collagen in the body:

Type I—This type accounts for 90% of your body's collagen and is made of densely packed fibres. It provides structure to skin, bones, tendons, fibrous cartilage, connective tissue, and teeth.

Type II—This type is made of more loosely-packed fibres and is found in elastic cartilage, which cushions the joints.

Type III—This type supports the structure of muscles, organs, and arteries.

Type IV—This type helps with filtration and is found in the layers of your skin. (55)

Simply put, collagen is said to be the "glue" that holds our bodies together. In our youth, our body produces all the collagen it needs, allowing for firm skin, supple joints, and strong bones. However, production levels start decreasing after you turn 30, gradually leading to physical signs like older-looking skin, thinner hair, brittle nails, stiff joints, and slower recovery from physical activity. Therefore, supplementing with a high-quality collagen supplement is a steadfast way to get ahead of the most common signs of ageing. In an ideal world, we would be getting doses of collagen from our diets. Collagen is abundantly found in animal connective tissue, skin, bones, and cartilage (bovine—cow collagen), however, very rarely do we consume adequate amounts of these sources. Thankfully, there is a better, simpler solution that makes it even easier to get more collagen in your diet—by getting it in supplement form.

What about marine collagen? Marine collagen has gained popularity in recent years and can be a great alternative to animal-sourced collagen for people who do not eat animal products. Marine collagen comes from fish—either the skin, bones, or scales. If you're a pescetarian and want to consume collagen, this is the type for you. Marine collagen boosts types I and II collagen, whereas bovine has been found to increase types I and III collagen. (56)

In his book, *The Collagen Cure: The Forgotten Role of Glycine and Collagen in Optimal Health and Longevity,* author and renowned cardiovascular research scientist, James DiNicolantonio emphasizes the importance of consuming adequate amounts of collagen, glycine, and other essential nutrients to support overall health and well-being. Collagen and glycine are critical for collagen turnover in the body, and low levels of these compounds can lead to a range of health issues. Glycine is also required for the synthesis of glutathione, creatine, and heme, making it a crucial nutrient for overall health. However, most people do not consume enough glycine in their diet and may be deficient in this essential amino acid. To properly absorb glycine and other essential nutrients, it is also important to consume adequate amounts of vitamin C. DiNicolantonio recommends a daily intake of 10-20 grams of collagen, 10-15 grams of glycine, 6-15 grams of glutamine, and 1-3 grams of taurine, divided into several smaller doses throughout the day. By ensuring adequate intake of these important nutrients, individuals can support optimal health and wellness. (57)

Magnesium

Magnesium is an essential mineral whose health benefits are often overlooked. This mineral is used by every organ in your body, especially your heart, muscles, bones, and kidneys. Researchers have recently found over 3000 magnesium binding sites on human proteins and have also found it in more than 300 different enzymes in the body which are responsible for: (58)

- Creation of ATP (energy)
- Formation of healthy bones and teeth
- Relaxation of blood vessels
- Promotion of proper bowel movements
- Regulation of blood sugar
- Detoxification processes

In North America, magnesium intakes fall short of dietary recommendations for a large segment of the population. Causes of magnesium deficiency may be related to poor diet, high caffeine or alcohol consumption, hormonal imbalances, exposure to pesticides, and the regular use of diuretics and antibiotics that prohibit the proper absorption of the mineral.

Magnesium influences muscle performance by participating in energy metabolism and maintenance of muscle contraction and relaxation. Research further shows that magnesium deficiency can lead to a disruption of neuromuscular function and that high levels of physical activity increase the body's demand for magnesium.

When monitoring your magnesium levels, it is crucial to focus on red cell magnesium instead of solely relying on serum magnesium. The serum magnesium test measures the level of magnesium in the liquid portion of the blood, known as serum. It is a common test that evaluates the concentration of magnesium ions circulating in the bloodstream at the time of the test. Serum magnesium levels can fluctuate rapidly, as the body tightly regulates levels to maintain normal physiological function.

On the other hand, red cell magnesium measurements provide a more accurate reflection of your body's magnesium status. This test assesses the level of magnesium within red blood cells (erythrocytes). It measures the amount of magnesium that is bound to the red blood cells and provides an estimate of the body's magnesium stores over a longer period.

Red blood cells have a higher concentration of magnesium than serum, and measuring magnesium within them can give a better indication of intracellular magnesium levels. It is often used when there is suspicion of chronic magnesium deficiency or to monitor magnesium levels in individuals with certain conditions.

There are many different forms of magnesium available, each with its own specific role and benefits. For example, magnesium glycinate is known for its ability to promote restful sleep and relaxation, while magnesium malate is often used to support energy production and combat fatigue. Magnesium threonate has been shown to cross the blood-brain barrier (BBB) more effectively than other forms of magnesium, due to its unique molecular structure. It has been shown to support cognitive function and improve memory, while magnesium bicarbonate is crucial for maintaining pH balance in the body. Other forms, such as magnesium taurate, chloride, citrate, and sulphate, each have unique properties and benefits, ranging from regulating blood pressure to improving digestion and combating constipation. Some supplements contain a combination of different forms of magnesium to ensure that all of the body's magnesium needs are met. Avoid taking magnesium with zinc as it may reduce absorption.

SMART CONSIDERATION

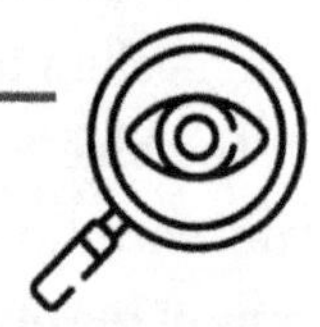

Transdermal Magnesium

For individuals with compromised gut health, including those with intestinal permeability or malabsorption issues, oral magnesium supplements may not be efficiently absorbed by the body. In such cases, the intended benefits of supplementation may not be fully realized, leading to suboptimal magnesium levels. Transdermal magnesium, or the absorption of magnesium through the skin, is an alternative method for supplementing this essential mineral. It offers a way to bypass the digestive system, allowing for direct absorption into the bloodstream and tissues. Epsom salts, or magnesium sulphate, can be dissolved in warm water, allowing the body to absorb magnesium during a relaxing bath. This absorption occurs mainly through the hair follicles and sweat glands on the skin. (59) There are also several topical transdermal magnesium products available. We recommend the MagSol gel from epsomgel.ca as a convenient way to provide the body with a readily absorbable source of this vital mineral.

Creatine Monohydrate

Creatine is a peptide, which is a compound consisting of two or more amino acids linked in a chain—in this case, L-arginine, glycine, and methionine. Creatine is naturally produced in the body in small amounts. The kidneys use glycine and arginine to create guanidine-acetic acid (GAA) which is then transported via the bloodstream to the liver where it is then converted into creatine. From there, the creatine is once again carried around by your bloodstream, primarily to skeletal muscle, but also to other target tissues—one notable one being the brain.

Just like in humans, creatine is also produced naturally in other animals which is why consuming animal protein is an excellent source of creatine.

When the body utilizes energy in the form of ATP, it transforms into ADP (adenosine diphosphate) as it loses a phosphate group. Creatine, which has its own phosphate, can replenish ADP by donating its phosphate, transforming it back into ATP, enabling the body to use it for energy again. This can result in improved pre-workout energy.

Isn't creatine just used for bodybuilding? No. Recent research also supports the consumption of 5 g of creatine per day for brain health and cognitive function, especially in people who follow a meat-free diet. (60)

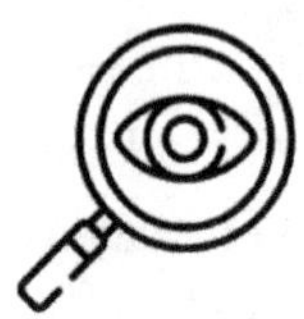

SMART CONSIDERATION

Go Green

Incorporating greens supplementation into your diet can be an effective means of addressing nutrient shortcomings. Often referred to as "green superfood powder," these supplements consist of a blend of dried greens, algae, berries, and herbs. These ingredients have earned the title of "superfoods" due to their high levels of nutrients, including phytochemicals, antioxidants, and other beneficial compounds. By incorporating these supplements into your daily routine, you can boost your intake of essential vitamins, minerals, and antioxidants.

It's worth noting that some people may experience adverse reactions to high-oxalate greens like spinach, kale, and chard, which can hinder nutrient absorption. These oxalates are commonly referred to as "anti-nutrients," and it's crucial to be mindful of their effects. For those who are sensitive to oxalates or at risk of kidney stones, low-oxalate greens drinks can be an excellent alternative. Opting for greens like arugula, broccoli, Brussels sprouts, and Bok choy, along with low-oxalate fruits like blueberries, kiwi, and grapes, can provide added nutrients and flavour to the greens drink.

SMART PROTOCOL

Foundational Supplements - $ to $$

Try your best to integrate these foundational supplements into your daily routine:

- Vitamins D (if your tested levels are low)
- Omega-3 fatty acids
- Collagen (with glycine & Vitamin C)
- Magnesium and creatine monohydrate.

Other Sources Of Fuel And Energy

It has been said that we are portable electronic devices, and we get our charge from the sun and from the electrons in the ground. Our ancestors certainly spent a lot of time with large amounts of their skin exposed to the sun and their bare feet on the ground. When you are grounded, electrons move from the Earth into your body and from your body into the

Earth. The theory is that this helps maintain the body's negative charge electrical potential. Among the many benefits are lowered oxidative stress and inflammation.

Grounding, also known as earthing, is the practice of connecting with the Earth's natural energy by direct physical contact. This can be achieved by simply walking barefoot on the grass, sand, or soil, or by using grounded products such as mats or sheets. Grounding has been found to offer a wide range of benefits, both physical and psychological, and has been gaining popularity as a complementary therapy for various health issues.

One of the most well-known benefits of grounding is improved sleep quality. Grounding has been found to reduce cortisol levels and promote the production of melatonin, which helps regulate sleep patterns. This can lead to better, more restful sleep and a reduction in symptoms of insomnia.

Studies have shown that grounding can help regulate our circadian rhythm, the internal biological process that controls our sleep-wake cycle. (61) This is because the earth's negative electrons can help neutralize the positive charges in our bodies that can disrupt our sleep patterns. As a result, grounding can help us fall asleep faster, sleep deeper, and wake up feeling refreshed.

Depending on where you live, and the climate or season, it may not be easy to just pop out the door and walk barefoot in the backyard so grounding mats are a great way to reap the health benefits when weather or circumstance is prohibitive. These mats are made of conductive materials that allow you to connect with the earth's surface. By placing a grounding mat under your sheets, you can absorb the earth's electrons throughout the night, promoting deeper and more restful sleep.

Another great benefit of grounding is that it can help protect the body from electromagnetic fields (EMFs) emitted by electronic devices such as cell phones, computers, and Wi-Fi routers. By grounding oneself, it is believed that the body can absorb electrons from the earth, which can help neutralize the effects of EMFs and restore the body's natural electrical balance. (62)

SMART PROTOCOL

Grounding - $0

Spend time outdoors in nature—make an effort to spend time in green spaces like parks, forests, and gardens. Try to walk barefoot on natural surfaces such as grass, sand, and dirt as often as possible. Unfinished concrete can be a suitable option for those living in snowy and cold climates.

SMART UPGRADES

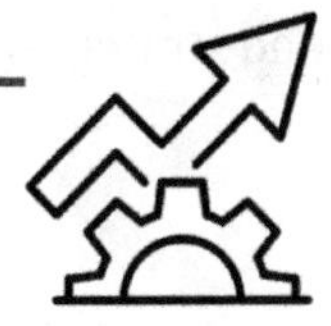

Get Grounded

Consider purchasing a grounding mat for your sleep mattress or for the area where you stand while working. A reliable resource with good information: earthing.com. This can help to transfer the earth's energy into your body. Earthing shoes, also known as grounding shoes, are designed to help individuals connect with the earth's natural energy by allowing electrons to flow from the ground to the body. These shoes are made with conductive materials, such as copper, that allow for the transfer of electrons from the ground to the body, promoting the health benefits of earthing or grounding.

Section Wrap-Up

Hydration and proper nutrition are the foundations upon which our health and vitality are built. Fueling our bodies with the right nutrients is crucial for sustained energy levels, healthy metabolism, and the prevention of chronic diseases; however, the journey to holistic well-being doesn't stop here. In Section 3—Movement, Exercise & Detoxification, we will delve into another vital aspect of a healthy lifestyle: exercise, movement, and detoxification. Just as hydration and nutrition nourish our bodies from within, exercise and movement serve as essential catalysts for our physical well-being. We will explore effective strategies to build athletic endurance, outline a variety of exercises that can be incorporated into your routine, and strategies to aid detoxification.

PROTOCOLS QUICK REFERENCE CHECKLIST:

PROTOCOL—Daily Water Intake - $0 to $

☐ *Currently doing* ☐ *Want to integrate* ☐ *Not for now*

PROTOCOL—Exercise Hydration - $0 to $

☐ *Currently doing* ☐ *Want to integrate* ☐ *Not for now*

PROTOCOL—Electrolytes Replenishment For Heavy Sweating - $

☐ *Currently doing* ☐ *Want to integrate* ☐ *Not for now*

PROTOCOL—Daily Protein Intake - $

☐ *Currently doing* ☐ *Want to integrate* ☐ *Not for now*

PROTOCOL—Daily Fat Intake - $

☐ *Currently doing* ☐ *Want to integrate* ☐ *Not for now*

PROTOCOL—Daily Fermented Food Intake - $

☐ *Currently doing* ☐ *Want to integrate* ☐ *Not for now*

PROTOCOL– Oil Pulling - $

☐ *Currently doing* ☐ *Want to integrate* ☐ *Not for now*

PROTOCOL—Pantry Clean-Up Time - $0

☐ *Currently doing* ☐ *Want to integrate* ☐ *Not for now*

PROTOCOL—Eat Your Food In This Order - $0

☐ *Currently doing* ☐ *Want to integrate* ☐ *Not for now*

PROTOCOL—Time-Restricted Eating - $0

☐ *Currently doing* ☐ *Want to integrate* ☐ *Not for now*

PROTOCOL—Foundational Supplements - $ to $$

☐ *Currently doing* ☐ *Want to integrate* ☐ *Not for now*

PROTOCOL—Grounding - $0

☐ *Currently doing* ☐ *Want to integrate* ☐ *Not for now*

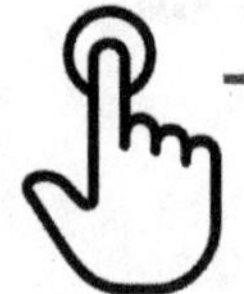

SMART RESOURCES

- Vivoo strips—(water, magnesium, calcium, Vitamin C, ketone, pH, sodium, free radicals and protein) vivoo.io
- OmegaQuant (omega-3/omega-6 index)—omegaquant.com
- Blood glucose monitor (BGM)—dexcom.com or levelshealth.com
- Transdermal Magnesium—epsomgel.ca
- Ketone strips blood (Free Style Precision)
- Ketone Ester—hvmn.com, or ketone salts—pruvitnow.com

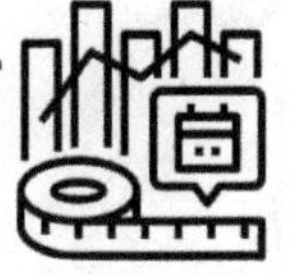

SMART TOOLS AT A GLANCE

- GI Assessment—diagnosticsolutionslab.com/tests/gi-map, gdx .net/products/gi-effects
- Nutritional Assessment Tool from Genova Diagnostics— gdx.net/products/nutreval, gdx.net/products/metabolomix
- Organic Acid Test from Mosaic Diagnostics—mosaicdx.com
- Grounding mats (Clint Ober)—ultimatelongevity.com/earthing-grounding/products

Section 3—Movement, Exercise & Detoxification

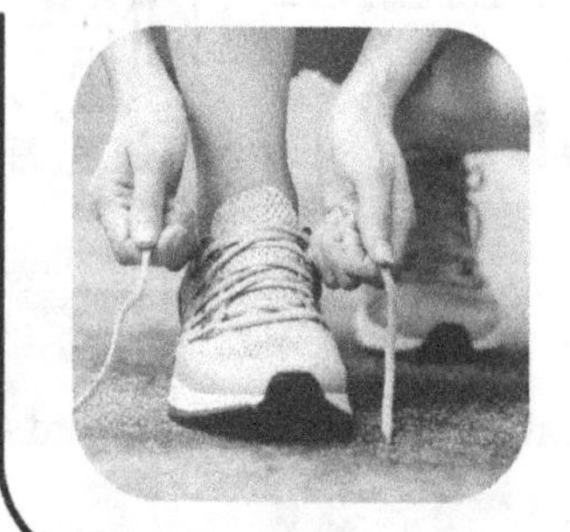

"The only bad workout is the one that didn't happen."

—Unknown

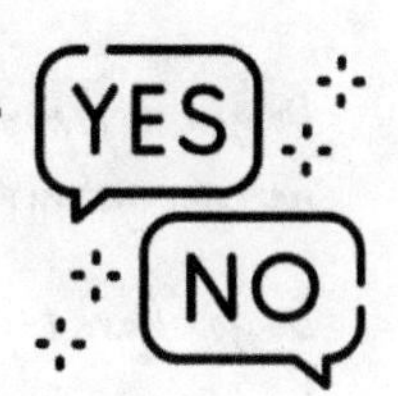

SELF EVALUATION-DISCOVERY QUESTIONS

Question	Y	N
Do you have a strength training practice?	Y	N
Do you have a muscular endurance practice?	Y	N
Do you have an aerobic training practice?	Y	N
Do you have an anaerobic training practice?	Y	N
Do you have full and pain-free joint and spine mobility?	Y	N
Do you walk at least 10,000 steps per day?	Y	N
Do you have a daily basic movement routine?	Y	N
Can you get up from the ground without using your elbow or hands?	Y	N
Do you integrate good breathing techniques into your exercise routine with attention to breathing gear?	Y	N
Do you do any weekly advanced breathwork or simulated altitude training?	Y	N

Question	Y	N
Do you do a post-workout breathing routine to rebalance your nervous system?	Y	N
Do you have 1-2 bowel movements per day?	Y	N
Do you sweat at least 4 or 5x times a week? (sauna or exercise)	Y	N
Do you eat organic/non-GMO most of the time?	Y	N
Do you buy natural beauty products most of the time?	Y	N
Do you buy natural cleaning products most of the time?	Y	N
Do you use non-toxic cookware?	Y	N
Do you use a HEPA filter system for your house?	Y	N
Do you use a water filtering system for your house's tap water?	Y	N
Do you have strategies to mitigate EMFs?	Y	N
Do you use detox supplements/botanicals on a regular basis?	Y	N
Have you ever done a genetic test to look at your SNPs to determine if you have slower detoxification pathways?	Y	N

Do you have a quick daily lymphatic drainage routine? Y N

Do you have a more extensive weekly lymphatic drainage routine to detox more in-depth? Y N

You can "cheat" on your nutrition but you can't cheat on exercise. For example, if you have the resources, you can have someone cook excellent meals for you, do the work to eliminate refined and processed foods, and make it all tasty. You can use high-quality greens supplements to make up for a lack of veggies on a particular day. You can support your nutrition with vitamins, minerals, and even fibre supplements.

You can't cheat on exercise. You own it. When you see someone who has dedicated themselves to working out regularly you can tell by their posture, by their look, the way they move. And you know that they have put the work in, not somebody else.

Of all the things an individual can do and not do in the name of health and longevity, exercise is the most important, and its benefits can not be made up for in any other way. Resistance exercise and strength training is the number one way to combat neuromuscular ageing, and the ability to engage in movement is the key to independent living.

The best sleep medication: EXERCISE
The best medicine to regulate blood sugar: EXERCISE
The best longevity drug: EXERCISE
The best way to increase healthspan: EXERCISE

Building A Strong Foundation

As we age, we begin to lose muscle mass with each passing year. This muscle loss is a condition known as sarcopenia, which typically starts around age 30 and accelerates after age 60. Once you reach the age of 40, you begin to lose muscle mass at a rate of approximately 1% every year, depending on the individual. According to a study published in *Current Opinion in Rheumatology*, adults can lose between 3% to 8% of their muscle mass each decade after 30. (1) Resistance and strength training has been proven to slow down this process, and as we discussed in Section 2—Hydration, Fuel & Foundationals, eating plenty of high quality protein also helps to combat sarcopenia. (2)

It is equally important to consider the decline in strength and power as we age, which can range from 3% to 5% per year after age 40. A review in the *Journal of Gerontology* noted that, on average, strength declines about 15% per decade in our 60s and 70s, and about 30% per decade after that. (3) It's not solely the process of ageing that leads to a decline in functionality, but rather the loss of movement and lack of training. The good news is that it's never too late to start addressing this issue. According to neuroscientists, the reason we have a large brain is to direct movement. Our bodies are tuned to move, often and rigorously.

In addition to the decline in strength, power and muscle mass, there is also an 8-10% decrease in speed every year after age 40. This rate of decline seems quite high. While it is true that speed, measured as sprint speed or reaction time, tends to decline with age, the exact rate can be variable. A study on master athletes found that sprint speed declines at about 0.7–0.8% per year after the age of 25. (4) The decline would likely be more pronounced in non-athletes and older individuals, but an 8-10% annual decrease may overstate the average rate of decline.

Individual rates of decrease in muscle mass, strength, power and speed can vary based on a range of factors including diet, exercise, genetics, and overall health status. The message to take away is two-fold. Number one, it is never too late to halt or reverse this decline with good diet and exercise. Number two, if you are younger than 40 years of age, build the greatest base of all of these parameters of fitness while it is easier to do so. Your future older self will be grateful.

This isn't your parents' era of exercise. Our ancestors had to engage in vigorous activities to sustain and safeguard themselves, and our bodies have evolved accordingly. Exercise impacts numerous aspects of health and well-being, encompassing joint and musculoskeletal health, cardiovascular and respiratory health, metabolic health, mental health, and even learning and behaviour. It also increases both blood flow to the brain and the production of a protein called Brain-Derived Neurotrophic Factor (BDNF), which plays a crucial role in promoting neural connections and enhancing cognitive functions. In fact, exercise can help overcome a great many lifestyle "sins," most notably helping our body regulate blood sugar.

Exercise has a very low barrier to entry—anybody can do it, and it costs nothing to get started. When Dr. Nathalie's patients give her excuses as to why they can't exercise, she says, "Do you own a floor?". At its simplest, the cost involved is your time and effort - and literally, your sweat! For maximum benefit, you need to work hard. Notice we said for maximum benefit. Any movement for any amount of time is better than none, and the benefits scale according to the time and effort one applies.

Exercise is not one thing but many things. It should encompass strength, hypertrophy (increasing or at least maintaining muscle size), muscle endurance, and aerobic and anaerobic capacity. Strength is the ability to lift a heavy object, and involves both the muscle and the nervous control of the muscle. Hypertrophy refers to the size of the muscle (think bodybuilders) and is related to but not the same as strength. Muscle endurance refers to the muscles ability to keep contracting over longer periods of time, as is the case with postural muscles. Aerobic capacity refers to the ability of the body to keep moving with an adequate supply of oxygen to the cells, as in a long jog or run. And anaerobic capacity refers to the ability of the body to keep moving in the absence of oxygen, as in the case of sprinting.

Drs. Andy Galpin and Andrew Huberman, in their collaboration series, aired on the popular Huberman Lab podcast, delineate nine adaptations to exercise. (5) They include skill and technique, speed, power, strength, muscular hypertrophy, muscular endurance, anaerobic capacity, aerobic capacity, and overall body endurance.

Training to encompass the nine adaptations is a complex endeavour. This Section will give you an excellent current science-based framework for designing a program to work on overall health, even if you are quite experienced in the gym or in other areas of training. It is not, and indeed cannot, take you from zero knowledge to even beginner or intermediate if you have no training background. We have made every effort to keep terminology basic. If you find yourself repeatedly unfamiliar with what we are talking about, you need to engage a good strength and conditioning coach to help you—it will be one of the best investments you can make in yourself.

In order to design an exercise program that optimizes both your health and the use of your valuable time, each of these adaptations needs to be considered. Which ones should you focus on, and what ratio of each should you do? To answer that question is the old adage "test, don't guess". Here are a variety of ways to accomplish that. Whenever possible, low or no-cost methods are included.

1. Skill And Technique

Learning to move with more efficiency, and the ability to achieve a specific position, timing or sequence, are critical for moving and exercising safely.

The best route here is to have a movement assessment done by a good strength and conditioning coach, athletic therapist, chiropractor, or physiotherapist. They will assess movement patterns and the range of motion of each relevant joint. Look for one of the above-mentioned professionals who are certified in a validated assessment system like Functional Movement Systems™. The basis of these types of assessments is that if you are unable to attain a certain position or range of motion with body weight or unloaded, you certainly should not be adding weight, let alone performing repetitions.

If you must do this assessment yourself, here is a great self-test we have designed that can provide valuable insight into your stability and mobility levels.

SMART PROTOCOL

Stability And Mobility Self Evaluation - $0

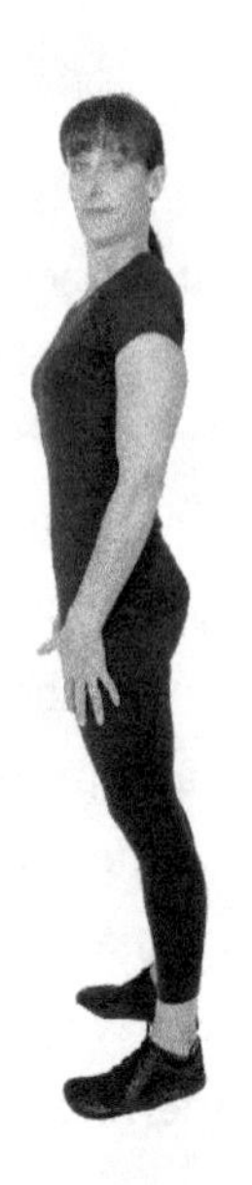

NECK ROTATION

While standing 90 degrees to a mirror, assume the starting position by standing erect with feet together and toes pointing forward. Rotate the head as far as possible to the right using the nose-to-chin line as your reference, and view your head rotation in the mirror. The line from your nose to your chin should reach mid-clavicle or 80 degrees. Change your stance position to view yourself in the mirror on the other side and then rotate the head as far as possible to the left and view your result in the mirror.

- 2 POINTS IF YOU CAN TURN TO MID-CLAVICLE OR 80 DEGREES TO THE LEFT
- 1 POINT IF YOU CAN REACH TO MIDLINE (STERNAL NOTCH) TO LEFT
- 2 POINTS IF YOU CAN TURN TO MID-CLAVICLE OR 80 DEGREES TO THE RIGHT
- 1 POINT IF YOU CAN TURN TO MIDLINE (STERNAL NOTCH) TO RIGHT

SHOULDER MOBILITY TEST

Assume the starting position by standing erect with feet together and toes pointing forward. (a) Reach overhead with the right arm in a "combing hair" motion, trying to touch the left shoulder blade. (b) Reach behind your back with your right arm, trying to touch the bottom of your left shoulder blade. Repeat on the other side.

- 2 POINTS IF YOU CAN REACH YOUR LEFT ARM OVERHEAD AND TOUCH THE RIGHT SHOULDER BLADE
- 1 POINT IF YOU CAN REACH YOUR LEFT ARM TO TOUCH THE TOP OF YOUR HEAD
- 2 POINTS IF YOU CAN REACH YOUR RIGHT ARM OVERHEAD AND TOUCH THE LEFT SHOULDER BLADE
- 1 POINT IF YOU CAN REACH YOUR RIGHT ARM TO TOUCH THE TOP OF YOUR HEAD
- 2 POINTS IF YOU CAN REACH YOUR LEFT ARM BEHIND YOUR BACK AND TOUCH THE BOTTOM OF YOUR RIGHT SHOULDER BLADE
- 1 POINT IF YOU CAN REACH YOUR LEFT ARM BEHIND YOUR BACK ABOVE YOUR BELTLINE
- 2 POINTS IF YOU CAN REACH YOUR RIGHT ARM BEHIND YOUR BACK AND TOUCH THE BOTTOM OF YOUR LEFT SHOULDER BLADE
- 1 POINT IF YOU CAN REACH YOUR RIGHT ARM BEHIND YOUR BACK ABOVE YOUR BELTLINE

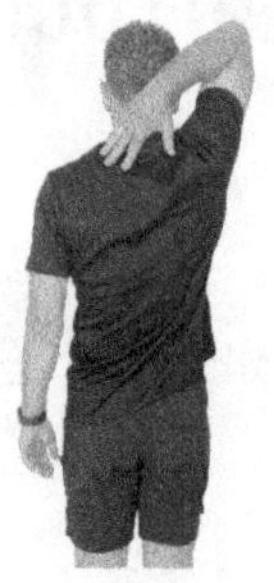

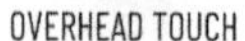

OVERHEAD TOUCH

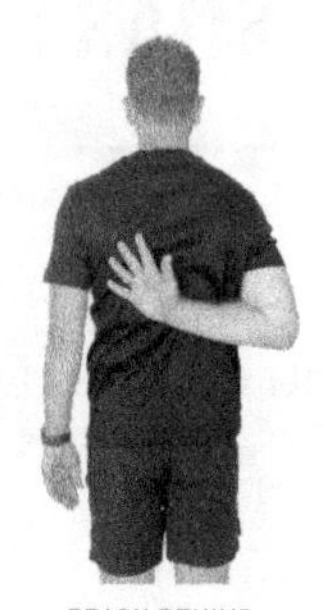

REACH BEHIND

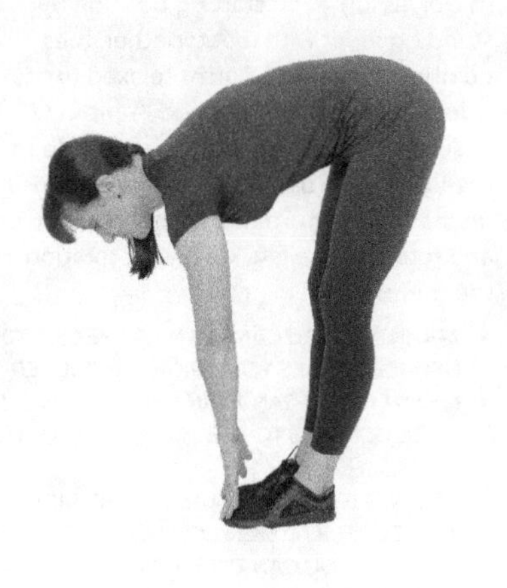

SPINAL FLEXION

Assume the starting position by standing erect with feet together and toes pointing forward. Bend forward from hips reaching down to touch the ends of your fingers to the tips of your toes without bending your knees.

- 4 POINTS IF YOU CAN TOUCH YOUR TOES WITH YOUR KNEES STRAIGHT
- 2 POINTS IF YOU CAN TOUCH YOUR TOES WITH A SLIGHT KNEE BEND

SPINAL EXTENSION

Assume the starting position by standing erect with feet together and toes pointing forward. Reach both arms straight up over your head. Keeping your balance with your feet remaining flat on the ground, bend backwards as far as you can.

- 2 POINTS IF THE FRONT OF YOUR HIPS GETS FURTHER FORWARD THAN YOUR TOES
- 2 POINTS OF YOUR SHOULDER BLADES GET FURTHER BACK THAN YOUR HEELS

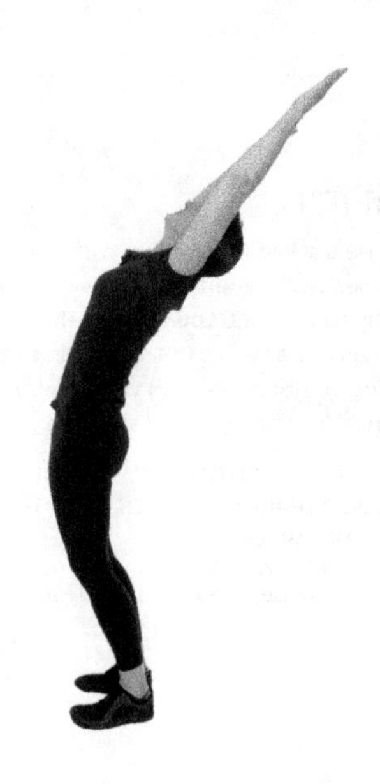

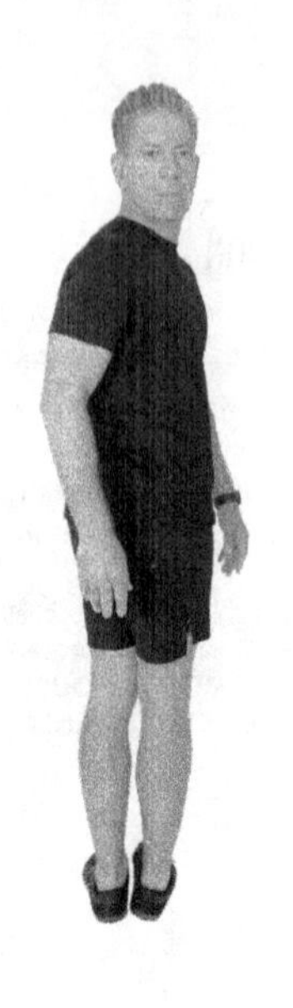

SPINAL ROTATION

Stand with your back facing a full-length mirror, assume the starting position by standing erect with feet together, toes pointing forward and arms relaxed to the sides. Rotate your entire body—hips, shoulders and head—as far as possible to the right while the foot position remains unchanged. Return to the starting position, and rotate to the left. View your rotation in the mirror.

- 2 POINTS IF YOU CAN TURN TO THE LEFT 100 DEGREES TO SEE YOUR RIGHT SHOULDER
- 1 POINT IF YOU CAN TURN PERPENDICULAR OR 90 DEGREES TO THE MIRROR TO YOUR LEFT
- 2 POINTS IF YOU CAN TURN TO THE RIGHT 100 DEGREES TO SEE YOUR LEFT SHOULDER
- 1 POINT IF YOU CAN TURN PERPENDICULAR OR 90 DEGREES TO THE MIRROR TO YOUR RIGHT

SQUAT TEST

Assume a standing position with your feet shoulder-width apart. Your toes may be slightly turned out. Lower yourself into a squat as low as you can and return to the starting position, keeping your heels on the ground. Your back should stay straight.

- 4 POINTS IF YOU CAN GET YOUR HIPS LOWER THAN YOUR KNEES (YOUR THIGHS BREAK PARALLEL)
- 2 POINTS IF YOU CAN GET YOUR HIPS TO THE SAME HEIGHT AS YOUR KNEES (YOUR THIGHS REACH PARALLEL)

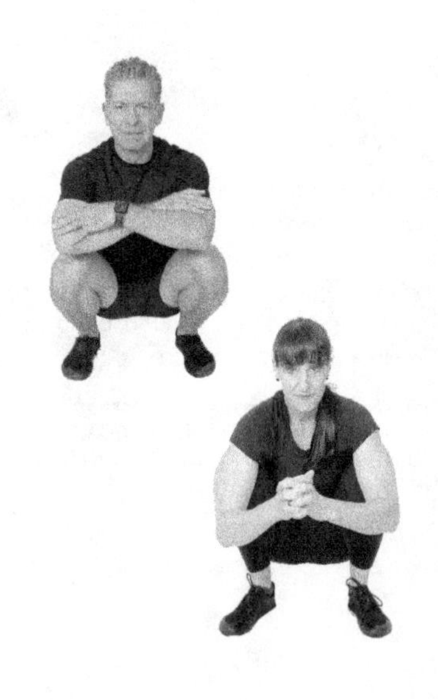

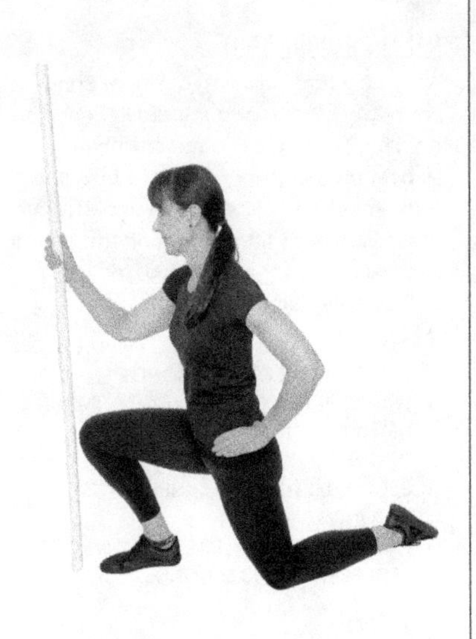

ANKLE MOBILITY

Assume a standing position in front of a wall, with the big toe of your right foot one hand width from the wall. Push your right knee forward attempting to touch the wall with your right heel on the ground. Repeat on the left.

- 2 POINTS IF YOU CAN TOUCH YOUR RIGHT KNEE TO THE WALL WITH THE TOE ONE HAND WIDTH FROM THE WALL
- 1 POINT IF YOU CAN TOUCH YOUR RIGHT KNEE TO THE WALL WITH THE TOE ½ OF ONE HAND WIDTH FROM THE WALL
- 2 POINTS IF YOU CAN TOUCH YOUR LEFT KNEE TO THE WALL WITH THE TOE ONE HAND WIDTH FROM THE WALL
- 1 POINT IF YOU CAN TOUCH YOUR LEFT KNEE TO THE WALL WITH THE TOE ½ OF ONE HAND WIDTH FROM THE WALL

TOE MOBILITY

Stand with your bare feet shoulder-width apart. Try to lift your big toes off the ground without lifting the other four toes, either both at the same time or separately. Then try to lift the other four toes off the ground, without lifting your big toes.

- 2 POINTS FOR EACH SIDE THAT YOU CAN LIFT THE LARGE TOE WITHOUT RAISING THE OTHER 4
- 2 POINTS FOR EACH SIDE THAT YOU CAN RAISE THE 4 TOES WITHOUT RAISING THE BIG TOE

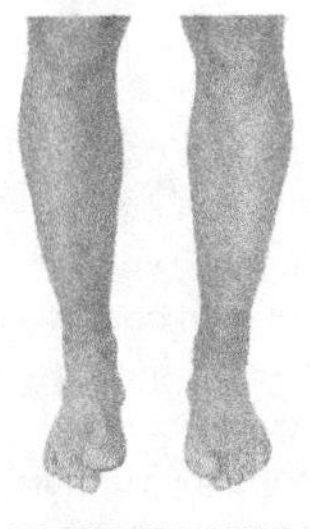

BIG TOES OFF GROUND

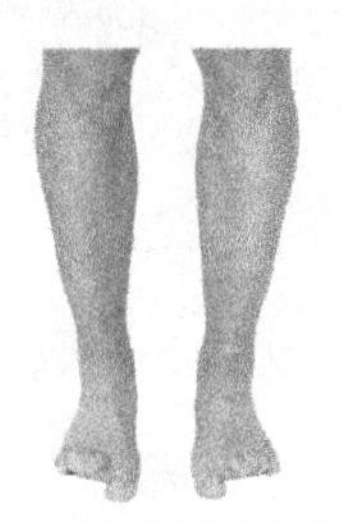

FOUR TOES OFF GROUND

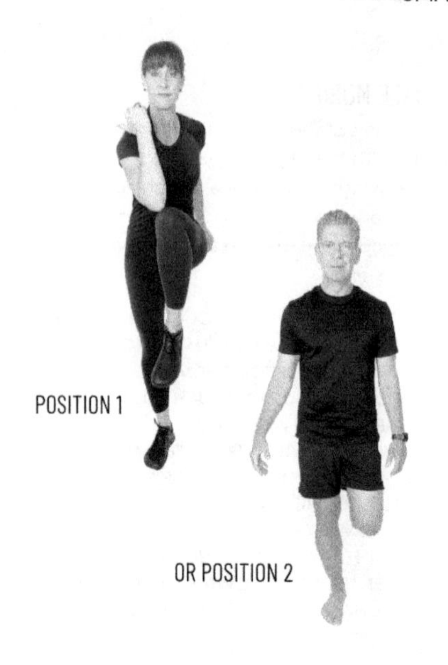

BALANCE/CORE TEST

Assume a firm standing position. Bring your right elbow to your lifted left knee and hold for 2 seconds without stumbling. Repeat on the other side (left elbow and right knee). If you are unable to perform that test, simply lift one foot off the ground and balance on the other foot for 10 seconds. Repeat on the other side.

- 2 POINTS IF YOU CAN HOLD RIGHT ELBOW TO LEFT KNEE FOR 2 SECONDS
- 1 POINT IF YOU CAN BALANCE ON YOUR RIGHT FOOT FOR 10 SECONDS
- 2 POINTS IF YOU CAN HOLD THE LEFT ELBOW TO THE RIGHT KNEE FOR 2 SECONDS
- 1 POINT IF YOU CAN BALANCE ON YOUR LEFT FOOT FOR 10 SECONDS

SIT TO STAND WITHOUT HANDS

Assume a ground position with the legs crossed. Stand up without using your hands and arm or knees to help boost you up in a standing position. According to a Brazilian study, those who are able to spring up and down without any support live longer than those who need to use both hands and knees to get up and down.

- 4 POINTS IF YOU CAN SIT FROM A CROSS-LEGGED POSITION TO STAND WITHOUT YOUR HANDS

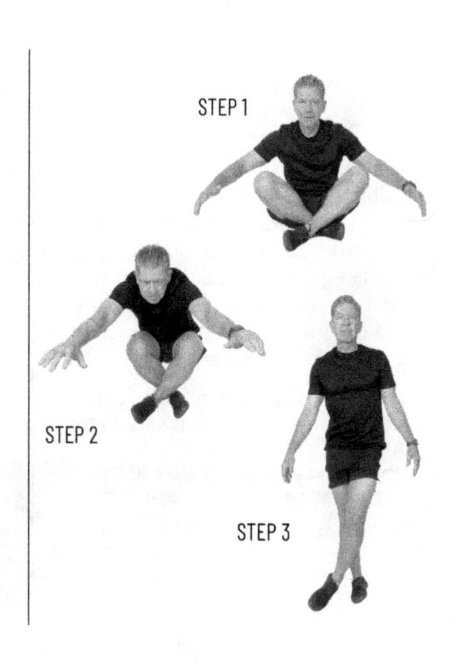

Tally Your Score

Add up all your points from the 10 tests outlined above to find your total score. Where do you rank? In which area(s) could you improve?

0 to 10 Points—You have a severe decrease in overall stability and mobility.
11 to 20 Points—You have a moderate decrease in overall stability and mobility.
21 to 30 Points—You have a mild decrease in overall stability and mobility.
30 to 40 Points—You have good overall stability and mobility.
40 to 44 Points—You have excellent stability and mobility.

2. Speed

Speed refers to a higher velocity or rate of acceleration of movement. This is a test that is likely not required unless you are a serious athlete performing a particular sport, and does not impact the safety of exercise and movement. If you are engaged in a sport in a serious fashion, your coach will be tracking speed as a metric. For everyone else, speed will be a component of the power adaptation.

3. Power

Power is a fundamental concept in physics and sports that involves the combination of speed and force. When it comes to physical activities, power is a crucial attribute that determines an individual's ability to generate force quickly. The standing broad jump is a simple and effective test used to assess power. It involves jumping forward from a standing position and measuring the distance covered. Measure from the toes to where the heels land.

SMART PROTOCOL

Standing Long Jump - $0

For males, a general guideline suggests that they should be able to jump their own height. This means that if a male is, for instance, 6 feet tall (72 inches), he should ideally be able to cover a distance of 72 inches in the standing broad jump. In the case of females, the guideline suggests subtracting 15% from their height before determining the expected distance. This adjustment is made to account for average physiological differences between males and females. For example, if a female is 5 feet tall (60 inches), she should aim to jump a distance of 60 inches minus 15%, which equals 51 inches.

4. Strength

Strength is the foundation for various physical activities and plays a vital role in everyday tasks, sports performance, and overall functional movement. At its core, strength can be defined as the ability to move or overcome resistance. It involves the recruitment of muscle fibres to generate force and overcome the load or weight being lifted. The greater the force an individual can produce, the stronger they are considered to be.

SMART TOOLS

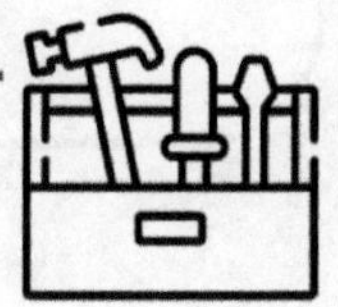

Grip Strength Measurement

Grip strength is easily tested and has been validated as an objective measure of upper body strength and overall physical function. (6) Greater grip strength has been associated with better cognitive functioning, higher life satisfaction, greater subjective well-being, and reduced depression and anxiety symptoms. (7) Grip strength can be assessed in a couple of ways. Hand Dynamometers are handheld devices that can be purchased for around $20 USD. See Smart Tools At A Glance at the end of this Section for options.

SMART PROTOCOL

Strength Test Novice - $

Using a hand dynamometer, a male should have a minimum grip strength of 40 kg and a female 35 kg, with a variation between the two sides of less than 10%. However, grip strength should be trained if it is below 50 kg for a male or 45 kg for a female.

SMART PROTOCOL

Strength Test Intermediate - $0

Grip strength can also be inferred from doing a dead hang with an overhand grip from a chin-up bar. A minimum should be 30 seconds for men and women, but it should be trained if less than 60 seconds.

SMART PROTOCOL

Strength Test Advanced - $

On a leg extension machine in the gym, you should be able to lift your weight minus 10% per decade beyond age 40. In a front or goblet squat position (see the following picture) you should be able to hold ⅓ of your body weight for 30 seconds and ideally ½ your body weight for 45 seconds. The ultimate testing of strength is the one repetition maximum, or one rep maximum (1RM). Once an individual has some lifting experience 1RM is tested and programming is often based on a percentage of 1RM. 1RM should never be tested unless you are certain you are technically proficient with any lift being tested.

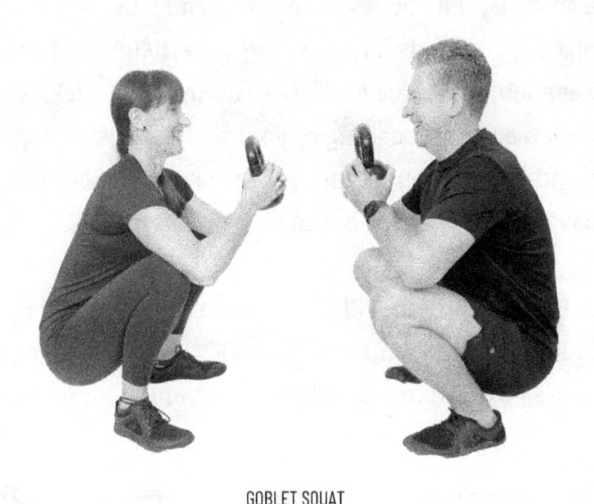

GOBLET SQUAT

5. Hypertrophy

Hypertrophy refers to muscle size. As mentioned earlier, it is related to but not synonymous with strength. What we are really measuring here is how much muscle you have. There are some crude but commonly used measures related to this such as the Body Mass Index or BMI which is simply a height and weight formula without consideration of body type or conditioning. A well-muscled individual with a very low body fat percentage could be labelled overweight or even obese by the BMI. Measuring body fat percentage is better, but in rare cases of malnutrition or disease states involving lean tissue wasting it can be misleading.

A calculation of fat-free mass index or FFMI is much superior. Lean body mass, also known as fat-free mass, is the weight of all tissues minus the fat. This includes organs, skin, bones, body water and muscle. To calculate your FFMI you will need your body fat percentage, age, height and weight to enter in a readily available and free online calculator. The trickiest part about this is getting an accurate reading of your body fat percentage. Someone experienced with the calliper method, or the use of a bioelectric impedance scale, will have an error of plus or minus 3-5% or more.

According to Dr. Andy Galpin, FFMI for a male should be 20 or greater, and for a female, 18 or greater. A male with an FFMI of less than 17, or a female below 15 is at risk for severe physiological detriment for low muscle mass.

SMART PROTOCOL

Determine Your FFMI - $0

Figure out your FFMI by using one of the following free online calculators.

ffmicalculator.org
omnicalculator.com/health/ffmi
fitnessvolt.com/ffmi-calculator

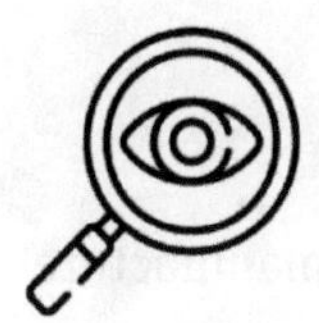

SMART CONSIDERATION

Skinfold Calliper

Skinfold callipers are commonly used to assess body composition by measuring skinfold thickness at standardized sites on the body. These measurements help estimate overall body fat percentage using specific equations or models. To perform the measurement, the practitioner gently pinches the skin and subcutaneous fat at the designated site using the callipers, which apply consistent pressure for accuracy. While skinfold callipers are affordable and portable, they have limitations. Factors like practitioner skill, fat distribution variations, and measurement errors due to skin thickness or hydration levels can affect accuracy. Despite these limitations, skinfold callipers are widely used in research, sports science, and clinical practice for cost-effective body fat estimation. However, caution is advised, and complementary methods like Bioelectrical Impedance Analysis (BIA) or DEXA should be considered for a more comprehensive assessment.

SMART TOOLS

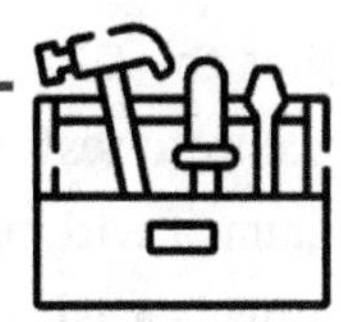

Portable Body Fat Monitor

Omron, Tanita, and Withings are well-known brands that manufacture a range of body fat monitors, each with its own unique features and technologies. These devices typically use bioelectrical impedance analysis to estimate body fat percentage. BIA works by sending a low-level electrical current through the body and measuring the resistance encountered. Since fat, muscle, and other tissues conduct electricity differently, the device can estimate the amount of fat in the body based on the resistance measured. However, remember that these monitors may not be as accurate as more sophisticated methods and should be used as trend trackers rather than sole measurements. They can be accurate enough, and will certainly tell you if body fat is increasing or decreasing.

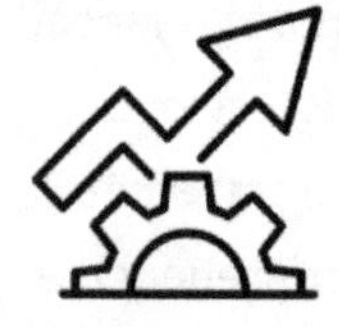

SMART UPGRADES

Accurate Assessment Of Body Fat With DEXA Scan

Of the many ways of getting your body fat tested, most experts agree that the DEXA (Dual-Energy X-ray Absorptiometry) scan is the most accurate testing technology available. (8) These scans are available in Canada without a prescription and cost under $200 CDN. These scans provide a wealth of information including body fat percentage, visceral fat, body water, FFMI and even appendicular (arms and legs) lean mass which removes organs from the equation.

6. Muscular Endurance

Muscular endurance is a fundamental component of physical fitness that pertains to the specific capability of a muscle or a group of muscles to sustain contractions or maintain a position over an extended period. It focuses on the capacity to perform repetitive movements or hold static positions without succumbing to fatigue. Enhancing muscular endurance involves specific training techniques that target both slow-twitch muscle fibres (Type I fibres) and fast-twitch muscle fibres (Type II fibres) in the muscle groups being trained. Slow-twitch fibres are characterized by their endurance-oriented characteristics, such as a high resistance to fatigue and a greater reliance on oxygen for energy production. On the other hand, fast-twitch fibres are responsible for generating force and power but fatigue more quickly due to reliance on glycolytic energy production. Improving muscular endurance also enhances the capacity of mitochondria to efficiently utilize oxygen for energy production.

There are several ways to test muscular endurance, with each level building upon the previous. If you are at an intermediate level, you should be able to complete the novice protocol, and if advanced, you should be able to complete both the novice and intermediate protocols as well.

SMART PROTOCOL

Muscular Endurance Novice - $0

Hold a front plank for 60 seconds. Hold a side plank for 45 seconds. Ensure proper form for the duration.

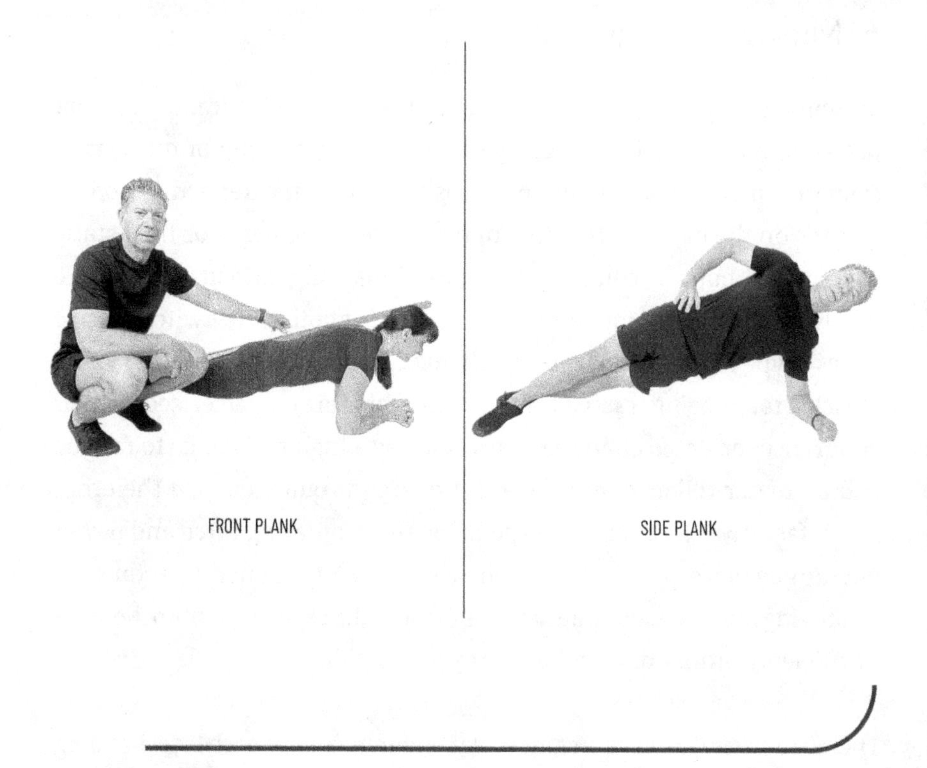

FRONT PLANK

SIDE PLANK

SMART PROTOCOL

Muscular Endurance Intermediate - $0

In addition to the front and side plank holds, complete quality, full range-of-motion push-ups. For males, 10 repetitions is a minimum and should be trained if less than 25 can be completed. For females, 5 repetitions are the minimum and should be trained if less than 15 can be done.

SMART PROTOCOL

Muscular Endurance Advanced - $

Only to be done if you are an experienced lifter. Take 75% of your 1 rep maximum, and see if you can perform 8-12 good repetitions at that load. This is good endurance. If you can perform more than 12 repetitions, that would be an indication that may not be a true 1-rep maximum for you.

7. Anaerobic Capacity

This is referring to an all-out effort of short duration. It is the ability of your cells to resynthesize the energy source ATP via anaerobic (without oxygen) metabolism.

Anaerobic capacity is defined as the maximal amount of adenosine triphosphate (ATP) resynthesized via anaerobic metabolism during a specific short-duration maximal exercise. This is a difficult adaptation to get a quality metric on. If you are in a lab, or a sophisticated gym setting, the most commonly used test is the Wingate Anaerobic Test (WAT). The WAT is an all-out cycle ergometer ride for 30 seconds against a resistance based on body weight. You can do an internet search for a gym in your area that will perform this test on you.

To get an estimate of your anaerobic capacity, you can use heart rate recovery (HRR). To do this you will perform high-intensity work sufficient to reach your maximum heart rate (HRmax), and then track your heart rate as it lowers for 3 minutes post-exercise.

A procedure for hitting the maximum heart rate is laid out on the website of the Norwegian University of Science and Technology (ntnu.edu/cerg/hrmax). This page also has a predictor of maximum heart rate that is slightly more sophisticated than the crude "220-age". This procedure is used in the protocol below. Please note: DO NOT attempt to hit your true maximum heart rate without your medical physician examining you and telling you that you are healthy enough to do so.

According to Dr. Galpin, you are looking for your heart rate to decrease by ½ beat per second. At 1 minute, you should be HRmax-30. At 2 minutes you should be HRmax-60, and at 3 minutes, you should be HRmax-90.

As a comparison and giving you a bit of a range, a 2014 study found that a heart rate recovery of 15-20 beats per minute after one minute of rest was considered about average for heart health and anything faster than that was considered to be good heart health. (9) A 2017 study of elite athletes found the average one-minute heart rate recovery to be 23 beats per minute, the average two-minute heart rate recovery to be 58 beats per minute, and the average three-minute heart rate recovery to be 82 beats per minute. (10)

SMART PROTOCOL

Assess Heart Rate Recovery - $0 to $$

Warm up thoroughly so you start sweating. Do two intervals, each four minutes long. This could be running or on a bike or any other piece of equipment where you can get your heart rate high enough. During the intervals, you should be too short of breath to talk. Intersperse each interval with three minutes of active rest. Start the third interval, but two minutes in, and increase your speed even further until you're too exhausted to continue. Your HRmax will be the highest heart rate you reach. The heart will reach a plateau at which it cannot beat any faster, regardless of how much you increase the workload. Track and record your heart rate as you recover over a three-minute period, and compare it to the values listed above.

SMART TOOLS

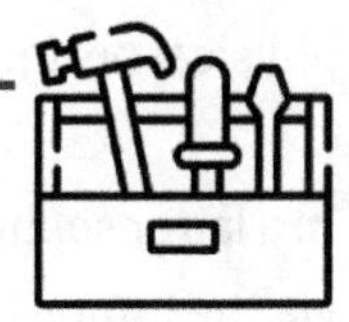

Polar H10

The Polar H10 heart rate monitor is a popular device for accurate heart rate tracking during physical activities. It consists of a chest strap with built-in electrodes that detect heart signals and wirelessly transmit data to a compatible device like a smartphone or smartwatch. With advanced sensor technology and algorithms, it provides real-time heart rate data for confident monitoring during workouts. Paired with apps like Polar Beat, it offers training programs, personalized guidance, and performance analysis tools, enabling users to optimize workouts, set goals, and track progress.

8. Aerobic Capacity

Aerobic capacity is the volume of oxygen your body can use per kg of body weight in a minute, usually expressed as ml/kg/minute. This is high-intensity work typically lasting 8 to 15 minutes, approaching maximum heart rate. Increasing aerobic capacity provides several benefits, such as improving ATP and mitochondrial function, enhancing oxygen utilization in muscles and the brain, and increasing lung capacity for better overall physical performance.

In a lab or sophisticated gym setting, your aerobic capacity will be measured via the famous VO2 Max test. VO2 max, or maximal oxygen consumption, refers to the maximum amount of oxygen that an individual can utilize during intense or maximal exercise. It is expressed in ml/kg/min. This measurement is generally considered the best indicator of cardiovascular fitness and aerobic endurance. Dr. Galpin believes VO2 max should be a minimum of 35 ml/kg/min for males and ideally over 55 ml/kg/min, and a minimum of 30 ml/kg/min for females and ideally over 50 ml/kg/min. You can do an internet search for a gym in your area that will test your VO2 Max.

However, there are a couple of well-validated techniques for estimating VO2 max yourself.

SMART PROTOCOL

Novice VO2 Max Assessment - $0

If you have difficulty running, use the Rockport Walk Test. Walk 1 mile, as fast as you can but avoid jogging, and record the time in decimals (minutes in seconds/60) and your heart rate when finished. Enter this and your weight and age in decimals (years in months/12) in an online calculator, or use the formula: 132.853 - (0.0769 x weight in lbs) - (0.3877 x age) + (6.315 if male or 0 if female) - 3.2648 x time) - (0.1565 x heart rate) (11)

SMART PROTOCOL

Intermediate VO2 Max Assessment - $0

Cooper 12-minute Run Test. Just as it sounds, you run as far as you can in 12 minutes. This is likely to be between 1 and 2 miles unless you are very well trained. Enter the distance you cover into an online calculator or use the formula: (35.97 x miles) - 11.29 or (22.351 x kilometres) - 11.288 (12)

SMART PROTOCOL

Advanced VO2 Max Assessment - $$

Find a gym or facility in your area that offers VO2 Max testing for a more accurate assessment. These facilities often offer the use of more advanced equipment, such as metabolic carts or portable gas analyzers, which provide real-time data during the test. These devices accurately measure oxygen consumption and help professionals determine the exact point at which you reach your maximal effort. Additionally, the equipment may offer additional insights into breathing patterns, heart rate response, and other physiological variables, enhancing the overall assessment.

9. Steady-State Endurance

Steady-state endurance, also known as aerobic endurance, refers to the capacity of an individual to sustain sub-maximal exercise for an extended period. This is full-body cardiorespiratory endurance. This endurance type typically involves activities performed at a moderate intensity level that can be sustained for 20 minutes or more.

This would correspond most closely to "Zone 2" training. This is commonly defined as 60-75% of true maximum heart rate. If using a lactate monitor, you would be below 2.0 mmol lactate. So if you were to measure lactate after your training session and it was 1.7-1.9 mmol, you were in Zone 2.

According to Dr. Inigo San Milan, a researcher interviewed by Dr. Peter Attia, this is how you exercise your mitochondria. (13) His research shows that Zone 2 work increases both the efficiency and number of your mitochondria. Two things occur when you train in Zone 2. First, your slow twitch fibres are increasing mitochondrial density, and they are learning to sustain long periods with high-fat oxidation (they are burning fat). Second, your fast twitch fibres are generating a slow trickle of lactate so that your slow twitch fibres are consuming the lactate, thus training to dispose of it.

San Milan believes this is the most important exercise for metabolic health, to which Dr. Peter Attia agrees. They believe this training helps to prevent cancer, heart disease, and neurodegenerative conditions. It is further how we build an aerobic base, which supports all other types of exercise and activity. San Milan believes Zone 2 should optimally be done in 1-hour bouts and needs to be done 2-3 times a week for maintenance and ideally 4-5 times a week to make gains.

This seems to largely agree with a 2018 study suggesting the "Goldilocks Zone" of physical activity may consist of 150 minutes per week of moderate-intensity aerobic activity or 75 minutes per week of vigorous-intensity aerobic activity, but no more than 4 to 5 cumulative hours per week of vigorous exercise (heart-pounding, sweat producing), especially for those over 45 years of age. Furthermore, the study concluded that taking at least one day off from vigorous exercise per week was beneficial. (14)

SMART PROTOCOL

Novice Aerobic Endurance Test - $0

Using your rate of perceived exertion is the most practical way to assess whether you are in Zone 2. You are there if you can sustain the exercise while nasal breathing and talk in complete sentences, but talking would be annoying. You should be able to sustain this pace for 20 minutes.

SMART PROTOCOL

Advanced Aerobic Endurance Test - $$ to $$$

Purchase and learn how to use a lactate monitor. This involves using a lancet to produce a drop of blood from your finger which is put on a test strip and assessed via a small device. More practically, find a gym or lab in your area that will do this assessment for you.

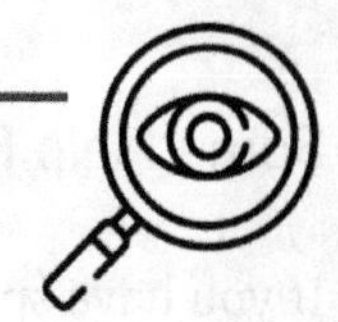

SMART CONSIDERATION

Overall Fitness Testing

Perform the tests explained above on yourself, over a 4-day period, to see where you need to focus your attention for training adaptations. A good split for these tests would be:

Day 1—Body composition and FFMI—These should be done on 48 hours of rest, so exercise, hydration levels and inflammation do not interfere. The movement testing and/or screening could be done on this day as well.

Day 2—Power, lower body strength, lower body muscular endurance, upper body strength, upper body muscular endurance.

Day 3—Steady state endurance, and following that the procedure for reaching HRmax and measuring heart rate recovery.

Day 4—VO2 max testing. Any of the methods are taxing and probably require a dedicated day.

SMART CONSIDERATION

Some Help Ranking Adaptations

If you have specific goals, or you have some experience in all areas and want to refine the way you go about your workouts, this kind of ranking will be a great tool for you to use.

If you are starting out, maybe a little (or a lot) de-conditioned, and your focus is to be the healthiest you can be, congratulations! This will make a bigger change in your healthspan and lifespan than anything else you might do. In this case, keep it simple, and focus on three things.

Number one, build your base of steady state (Zone 2) endurance. That might be starting out as a walk for 20-30 minutes, it might be a jog or cycling, anything that works for you. Work your way up to at least an hour, three times a week.

Number two, do some resistance training. Three times per week, work on strength, power and speed for a quarter, then hypertrophy for a quarter, back and forth.

Number three, at least once a week get your heart rate up higher. Simulated altitude may be a great place to start, then maybe after weeks to months, throw in a timed mile, or some of the other suggestions in developing adaptations below. This will ultimately become your development of VO2 Max.

Building a great base of these three areas will set you up for a lifetime of effective and efficient healthspan-enhancing exercise.

SMART PROTOCOL

Figure Out Your Fitness Priorities - $0

After testing yourself in the 9 adaptations with the methods outlined above, use the chart below to rank your fitness priorities based on your personal results—1 being the area you need to focus the most on and 9 being the area you require the least amount of improvement in. Refer back to this chart and re-test yourself as you develop skill and endurance in each area, and update your ranking as necessary.

Rank your fitness priorities here:	Re-order from 1 to 9 here:
☐ *Skill and Technique*	______________________
☐ *Speed*	______________________
☐ *Power*	______________________
☐ *Strength*	______________________
☐ *Muscular Hypertrophy*	______________________
☐ *Muscular Endurance*	______________________
☐ *Anaerobic Capacity*	______________________
☐ *Aerobic Capacity*	______________________
☐ *Steady State Endurance*	______________________

Now that we have covered how to test these 9 adaptations, the following sections will provide you with strategies to develop proficiency in each area.

Developing Skill And Technique

In this area, you need to do an honest self-appraisal. If you have no real experience and do not have the patience or desire to spend a lot of time watching quality videos and learning proper techniques, you need help. Engage a chiropractor or physiotherapist to assess your movement and help you with corrective exercises if necessary. Then a good strength and conditioning coach will help you to lift properly once your movement quality is good.

Some examples of good-quality movement and exercise videos are Athlean-

X on YouTube, ericcressey.com, functionalmovement.com, and foundationtraining.com.

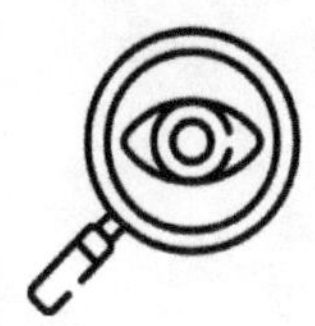

SMART CONSIDERATION

Warm-Up For Resistance Training (Strength, Power, Speed, Hypertrophy)

Contrary to popular belief, it is best to avoid static stretching prior to working out. Why? Static stretching can reduce the activity of muscle spindles, which, in turn, can lead to a decrease in the activity of the stretch reflex. Additionally, there can be a decrease in the sensitivity of nociceptors (pain receptors) and joint receptors, both of which are crucial mechanisms that protect the structures involved in movement. This can affect your overall workout performance. For general purposes, a dynamic warm-up involving different planes and ranges of motion is ideal. 5-10 minutes should be sufficient. The possibilities are endless. Here's a great example:

Warm The Intercostal Muscles—The intercostal muscles are the muscles located between the ribs, and they play an essential role in breathing. To warm up the intercostal muscles before exercise, take a deep breath through the nose, inhaling as deeply as you can and feeling the rib cage expand. Hold the breath for a few seconds before exhaling. Repeat this for several breaths to fully warm up the muscles.

Skip/Bike/Jog For 2-3 Minutes—Start your warm-up with easy skipping, biking, or jogging for 2-3 minutes to increase your core temperature.

BAND OR DOWEL DISLOCATES

Stand with feet shoulder-width apart, core engaged, and grip a band/dowel wider than shoulder-width. Maintain a slight elbow bend to avoid hyperextension and start with the band/dowel at hip level. Lift the band/dowel overhead in an arched motion until it's behind you, keeping your arms straight and shoulders engaged. Pause briefly to feel a chest and shoulder stretch. Reverse the motion to return to the start. Repeat for 10-20 reps, stopping if there's pain or discomfort and consulting a professional. Perform two sets.

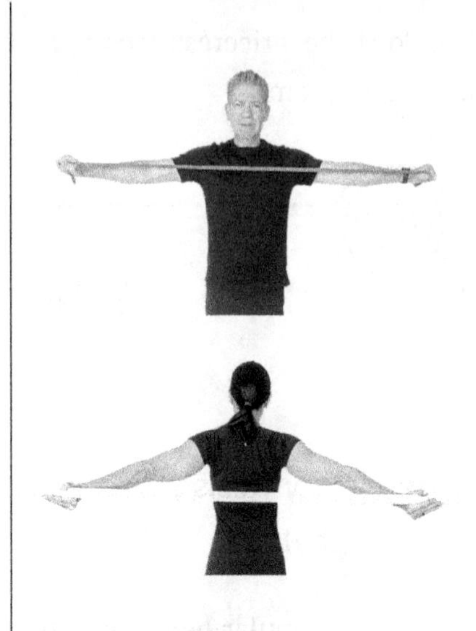

BAND PULL-APART

FACE PULLS

BAND PULL-APART OR FACE PULLS

Band Pull-apart: Stand with feet shoulder-width apart, holding a resistance band in front of you. Keep arms straight, shoulder-width apart, palms down. Squeeze shoulder blades, and pull the band apart until it reaches the chest or arms parallel to the ground. Release slowly and return to start. Repeat for 2 sets of 10-20 reps.

Face-pulls: Stand facing the band, overhand grip, hands shoulder-width apart. Step back to create tension. Pull the band towards the face, keeping elbows high and out. Hold when the band is near the forehead, then slowly release. Repeat for 2 sets of 10-20 reps

90/90 HIP WINDSHIELD WIPERS

The name "90/90" refers to the position of the legs during the exercise, resembling 90 degrees on each side. Lay on the floor propped on your hands, legs raised creating 90-degree angles at hips and knees, calves parallel to the floor. Engage your core and lower legs to one side, pausing at the bottom to feel the stretch. Return to the start and repeat on the other side. Complete this alternating movement in 2 sets of 10-20 reps each way.

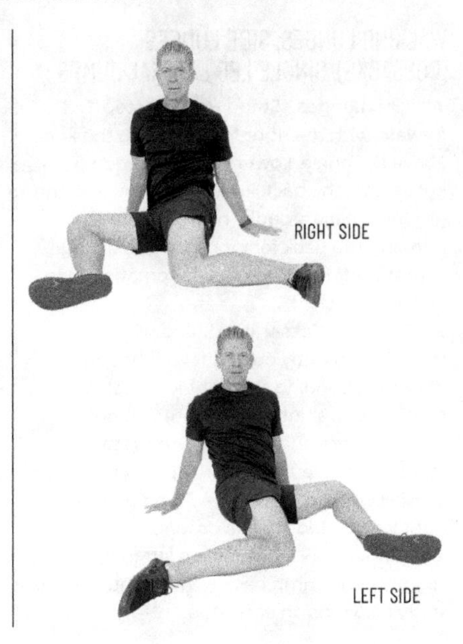

STEP 1

STEP 2

BOTTOM SQUAT

Start in a standing position with feet shoulder-width apart, toes slightly turned out. Squat as low as you can, maintaining a straight back and heels grounded. Rotate in a clockwise and counterclockwise direction, pushing your ankle flexibility. Do this 10 times each way, then return to the start.

WALKING LUNGES, SIDE LUNGES (COSSACKS), SINGLE LEG LATERAL JUMPS

Walking Lunges - Stand upright, step forward with the right foot, aligning the knee above the ankle. Lower body by bending knees until the back knee nearly touches the ground. Push through the front heel, bringing the back foot forward into a lunge with the left foot. Continue, alternating legs for 5 reps each.

Side Lunges (Cossacks) – Stand wide, toes forward or slightly out. Shift weight to the right side, bending the right knee, left leg straight. Lower into a right lateral lunge, chest up, core engaged. Return to start and repeat on the left side for 5 reps each.

Single Leg Lateral Jumps – Stand on the right leg, left foot off the ground. Jump laterally left, landing softly on left foot, knee slightly bent. Jump back to the right, landing softly for 5 reps on each side.

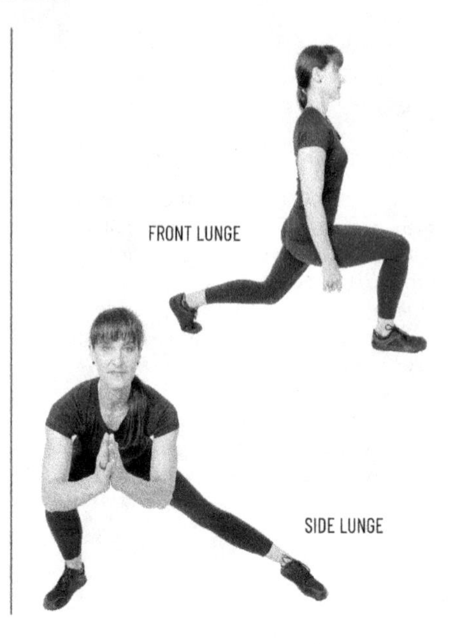

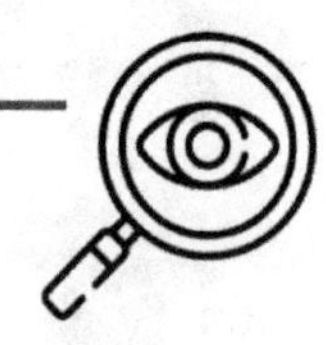

SMART CONSIDERATION

Stretch Smart—Prioritize Core Engagement

Stretching can be overrated if it's not accompanied by proper core engagement and joint stability. Without these foundations, your muscles may not be able to achieve their full range of motion (ROM) during stretching. If you decide to stretch, it's best to do so after your body is warmed up to prevent injuries and allow for better flexibility.

However, instead of advocating widespread stretching, it is more beneficial to prioritize addressing functional movements first. If individuals have specific issues that require attention, then targeted stretching may be recommended to address those particular concerns.

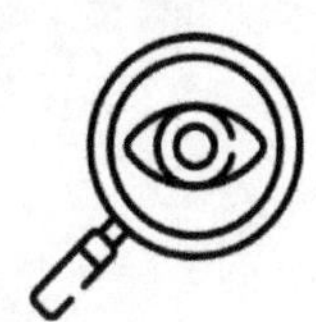

SMART CONSIDERATION

Free Your Feet

We have a greater density of sensory receptors in our feet than any other part of our body and the brain power needed to process all the sensory information from your feet uses more of your sensory cortex than your entire torso. (15) That means your feet are extremely sensitive to touch, pressure, temperature and pain. We are built to sense the ground we move on and make adjustments accordingly, but we cover our feet with an inch of padding practically from birth, and we lose that sensory ability. We feel it is a great practice to work out in bare feet, or use barefoot shoes, and let your body use your feet as the sensory instruments they were meant to be. Safety is a primary consideration so if the surface is not clean and free of debris or anything else that might cut your feet, barefoot shoes are a necessity. If you are interested in using barefoot shoes for running or jogging, make this change gradually and preferably under the supervision of a chiropractor or physiotherapist who understands barefoot running mechanics.

SMART TOOLS

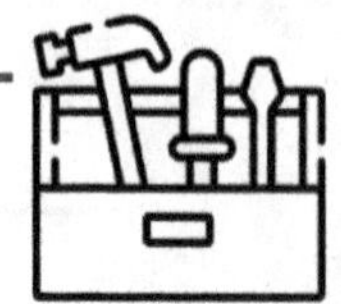

Barefoot Footwear

Barefoot shoes, also known as minimalist shoes, offer a unique approach to footwear by providing a natural and unrestricted walking experience that closely mimics being barefoot. These shoes are designed to promote a more natural gait and foot movement, allowing the feet to engage muscles and tendons while providing protection from the elements. When it comes to top-notch barefoot shoe brands, Vivobarefoot, Xero Shoes, and Lems Shoes stand out as leading contenders in the industry. Links are provided at the end of this Section.

Developing Strength, Power, And Speed

Unless you are working with a coach on a very specific adaptation, strength, power and speed can be grouped together. The primary driver for these adaptations is the intensity of work.

Dr. Galpin favours the "3-5" rule: 3-5 days per week, choose 3-5 exercises, perform 3-5 working sets of 3-5 reps per exercise, and rest 3-5 minutes between sets. (16) Note that working sets do not include the warm-up for a particular exercise—an example would be bench press, 5 reps with the bar, 5 reps with 40% 1RM, 5 reps with 50% 1RM, 5 reps with 60% 1RM. and then your 3-5 working sets.

This may look as simple as an upper body push, upper body pull, lower body push, lower body pull and a rotation in each workout. A sample would be:

This is an example of what a week could look like:	Upper Push	Upper Pull	Lower Push	Lower Pull	Rotation
Monday	Bench press	Lat pulldown	Back squat	Romanian deadlifts	Cable core rotation
Wednesday	Incline dumbbell press	Bent over dumbbell rows	Walking lunges	Deadlift	Medicine ball rotational throws
Friday	Military press	Pull-ups	Goblet squat	Cable pull through	Paloff press (anti-rotation)

Understanding The Phases Of Movement—Concentric And Eccentric

Concentric and eccentric exercises represent distinct phases in muscle movement, each serving a unique purpose in physical training and muscle development.

In the concentric phase, the muscle shortens as it contracts to move a limb or a weight against the force of gravity, while the eccentric phase involves lengthening the muscle as it contracts, often while controlling the descent of a weight or the body against gravity.

Concentric training can be beneficial for improving mitochondrial biogenesis, which is the process by which new mitochondria (the powerhouse of cells) are formed within muscle cells. (17) Mitochondria play a vital role in energy production, and an increase in their numbers can lead to improved endurance and overall energy metabolism.

Eccentric training is particularly effective for promoting strength gains, enhancing athletic performance, and stimulating muscle hypertrophy. The controlled tension placed on the muscles during eccentric exercises contributes to greater muscle fibre recruitment and overall muscle development.

SMART PROTOCOL

Power And Speed Bias - $0 to $

If you are trying to bias for power and speed, work in the 30-70% of 1RM range, and use plyometrics, medicine ball throws, sprints, Olympic lifts (if you are experienced), clapping push-ups, jump squats, box jumps, kettlebell swings. Try to move the weight with as much intensity and speed as possible. This type of work is not as fatiguing and could be done every day.

SMART PROTOCOL

Strength Bias - $0 to $

If you are trying to bias for strength, work in the 70%+ of 1RM range, and use compound movements like bench presses, pull-ups and row variations, squats and deadlifts. Lift cadence is 113, that is 1 second on the concentric (contracting) phase, 1-second pause, and 3 seconds on the eccentric (lowering) phase. If you are working close to maximum strength, a little more recovery before working the same muscle group is preferable—about 48 hours.

Your rest interval between sets when working for strength, power and speed should be long enough to allow you to perform the next set at high intensity. You can keep the "3-5" rule going and rest for 3-5 minutes between sets.

This illustrates the principle that it is not the exercise but the execution of the exercise that determines the adaptation. For power, and most especially for strength, start slow and own the quality of the movement first. Then aim to add 3-5% to the load per week.

Workouts should be challenging and focused but not excessively long. Aim to keep your strength training sessions within the range of 45 minutes to 1 hour. This time frame allows you to maintain a high intensity and focus during the workout without risking overtraining or diminishing returns. Keep in mind that the effectiveness of a workout is not solely determined by its length, but rather by the quality of exercises, proper form, and the targeted muscle groups. Always listen to your body and adjust the workout duration based on your individual fitness level and energy levels on any given day. Remember that consistency and progressive overload are key factors in achieving strength training goals.

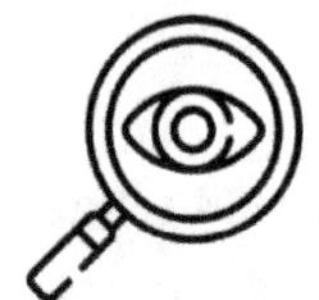

SMART CONSIDERATION

Progressive Overload

Progressive overload is a crucial component of training, but it needs to be done safely. Here is a checklist for each exercise to make sure you are ready to load it: (1) make sure you can do the movement perfectly with assistance (e.g., box squat); (2) make sure you can do the movement perfectly without assistance (e.g., air squat); (3) assess whether you can do the movement well with added load (e.g., goblet squat); (4) see that you can hold an eccentric position with a load while maintaining control for several seconds (e.g., goblet squat, hold the bottom with no sway, wobble or bounce); (5) now you can add speed and go to fatigue. Take as long as you need to perfect every movement before you load them so your training is not interrupted by injury. It is important to note that soreness is not a barometer of an effective or good workout! Yes, you want to feel the muscle group being worked, but your soreness level should never go higher than a 3 on a scale of 1-10. If you do find that you are uncomfortably sore, supplemental magnesium malate can help mitigate discomfort. Sodium bicarbonate, (aka baking soda) may also aid recovery. It is alkaline in nature, which can counteract the build-up of lactic acid in muscles during exercise. Just a pinch dissolved in water is enough—too much can cause gastric distress. Please refer to

Section 2—Hydration, Fuel & Foundationals for the recipe of a homemade electrolyte replenishment drink that includes sodium bicarbonate as one of the ingredients.

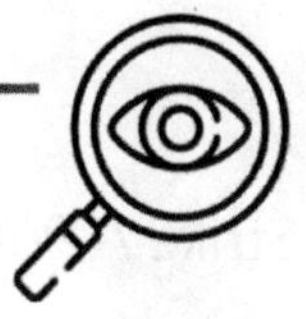

SMART CONSIDERATION

Build A Better Grip

Most resistance exercises, especially if you are using free weights, simultaneously strengthen your grip. If your grip strength tested below 45 kg as a female or 50 kg as a male, or you could not hang for 60 seconds, it would be wise to specifically train your grip. You can buy specialized tools to do this, but the easiest way is to add some heavy carries or gripping and holding a plate to your workout routine (see the following picture).

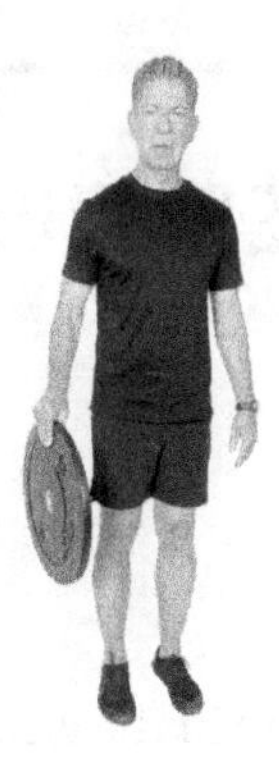

SMART CONSIDERATION

Strike A Pose

Though it is often ridiculed, "posing" or isolating and contracting a muscle that is being worked between sets can actually be beneficial to creating a good contraction during the working set. Your ability to make a strong contraction of a muscle without weight is a positive predictor of your ability to increase strength and hypertrophy of the muscle. A classic example of this is "making a muscle" with your biceps.

SMART CONSIDERATION

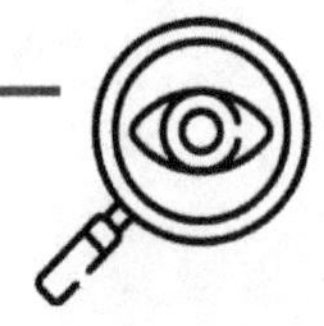

Support Full Motion Strength

You are only as strong as you are in the weakest part of a movement. The use of bands or chains on the bar is a great technique for making the weight heavier through the full-strength curve or range of motion. Use a slightly lower load (% of 1RM) because of the added tension.

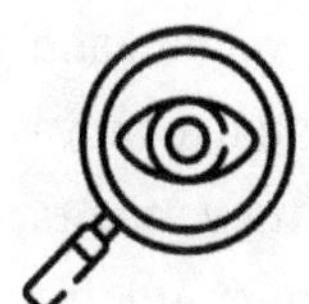

SMART CONSIDERATION

Belt It

Once you have become experienced and started lifting heavy, a valuable tool is the lifting belt. Especially when dealing with weights around 80% of your maximum capacity, the lifting belt proves to be highly beneficial. It enhances sensory feedback and boosts core activation, crucial factors for maintaining proper form and reducing the risk of injuries during challenging lifting exercises. With its provision of essential proprioceptive feedback, the lifting belt becomes a good ally in your quest for improved performance and safety. You should learn to lift safely and activate your core stabilizers without a belt first.

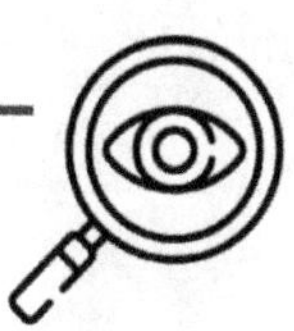

SMART CONSIDERATION

Don't Rely On Machines

Despite the convenience and accessibility of various gym machines, they do not challenge your ability to stabilize yourself the same way free weights do. While they can serve as a suitable introduction to resistance training, it becomes vital to include supplementary exercises with free weights and bodyweight movements as you progress. These exercises allow you to move in a more natural, functional manner, replicating real-life movements that occur in everyday activities, and are essential for enhancing joint stability and overall strength. Remember, life happens in 3D and not the limited planes of movement that these machines provide. So, while they can absolutely have their place in your fitness routine, incorporating free weights and bodyweight exercises will provide a well-rounded approach that better prepares you for the demands of everyday life and physical activities. Again, seek guidance from a qualified professional to suit your individual needs.

Developing Hypertrophy

If the primary driver of strength, power and speed is intensity, the primary driver of hypertrophy is volume. Here you will do 10-25 working sets per muscle group, performing 4-30 reps per set. The higher end is for very experienced lifters with a very high FFMI, who need a lot of stimuli to grow muscle.

SMART PROTOCOL

Build Muscle Size - $0 to $

You have a lot of latitude here, and you really just have to build up the volume. For most people, 10-15 working sets per muscle group per week, performing 8-15 repetitions per set will be more than sufficient. To maximize hypertrophy (and minimize the time you need at the gym), you want to select a weight that allows you to safely perform 8-15 repetitions, ending close to failure. To be very specific, you should be about 2 reps short of failure.

You could well use the same exercise selection method as was outlined for strength development. So let's say on each of Monday, Wednesday and Friday you select an upper body push, an upper body pull, a lower body push and a lower body pull. You will do 4 working sets of each compound movement 3 days a week for 12 working sets, right in the 10-15 sweet spot. So even if you are particularly rushed on one of your days and you do 2-3 working sets of each, you will still hit the 10 sets per week minimum.

Because of the leeway you have with repetition numbers, and the fact that you are really trying to maximize volume, you can keep your rest intervals to a shorter period, say 1-2 minutes. Suppose you pick a weight for one of your exercises that allows you to perform 12 good-quality repetitions, and be within a couple of reps of failure. If you rest for 1 minute and only get 10 or 11 reps on the second set, no problem. Maybe by the fourth set, you are only able to get 8 reps. Great. You are still in the sweet spot.

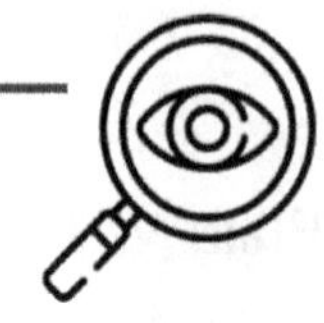

SMART CONSIDERATION

Keep It Cool

An emerging and very interesting concept for performance enhancement is cooling of glabrous (non-hairy) skin. These are specific areas of the body with specialized meshes of blood vessels known as arteriovenous anastomoses, which are adept at dissipating heat. The palms of hands, soles of feet, forehead, and ears are prime locations where these blood vessels are most accessible. To optimize your training, it is recommended to use cool water, slightly below your body temperature, before starting exercise and for 10 to 30 seconds between sets.This can be done with placing the palms of your hands into a water bath, or a cool towel to the forehead. This can help regulate body temperature, and delay fatigue. (18) After the cooling, you can resume your training for the next set. To maximize the benefits of this technique, gradually extend the duration of the cooling to 30 seconds to a minute. Ensure that the water used for cooling is not excessively cold or at freezing temperatures (don't use ice packs) as the blood vessels may constrict, which could impede the heat dissipation process and potentially reduce the benefits of this method on your exercise performance.

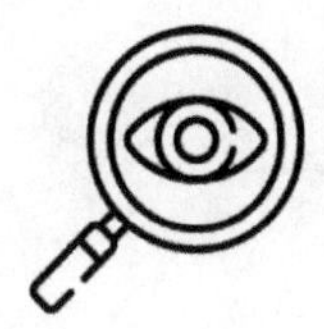

SMART CONSIDERATION

Depend On Your Diaphragm

The way you breathe while lifting is critically important for both safety and performance. Getting good activation and excursion of your diaphragm is what creates the intra-abdominal pressure that protects your lumbar spine. Learning to do this is covered in Section 1—Sleep, Rest & Recovery.

With a good diaphragmatic breath, there is little or no activation of the upper chest and neck muscles. You are "filling your belly" with air. It is a 360-degree expansion of your abdomen. Inhaling and holding your breath in this manner is known as a Valsalva manoeuvre.

For a 1RM lift or very heavy lift, it is best to Valsalva and hold throughout the repetition. In other words, big diaphragmatic inhale and hold, perform the repetition, and then exhale.

With multiple repetitions, you are going to need to breathe! If the weight is mild to moderate, inhale on the eccentric portion of the lift and exhale on the concentric contraction. Consider a squat - inhale on the way down, and exhale on the way up.

With a heavier weight, Valsalva and perform 1 or 2 reps, possibly 3, and then reset your breath. Find what works for you, but a very heavy compound lift like a squat or deadlift is going to require a breath every rep or you are going to risk passing out.

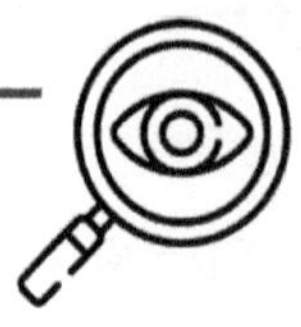

SMART CONSIDERATION

Know Your Gear

As we begin to talk about endurance, it would be useful to learn the system of breathing gears, as developed by Brian Mackenzie of *Shift Adapt.* (19) This refers to the cadence of your breathing, combined with whether you are breathing through the nose, mouth, or both.

Gear 1 is low-level aerobic, even cadence nasal in and nasal out.
Gear 2 is high aerobic, power nasal in and nasal out.
Gear 3 is pushing up against anaerobic threshold, power nasal in and power nasal out.
Gear 4 is low anaerobic, working very hard, power nasal in and mouth out.
Gear 5 is high anaerobic, with maximum effort, mouth in and mouth out.

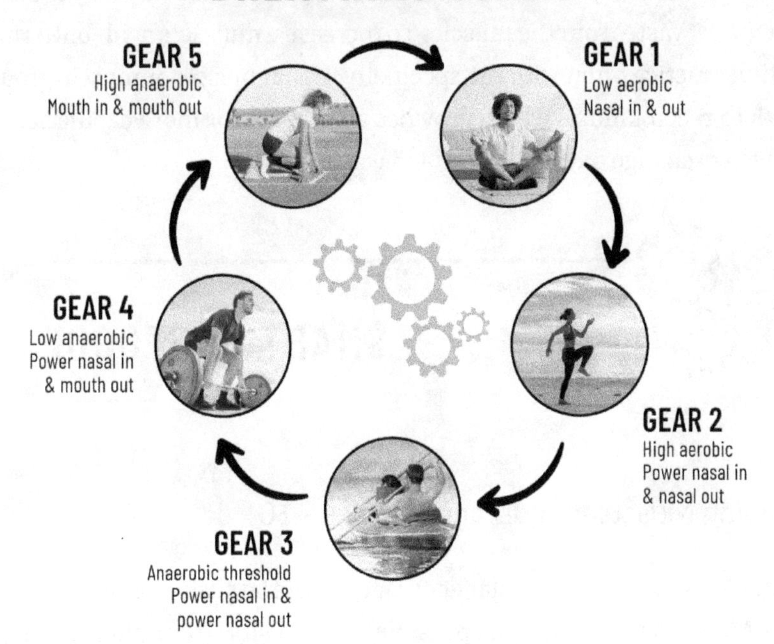

As discussed earlier in the book, nasal breathing is the desirable state most of the time. It is more healthy and efficient, oxygenates the tissues better, and activates the diaphragm. Most people make the mistake of initiating mouth breathing before they have to, and then never work back to nasal breathing as they can. This is hyperventilation and it will hinder your training response.

Developing Muscular Endurance

Muscular endurance is about the local muscle, not cardiovascular or systemic full-body endurance. How many reps of a movement can you do or how long can you hold a posture without breaking proper form? Generally, we are talking about 5-50+ reps but usually, it is in the 8-20 range. The limiting factor is typically acid (lactate) build-up or the inability to clear metabolic waste from the muscle. To increase a muscle's acid-buffering ability, practice often with the specificity of that muscle or muscle group. Work to reach failure, which provides a stimulus for more capillaries to grow to exchange oxygen, blood, and waste.

SMART PROTOCOL

Building Muscular Endurance Novice - $0

Examples of working muscular endurance would be push-ups or calf raises for AMRAP (as many reps as possible) or wall sits, front planks or side planks for as much time as possible, always considering good form. Try to increase by 1 or 2 reps per week, or several seconds more in a static postural hold.

SMART PROTOCOL

Building Muscular Endurance Advanced - $0

If you are experienced in lifting and used the test of being able to perform at least 8 repetitions at 75% of 1RM, you can apply the methodology to any lift you feel needs endurance work— pick a weight that allows you to do 8-12 repetitions and try to increase by 1-2 repetitions per week.

At this level of skill, you may also want to consider finishing your workout to failure for a final push. Perform push-ups to failure for the chest, wall sits or body squats to failure for legs, and pull-ups to failure for shoulders, or use machine exercises targeting the worked muscle groups. Ensure you are maintaining proper form and ample recovery for continued progress and to avoid overtraining.

You will generally work on muscular endurance once or twice per week. In developing muscular endurance, you are going to be in breathing gears 1 and 2, perhaps bumping into gear 3 at the most.

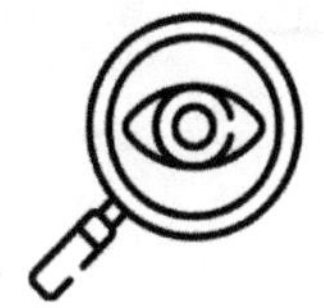

SMART CONSIDERATION

Emerging Research—Protein Timing And Fuel For Sports Performance

Recent research suggests that the timing of protein intake may not be as crucial as once believed. (20) Instead, the focus should be on meeting daily protein requirements while considering individual sport performance needs. Regarding carbohydrates, their timing plays a vital role in optimizing athletic performance, but it is not as simple as a formula based on body weight. It depends on factors like glycogen storage and the ability to use ketones as fuel.

Carbohydrates are the primary fuel source for athletic performance, especially during high-intensity activities. Properly timing carbohydrate intake is essential for maximizing glycogen stores and providing the energy necessary for optimal performance. Consuming carbohydrates before, during, and after workouts or events helps replenish glycogen stores, prevent fatigue, and support recovery. The specific timing and amount of carbohydrates vary depending on the sport, exercise duration and intensity, as well as individual preferences and tolerance.

Developing Anaerobic Capacity

Remember anaerobic capacity is a systemic adaptation, not a local one like muscular endurance. To develop it we want all-out maximal effort for a short period of time, followed by a recovery period and then repeat. This is sometimes referred to as HIIT or high-intensity interval training.

Choose a full-body movement that you are confident in producing maximum effort, with minimal injury risk. Stay away from heavy eccentric load movements like box jumps or downhill sprints. Some examples would be sprinting, bike/assault bike sprints, rowing, skipping, sled push or a similar exercise.

There are several anaerobic energy subsystems to consider here, and you can be pretty specific in working each one. Anaerobic training may be done once or twice a week.

SMART PROTOCOL

Developing Phosphagen Energy System - $0

To develop the Phosphagen energy system (also called the Adenosine Triphosphate—Phosphocreatine system): 5-10 seconds of all-out effort with a work: rest ratio of 1:12 to 1:20. An example would be 5 seconds all-out sprint, and 60 seconds rest.

SMART PROTOCOL

Developing Fast Glycolysis Energy System - $0

To develop the Fast Glycolysis energy system: 15-30 seconds of all-out effort with a work: rest ratio of 1:3 to 1:5. An example would be 20 seconds all out on the assault bike and 80 seconds rest.

SMART PROTOCOL

Developing Fast Glycolysis/Oxidative Energy System - $0

To develop the Fast Glycolysis/Oxidative energy system: (where you start to get some crossover into aerobic training) 1-3 minutes of hard effort (this will not be maximal effort, but the maximum you can do for the set time) with a work: rest ratio of 1:3 to 1:4. An example would be 2 minutes hard row, and 6 minutes light row recovery.

SMART PROTOCOL

Repeat Sprint Ability - $0

A very good way of developing anaerobic capacity is with a form of simulated altitude training known in Patrick McKeown's *Oxygen Advantage System* as Repeat Sprint Ability. It is adapted from the research of Dr. Xavier Woorons. (21) This is a 40-metre sprint on an exhale breath hold, with a 30-second nasal breathing rest and repeat.

From a standing position, take a breath in and out through the nose, pinch the nose, sprint 40 metres, stop, begin breathing nasally, rest 30 seconds, and repeat.

The hypoxic (low oxygen) hypercapnic (high carbon dioxide) condition that this creates enhances the cellular conditioning in anaerobic energy production.

Start with 5 repetitions, and increase to 8 repetitions over 4 weeks or so. Repeat Sprint Ability can be done 2-5 times a week, but it is a short alternative, only taking a few minutes to do. 8 repetitions can be done in under 10 minutes.

SMART PROTOCOL

Intermittent Hypoxic Hypercapnic Training - $0

Another very efficient way of performing anaerobic training is Simulated Altitude work, again by Patrick McKeown in his book, *The Oxygen Advantage.* (22) It is also known as Intermittent Hypoxic Hypercapnic Training (IHHT). This means bouts of low oxygen (hypoxic) and high carbon dioxide (hypercapnic) periods with recovery in between. This provides some of the physiological benefits of training at altitude without being at altitude.

This can be done inside by going around in circles or back and forth, or outside. Take a normal breath in through your nose and a normal breath out through your nose. On completion of the exhalation, pinch your nose to hold your breath and start walking, after a few paces start jogging, and after a few paces go as fast as you can, even sprinting. Count your steps. When you can't go any further stop, resume breathing through your nose, and recover for about 15 breaths, or 45-60 seconds. Repeat for 5 or 6 reps. See if you can increase the number of steps you take. To prolong the effect once you become experienced, try to limit the first 5 or so breaths during recovery to just a sip of air in and out.

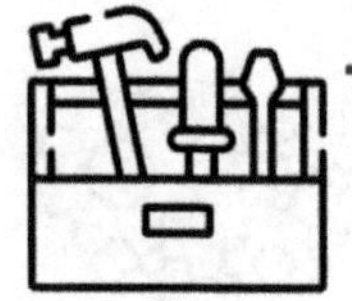

SMART TOOLS

Pulse Oximeter

A pulse oximeter clips onto the end of your finger in a non-invasive manner. Pulse oximetry is the measure of blood oxygen saturation or SpO2. This is a measure of the percentage of hemoglobin in the blood that is saturated with oxygen. It is expressed as a percentage, with normal values typically ranging between 95% and 100%. If you are performing simulated altitude training, you should see your SpO2 drop to 92% or below for a few seconds between repetitions. There are decent pulse oximeters available for about $50. When it comes to choosing a pulse oximeter, quality is important. The authors of this book recommend choosing devices from reputable brands such as Nonin. Dr. Sly is a certified Oxygen Advantage® Master Instructor and frequently uses these products with his clients. These companies have earned a solid reputation for reliable and accurate pulse oximeters, making them trusted choices for healthcare professionals and those seeking precise oxygen saturation monitoring.

Developing Aerobic Capacity

Developing aerobic capacity is a 5-15 minute effort, as hard as you can maintain. This may be a run, bike, row, swim or any similar activity. This is the development of VO2 Max, and oxygen demand takes the most prominent role here.

SMART PROTOCOL

Developing VO2 Max - $0

This could take the form of a timed mile run, which for the vast majority of people will be 6-8 minutes plus. It could be a 12-15 minute row as far as you can. Or this could take the form of intervals, 3-5 minutes of work with a work: rest ratio of 1:1 to 1:3. An example of this would be a 5-minute hard run, with a 10-minute walk, repeated 2 or 3 times.

This training initially may take you into breathing gear 4-5, but as you get better with your breathing, you may well be able to do this in gear 3. Your ability to breathe nasally will get better as you practice it, and your breathing will become much more efficient.

Aerobic capacity training may be done once or twice a week.

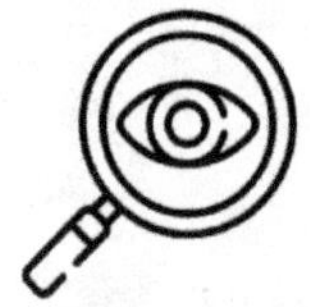

SMART CONSIDERATION

Breathe Your Way Back

After a few weeks of easing your way into producing max effort, you should be getting into breathing gear 5. While you don't want to baby yourself with the length of the rest period, it should be sufficient to get you back into gear 1-2 before the next interval of max effort. Rather than marry yourself to a strict amount of rest time, keep track of the time and be mindful of your breathing gear, you will find over time that you return to gear 1 faster.

Developing Steady State Endurance

As mentioned previously, the development of steady-state endurance involves prolonged submaximal work, for 20 minutes or more. This would refer to "Zone 2" cardio, or 60-75% of your maximum heart rate. Whereas high-intensity work burns carbohydrate stores in the body, this work taps into burning fat stores.

SMART PROTOCOL

Developing Steady State Endurance (Zone 2) - $0

A great way to stay in this zone is to focus on your breathing. If you are able to breathe nasally, preferably at the interface between gear 2 and 3, so that you could talk if necessary but it is uncomfortable, you are in a great place. Steady-state endurance training can and should be done several times a week and can include activities like jogging, biking, rowing, stand-up paddle-boarding, or "rucking"—hiking with a weighted backpack. If you are de-conditioned, start with bouts of 20-30 minutes and work your way up to an hour.

SMART TOOLS

Sports Mask

A sports mask can be used to take your training to the next level. The mask adds a load or resistance to your breathing, in particular your inspiration. This load forces the diaphragm to work harder, strengthening it in the same way weightlifting strengthens muscles. The Oxygen Advantage® Sportsmask is adjustable to create a variable load. It can be worn at any time, walking, working out, or performing simulated altitude training. There are many inspiratory training tools that fit in the mouth. These are not preferable as they encourage mouth breathing. The advantage of the mask is that you can maintain nasal breathing, and it also pools or traps more expired carbon dioxide, encouraging adaptations and reduced breathlessness. Plus, you look like a Hollywood villain!

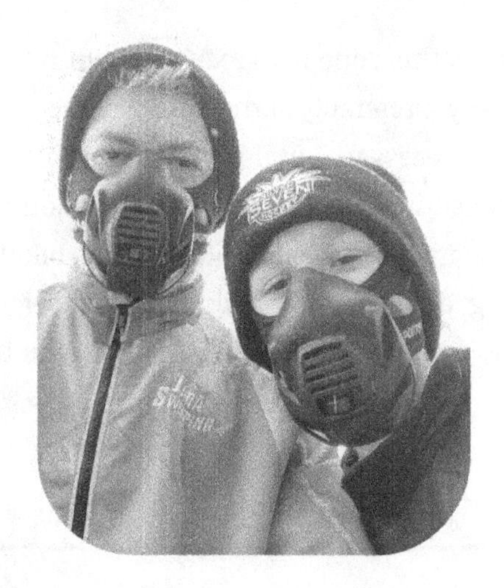

Putting It All Together

The possibilities for combining the 9 adaptations into your training are endless and limited only by your imagination. The top reasons that people fail to get results from an exercise program are lack of adherence (otherwise known as lack of willpower), not using a progressive overload strategy, and not sticking with a specified program long enough to see results.

A great way to combat these problems is to plan your year of workouts in yearly quarters and vary your exercise goals for each quarter. Pick one or two adaptations, based on your testing and priorities, and bias your workouts towards those adaptations. A great practice would be to work for 5 weeks on a consistent program, take a de-load week, and then 5 more weeks of the same program followed by another de-load. Then change your routine for the next quarter.

SMART CONSIDERATION

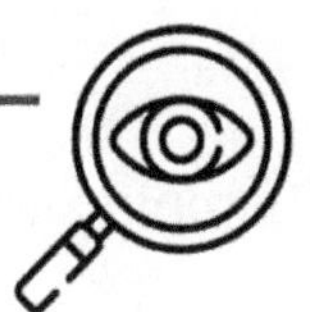

The Vital Role Of De-load Weeks In Training

The de-load is a critical piece of any training regime. It helps prevent overtraining, injury, and boredom. Your de-load week should be active but not difficult. You may choose to lift but keep it light, or you might do a lot of walking, stretching, and other movement practices. Above all else, focus on sleep and your favourite recovery modalities detailed earlier in this book. Gains are set up in the gym or on the track, field or road, but they are realized during rest!

Variety not only keeps it interesting, but it also mitigates against injury, especially overuse injury. Even if your main goal for the year is muscle hypertrophy, aiming to increase your FFMI, one quarter year of the kind of volume required for hypertrophy is plenty. So you might work on hypertrophy in quarters 1 and 3, and strength, power and speed in quarters 2 and 4. Sprinkle your aerobic and anaerobic endurance work in there and you have a nice complete program.

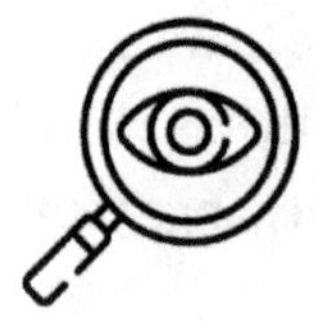

SMART CONSIDERATION

Sample Schedule

Following is a sample schedule for resistance training for strength/power/speed or hypertrophy plus endurance and aerobic/anaerobic work:

Sunday—Long endurance work 30-60 minutes. This could be any activity that takes you into breathing gear 2-3, "Zone 2". If you are just starting out, a brisk 30-minute walk will do this nicely. If you are more conditioned, you'll need to step it up a bit. If you are just starting out, unconditioned, a brisk 30-minute walk 5 times per week, until you can do it without getting out of breathing gear 2, would be the place to begin, and build to an hour.

Monday—Resistance work in the gym, 30-60 minutes. A good warm-up followed by a full body split, choosing an upper body push, upper body pull, lower body push and lower body pull exercise. If you are just starting out, working on power and speed first with the lighter weight that goes with it is great. If you are more experienced, this could be working on strength or hypertrophy as well.

Tuesday—Anaerobic capacity, 5 repetitions of Repeat Sprint Ability (about 6 minutes) followed by a VO2 Max workout - say a timed mile as fast as you can do (unless you are really well trained this will take between 8 and 15 minutes). If you are more advanced, your VO2 Max workout might consist of a 3-5 minute max effort bout with a 1:1 rest - say 3 minutes hard row with 3 minutes rest and repeat 4 times. If you are a beginner, this might be your 30-minute Zone 2 walk for the day.

Wednesday—Resistance work in the gym, 30-60 minutes. You will do the same adaptation as Monday, but you may have a different push and pull for each of the upper and lower body.

Thursday—Anaerobic capacity, 5 repetitions of Repeat Sprint Ability (about 6 minutes) followed by an anaerobic phosphatase adapted workout - 6 repetitions of 5-10 second all-out effort (this is short and really is maximal effort - sprint, assault bike, rower, sled push etc.) with a 60-90 second rest period between.

Friday—Resistance work in the gym, 30-60 minutes. You will do the same adaptation as Monday, but you may again have a different push and pull for each of the upper and lower body.

Saturday—Perhaps a rest and recovery day, or if you are beginning, this is another 30-minute brisk walk or another session in breathing gear 2-3, Zone 2.

Remember that this is a sample schedule. A 1000+ page book could be written detailing every possible permutation of combining training for the different adaptations detailed. On the low end of the above suggestions, you could be spending less than 3 hours per week. This is likely not enough to get optimal results. You need to be thinking in terms of an hour per day invested in your healthspan and lifespan.

Perhaps at certain times of the year, you enjoy playing a team sport—hockey, soccer, basketball or the like. Great! You are likely covering a part of your anaerobic and aerobic conditioning, maybe even some of your long endurance. And you are benefiting from the kind of social connection that we all need. Maybe for that quarter, you add in some other endurance work and you only hit the gym twice per week.

Then at other points in the year, when you are really focusing on strength or hypertrophy, you may be in the gym 4 or 5 times per week. Change it up! Variety in your programming goes a long way, but try to give it that 3-month period to allow for the adaptation you are focusing on to occur.

Even at an hour of exercise per day, don't consider that license to spend the other 15 on your derrière in front of a computer and/or television. We weren't designed for that.

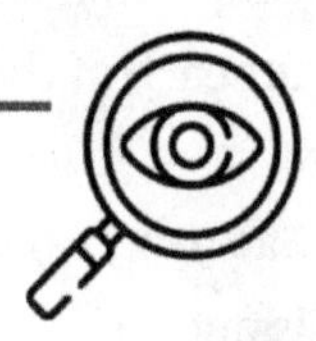

SMART CONSIDERATION

Step It Up

Are you getting enough movement throughout your day? If you sit in front of a computer for most of your day, likely you are not. A recent meta-analysis suggests that more steps per day are better for your overall health and that the benefit in terms of mortality risk levels off at around 6,000 to 8,000 steps for older adults and 8,000 to 10,000 steps for younger adults. Steps are now easily measured with most wearable devices. (23)

Post-Workout Breathwork—Balancing The Autonomic Nervous System

In the realm of post-workout recovery, breathwork has emerged as a powerful tool to promote relaxation and balance the body's autonomic nervous system. Intense exercise activates the sympathetic nervous system, responsible for the body's "fight or flight" response. This activation leads to increased heart rate, elevated blood pressure, and heightened alertness. While beneficial during exercise, prolonged activation of the sympathetic nervous system post-workout can hinder recovery. (24)

In Section 2—Hydration, Fuel & Foundationals, we talked about LSD breathing (light, slow and deep). It is a great practice to use 5 minutes of LSD breathing after your workout to downregulate your sympathetic nervous system, promoting optimal healing, muscle repair, and overall well-being.

SMART PROTOCOL

Post Workout Recovery Routine - $0

After your workout, find a comfortable, supported position without distractions. Take slow, deep breaths, focusing on expanding your belly while inhaling and releasing tension when exhaling. Use LSD breathing (light, slow, and deep) with a count of 4 in and 6 out. Repeat this pattern for 3-5 minutes.

Pre-Workout Optimization—Coffee, Electrolytes, And Essential Amino Acids

Achieving peak performance during your workouts requires strategic choices before you hit the gym. The natural caffeine found in coffee can enhance focus, endurance, and alertness during your workout. Coffee as a pre-workout drink works best if you are not caffeine adapted, or if you are not a regular caffeine drinker. Remember to consume it in moderation and be mindful of individual caffeine sensitivity.

Another key consideration is to maintain proper hydration and support muscle function by ensuring adequate electrolyte balance. Opt for natural, high-quality sources like LMNT or even a ¼ tsp of high-quality salt (Redmond Real Salt®, for example) per litre of water, which can be beneficial. To support muscle recovery and growth, be mindful of consuming all essential amino acids (EAAs). If you prefer to avoid extra calories, explore EAA supplements which offer a complete profile of essential amino acids. Unlike protein shakes, EAA supplements typically have a minimal calorie content. They are designed to provide amino acids without adding significant calories or other macronutrients. If you are consuming protein daily in the range of at least 1.2 - 1.6 g/Kg bodyweight from a high-quality (animal) source, additional EAA supplementation is not necessary.

An interesting addition to pre-workout supplements is Rhodiola Rosea. This is a herb that has a long tradition of use for its adaptogenic properties which include reduced stress and fatigue, as well as increased mental performance, particularly under stressful conditions. It has been shown to reduce perceived exertion during exercise. According to Examine.com dosage for acute usage is 288-680 mg.

Another noteworthy supplement to consider is beta-alanine, a non-essential amino acid commonly found in pre-workout formulations which increases carnosine levels in muscles. Carnosine acts as a buffer during intense exercise, regulating muscle pH levels. This helps neutralize the acidity caused by lactic acid, delaying muscle fatigue and boosting endurance during high-intensity workouts. However, its effectiveness may be limited for endurance-based activities like long-distance running, where carnosine's buffering effects are most prominent during short bursts of intense activity.

Typical pre-workout doses range from 2 to 5 grams daily. Some may experience harmless tingling (paresthesia) on the skin, which can be minimized by splitting doses or choosing sustained-release formulations.

Sports Drink Craze—Sugar, HFCS, And Electrolytes In Perspective

When it comes to sports drinks, it's crucial not to get caught up in the craze and to be mindful of a few key considerations. First and foremost, pay attention to the amount of sugar they contain. Many sports drinks have high sugar content, especially in the form of high fructose corn syrup (HFCS). HFCS has been associated with various health concerns, including obesity and metabolic issues.

Some glucose included in a pre-workout drink can be helpful for energy as long as it fits into your overall caloric plan. Opt for drinks that do not contain HFCS, and instead, seek out those with natural sweeteners or fruit extracts in moderation.

While electrolytes are essential for hydration and muscle function, it's worth noting that excessive electrolyte consumption may not be necessary for everyone. If you eat a whole food diet without a lot of added salt, add some quality salt such as Redmond Real Salt®, Boulder salt or a good quality Celtic sea salt to your water. See Section 2—Hydration, Fuel & Foundationals for more details.

Exercise And Movement—Boosting Your Body's Natural Detoxification Processes

As you focus on strengthening your body and improving cardiovascular health, it's equally important to consider the intricate interplay between movement, exercise and detoxification. Engaging in physical activity helps stimulate the lymphatic system, a key component of the body's natural detoxification process. By integrating movement and exercise and prioritizing the health of your lymphatic system, you can enhance your body's detoxification processes and its ability to eliminate toxins.

Unlike the circulatory system, which relies on the heart to pump blood, the lymphatic system relies on movement and exercise to circulate lymphatic fluids through the body. When we move our bodies through exercise, it causes the lymphatic vessels to contract and relax, which helps pump lymphatic fluids through the lymphatic system. This movement also helps to stimulate the lymph nodes, which act as filters, removing any harmful substances from the lymphatic fluids.

Exercise, particularly activities that involve a lot of movement and muscle contractions, such as running, jumping, and strength training, can help stimulate the lymphatic system and improve its efficiency. In contrast, a sedentary lifestyle can lead to the lymphatic system becoming sluggish and less effective at removing toxins from the body.

Lymph helps the body filter and clear toxins, debris and pathogens that accumulate in our circulatory system as a result of toxic environments, medications and an unhealthy diet. As the lymphatic fluid flows through the lymph nodes, immune cells identify and attack foreign substances, including bacteria, viruses, and toxins. The nodes act as filtering stations that move the lymph fluid to the surface of our skin near the neck, abdomen, armpits and groin. These nodes remove waste products, damaged cells, infectious organisms and foreign particles to prevent blockages and protect against infection. Ensuring the proper functioning of the lymphatic system is vital to the body's natural detoxification processes.

Toxic Load And Detoxification

Over the past few decades, our exposure to toxins has increased exponentially, from the air we breathe to the food we eat, and even the cleaning and personal care products we use. While our bodies all function in a similar way, our ability to handle toxins can vary greatly. Have you ever wondered why two people with similar lifestyles can have different responses to illness? The answer can be explained using the analogy of a bucket.

Think of your body as a bucket filled with liquid representing the toxins you've been exposed to throughout your life. If your bucket is half-full and your spouse's bucket is almost full, adding more liquid (toxins) will have a different impact on each of you. Your body may be able to handle it, but your spouse's body may not.

This analogy demonstrates how our individual toxic load, which is influenced by our past exposure to toxins, affects our susceptibility to illness and disease. The efficiency of our detoxification pathways and genetic factors also contribute to this complex situation. Some people may carry a lower toxic load than others, depending on their unique circumstances.

Why Should You Detox? Basics Of Detoxification

When toxins build up in the body, they can lead to a variety of health problems, including fatigue, headaches, and even chronic diseases. The long-term effects of these accumulative toxic chemicals in the body span everything from an increased risk of diabetes to hormonal imbalances, neurological and cognitive impairment, cancer, and the list goes on. The purpose of detoxification is to improve the overall functioning of the body, including digestion, circulation, and immune system health.

Even as you get a better understanding and fuller picture of your "toxic load," you'll need to address the organs in your body that are responsible for processing waste. These crucial organs are often the sites of hormone breakdown and production, so any disruptions to their functioning and pathways could lead to double trouble: the symptoms of a hormonal imbalance and the harmful effects of toxic chemical build-up. The only way forward is to try to limit your exposure to toxins the best you can and help your body detoxify itself.

There are many reasons why we should consider detoxifying our bodies. Some key benefits of detoxification: are improved digestion, increased energy, better immune system function, clearer skin, and weight loss.

Pathways Of Elimination

One essential aspect of detoxification is ensuring that our pathways of elimination are open and functioning correctly. Pathways of elimination refer to the body's various systems that help eliminate waste and toxins. The primary pathways of elimination include the liver, kidneys, lungs, colon, and skin (though our blood and lymphatic system are also involved). Each of these systems plays a critical role in removing toxins from our body, and when any of them aren't functioning correctly, it can hinder the detoxification process. Before embarking on any detox protocol, it is vitally important to ensure these pathways of elimination are functioning well, or else you run the risk of toxins released from your tissues recirculating, with no way out—this can make you feel pretty lousy in the process!

Liver

The liver is crucial for detoxification, filtering toxins and waste from the bloodstream, and aiding in digestion. It has two phases of detoxification: Phase 1 uses enzymes to make toxins easier to excrete, but can create toxic intermediate metabolites. Phase 2 conjugates these intermediates to make them less toxic and easier to eliminate. The liver distinguishes between nutrients and harmful substances like drugs and alcohol, and factors like genetics, age, diet, and toxin exposure can impact its efficiency. Imbalances in detoxification phases can lead to health issues.

Put simply, your liver is your body's processing plant, breaking down anything that you consume. It is your liver's job to distinguish between the nutrients you need to absorb like vitamins and minerals, and the dangerous or unnecessary substances that must be filtered out of your bloodstream like drugs, alcohol, pesticides, and chemical additives in food.

Kidneys

Similarly, the kidneys play an important role in detoxification. The kidneys help by maintaining the body's balance of fluids and electrolytes, regulating blood pressure, and removing waste and toxins from the body.

The kidneys are bean-shaped organs that are located in the lower back, just below the ribcage. Each kidney contains tiny structures called nephrons, which are responsible for filtering waste products from the blood and producing urine. As blood flows through the kidneys, waste products and excess fluids are filtered out and sent to the bladder for elimination. This process is controlled by a complex system of hormones and enzymes that work to maintain the proper balance of electrolytes in the blood.

When the kidneys malfunction, they can't effectively filter out toxins. This can result in a harmful accumulation of waste products in the body, potentially leading to kidney issues.

Lungs

The lungs are part of the body's respiratory system and play a vital part in detoxification by removing toxins and waste products from the body through the process of breathing.

When we breathe in air, it travels down our windpipe and into our lungs. Inside the lungs, the air is filtered, warmed, and humidified before it enters the bloodstream. One of the primary ways the lungs help with detoxification is by removing harmful pollutants and toxins from the air we breathe. The air we breathe can contain a variety of harmful substances, including pollutants, allergens, and other toxins. The lungs work to filter out these substances, preventing them from entering the bloodstream and causing damage to the body.

Additionally, the lungs play a role in the elimination of waste products from the body. When we exhale, we release carbon dioxide, a waste product produced by the body's cells. This process helps to remove excess carbon dioxide from the body, maintaining a healthy balance of gases in the bloodstream. To support the lungs in their detoxification role, it's important to maintain a healthy lifestyle that includes regular exercise and avoiding exposure to harmful substances in the air. Eating a healthy diet rich in antioxidants can also help to support lung function and reduce the risk of lung damage.

Intestines And Colon

The gut, and specifically the colon, plays an essential role in the body's detoxification process. When we eat food, it travels through the digestive tract, where it is broken down into its component parts. Nutrients are absorbed into the bloodstream and transported to the body's cells, while waste products are transported to the colon in the form of fecal matter, where they are stored until they can be eliminated from the body.

When waste products are eliminated from the body, they take with them any harmful substances that may have been present. Additionally, the colon contains trillions of bacteria that help to break down and eliminate harmful substances, further supporting the body's detoxification process.

When waste products and toxins accumulate in the colon, they can be reabsorbed into the bloodstream, leading to a range of health problems.

If there is dysbiosis (i.e. imbalances in the microflora), increased intestinal permeability, or inflammation, the liver is forced to work overtime. This means that good gut bacteria are not only important for gut health but for liver function, as well.

Heavy metals such as mercury, aluminum, and lead can damage the gut mucous membrane and tissues, causing them to become more permeable and allowing toxins to spread throughout the body. This is known to cause allergies, intolerances, and potential immune reactions. Toxins found in the gut need to be bound properly for excretion, or they will be recirculated in the body.

You need to ensure you are moving your bowels at least daily to prevent a backlog of toxic waste products.

Skin

The largest organ of the human body, the skin is responsible for protecting the body against external threats such as infections, physical injuries, and environmental toxins. Additionally, the skin plays a crucial role in the elimination of toxins from the body.

Sweat is produced by sweat glands located in the dermis layer of the skin. When we sweat, we release a variety of waste products, including salt, urea, and other toxins. This process helps to regulate the body's temperature and maintain a healthy balance of fluids in the body.

When the skin is not functioning properly, it can lead to a condition known as skin congestion. In this condition, the pores of the skin become clogged with dead skin cells, oils, and other debris, preventing the skin from properly eliminating toxins from the body.

To sum up, effective detoxification relies on a complex interplay of organs working together to eliminate toxins from the body. If one pathway of elimination is compromised, it can increase the burden on other organs, leading to a build-up of toxins in the body. Therefore, it's crucial to maintain the proper functioning of all organs involved in detoxification to ensure the efficient removal of toxins from the body.

Foods That Support Overall Detoxification

Supporting your body's detoxification process through your diet and lifestyle is crucial. It's important to prioritize all the organs responsible for detoxification. To support the liver's phase 1 and phase 2 detoxification, specific nutrients are needed, along with a high-fibre diet to promote proper bowel movement. A diet that is rich in plant phytonutrients, which can induce or inhibit specific enzymes, provide soluble and insoluble fibre and ensure the consumption of antioxidants is also beneficial. Incorporating a whole-food diet that includes fresh, local, and organic produce, as well as responsibly-raised meat (hormone-free and grass-fed), can provide your body with essential nutrients.

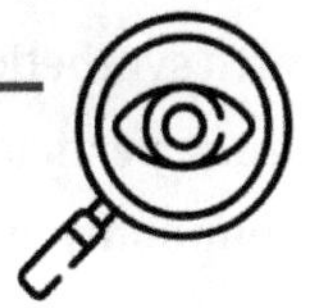

SMART CONSIDERATION

Detox Supportive Diet

There are several things you can implement immediately to support your body's detoxification process, including consuming foods high in sulphur (such as garlic, legumes, and onions), sources of water-soluble fibre (like apples, oat bran, and legumes), cruciferous vegetables (such as Brussels sprouts, cabbage, cauliflower, kale, and broccoli), artichokes, beets, carrots, and dandelion greens. Additionally, incorporating herbs and spices like turmeric, cinnamon, and licorice, and consuming green leafy vegetables, green tea, wheatgrass juice, chlorella, and spirulina can also support detoxification.

SMART CONSIDERATION

Choose Wisely

Choosing to eat organic foods is becoming more important as people become aware of the potential negative effects of consuming foods treated with synthetic chemicals. Organic foods are grown without synthetic fertilizers, pesticides, or GMOs, making them a healthier choice. Glyphosate, a commonly used herbicide, has been linked to cancer and ecosystem harm. By choosing organic, you can reduce your exposure to harmful chemicals and support sustainable agriculture. Each year, the Environmental Working Group releases its 'Dirty Dozen' and 'Clean Fifteen' lists. These lists highlight the top 12 most heavily sprayed produce crops that you should try to find grown organically, as well as the 15 'cleanest' produce items that, while conventionally grown, have the lowest amount of pesticides. Visit the website ewg.org or download their Healthy Living App for more resources on living a toxin-free lifestyle.

The Everyday Toxins All Around You

Regardless of your body's ability to process toxic chemicals, or how much of a tolerance or sensitivity you personally have, the sheer number of environmental toxins we're all exposed to does add to one's toxic load. Over time, these toxins accumulate and interact, stressing or debilitating the organs in charge of detoxification.

According to Dr. T. R. Morris, N.D., there are nine main toxic chemicals known as the 'toxic bunch'. (25) They include:

1. **Heavy Metals (lead, mercury, arsenic, and cadmium)**—Found in the foods we eat, due to pesticides, lead pipes, ceramics and glassware, batteries, dental fillings, and older imported toys.
2. **Polycyclic Aromatic Hydrocarbons (PAH)**—Can come from charred meats, exhaust fumes, smoke, trash incineration, and forest fires.
3. **Phthalates And Phenols**—Found in consumer products that use plastics, car interiors, mattresses, nail polish, processed foods, and more.
4. **Organochlorine (OC) Pesticides**—Specifically found in foods from countries where OCs aren't banned for growing produce or raising livestock.
5. **Organophosphate (OP) Pesticides**—Same as above.
6. **Polychlorinated Dibenzo-dioxin And Furans (PCDDs And PCDFs)**—Found in high-fat foods, as well as PVC production, paper production, and bleach products.
7. **Polychlorinated Biphenyls (PCBs)** — A toxic chemical and known endocrine disruptor found in farmed fish, also called "Atlantic salmon."
8. **Polybrominated Diphenyl Ethers (PBDEs)**—Used as flame retardants in furniture, foam, bedding, toys, electronics, and plastics.
9. **Polyfluorinated Compounds (PFCs)**—Used to make fast food grease-resistant and used in products like shampoos, and denture cleaners.

Xenoestrogens—Endocrine Disruption

Endocrine disruptors are chemicals that interfere with the normal functioning of our endocrine system. We are constantly bombarded by a myriad of environmental chemicals that mirror estrogen, also known as xenoestrogens. They can be found in a variety of everyday products, such as plastics, pesticides, cleaning products, and cosmetics. Just about every organ and tissue in the body has estrogen receptors. When estrogen circulates in the body, it binds to estrogen receptors and triggers certain effects in that organ or tissue. Xenoestrogens mimic our natural estrogen and attach to our estrogen receptors, potentially taking the place of a real estrogen molecule, or giving the cell the wrong signals. This disturbs our hormonal system and affects the entire body, leading to an increase in estrogenic activity.

Improve Indoor Air Quality

Poor indoor air quality can cause a wide range of health problems, including respiratory issues, allergies, and other illnesses. One of the easiest ways to improve indoor air quality is to increase ventilation. This can be done by opening windows and doors, using exhaust fans in the kitchen and bathroom, or installing a ventilation system. Dust, dirt, and other particles can accumulate in carpets, furniture, and other surfaces. Regular vacuuming, dusting, and wiping down surfaces can help to remove these particles. Air purifiers can help to remove pollutants and allergens from the air. There are many types of air purifiers on the market, including HEPA filters, activated carbon filters, and ionizers. Be sure to choose an air purifier that is appropriate for the size of the room.

High humidity can promote the growth of mould and other allergens, while low humidity can dry out the mucous membranes and make you more susceptible to respiratory infections. Keeping indoor humidity levels between 30-50% can help to maintain good indoor air quality.

Another way to improve indoor air quality is by adding plants to your environment. Peace lilies, snake plants, aloe vera, jade plants, and spider plants are all easy to care for and aid in removing formaldehyde, xylene, and benzene from the air. (26) Stop using synthetic air fresheners and paraffin candles and instead opt for natural beeswax or soy-based candles or diffuse essential oils.

SMART UPGRADES

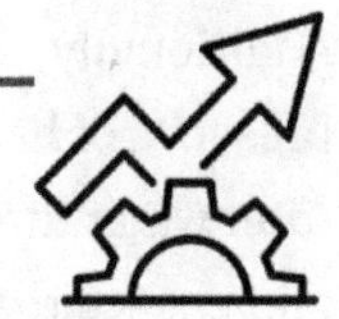

Air Purification

Consider upgrading your home with a reliable air purification unit to ensure cleaner and healthier air for you and your loved ones. Air purifiers, especially those fitted with HEPA filters, effectively reduce allergens like dust and pollen and capture harmful particles, including smoke and mold spores. Many also have activated carbon filters to neutralize odours and reduce volatile organic compounds from sources like paint, air fresheners, and household products. Some air purification units come equipped with UV or other sterilization technologies that can help neutralize certain pathogens. See Smart Resources at the end of this Section for links to companies that offer such products.

Watch Your Water Source

Water is an essential component for sustaining life, but even "clean" sources of water may not be safe for consumption. Municipal water often contains harmful contaminants, such as fluoride, pharmaceutical drug residue, and heavy metals, that can have adverse effects on our health.

Additionally, ageing pipes and infrastructure can also contribute to the presence of harmful contaminants in water. Therefore, it is important to filter water through a reliable filtration system to remove these impurities and ensure that you are drinking clean and safe water. There are many different types of filtration systems out there. Find one that fits your needs and budget. The Environmental Protection Agency (EPA) has a website (epa.gov/waterdata) where you can search for your local water system and access information about the quality of your drinking water. The website includes data on contaminants, violations, and compliance with drinking water standards. (Only available for U.S. municipalities.)

SMART UPGRADES

Water Testing

Consider testing your drinking water source through a company such as Tap Score (find link in Smart Resources). For a few hundred dollars, you can find out exactly what is in your drinking water, whether it be municipal, well water, rain or spring water.

Clean Up Cookware

Non-stick cookware, particularly those made with Teflon, has been a popular choice for many households due to its convenience in cooking and cleaning. However, over the years, there have been numerous health and environmental concerns associated with the use of Teflon cookware.

The main ingredient used in Teflon, polytetrafluoroethylene (PTFE), has been linked to several health problems when heated to high temperatures. When Teflon cookware is overheated, it releases toxic fumes that can cause flu-like symptoms, known as "Teflon flu." In severe cases, it can also lead to a condition called polymer fume fever, which can cause lung damage. Furthermore, some studies have shown that PTFE can leach into food and cause harmful effects on the body. (27)

Teflon and other non-stick cookware are made using perfluorinated chemicals (PFCs). PFCs, known as 'forever chemicals', are persistent in the environment and do not break down easily. Teflon production also requires the use of a highly toxic chemical called PFOS, which is classified as an organic pollutant and is linked to a number of health and environmental problems. Teflon and other non-stick cookware tend to have a limited lifespan, as the coating can start to deteriorate and flake over time. The non-stick coating is also prone to scratches and chips, which can also lead to the release of harmful toxic particles into the food being cooked.

While it may be convenient for cooking and cleaning, the potential health and environmental risks associated with Teflon make it a questionable choice. Instead, consider using cookware made with safer materials, such as cast iron, stainless steel, or ceramic, which are not only safer but also more durable and longer lasting.

Clothing

Much like the beauty products we put on our bodies, our skin also absorbs toxic compounds found in clothing and linens. Conventional clothing manufacturing practices involve the use of chemicals like formaldehyde and flame retardants, which can cause skin irritation, and allergies, and disrupt your hormones. Look for clothing and linens made with natural and organic fibres like cotton, wool, linen, and silk. In addition to the toxic compounds found in conventional clothing manufacturing, dyes used to colour clothing can also pose health risks. Synthetic dyes contain heavy metals, such as lead and cadmium, which can be absorbed through the skin and cause damage to the nervous system, reproductive organs, and kidneys. Organic and natural dyes, on the other hand, are made from plant-based materials and are much safer for both the environment and our health. Always wash brand-new clothing before wearing it.

Furniture

Furniture and mattress manufacturing is also a major source of toxin exposure that can be detrimental to our health. Polybrominated diphenyl ethers (PBDEs) are flame retardants that were widely used in the past. They are known to persist in the environment and accumulate in the food chain. Exposure to PBDEs has been linked to neurodevelopmental disorders, thyroid disruption, and cancer. (28) Formaldehyde is used as an adhesive in the manufacturing of furniture and mattresses and is a known carcinogen that can cause respiratory irritation, headaches, and dizziness. (29)

Perfluorinated compounds (PFCs) are used as stain and water repellents. These chemicals remain in the environment and have been linked to kidney and testicular cancer, as well as reproductive and developmental effects. (30)

Volatile organic compounds (VOCs) are released from the adhesives, paints, and finishes used in furniture and mattress manufacturing. These known carcinogens can cause eye, nose, and throat irritation, headaches, and dizziness. (31) Look for furniture that is certified low in VOCs whenever possible, and if space allows, store new furniture in a garage, or even better, somewhere outdoors for a day or two to allow harmful chemicals to off-gas outside, rather than in your home.

SMART PROTOCOL

Clean Your Beauty Products - $0 to $

Review your beauty products, such as toothpaste, shaving cream, deodorant, shampoo, moisturizer, and cosmetics, for harmful chemicals such as parabens, phthalates, sulphates, and formaldehyde. Seek out safer, natural alternatives to replace the products you currently use.

Websites like the Environmental Working Group's (EWG) ewg.org/skindeep, can aid in finding safe products and avoiding hidden toxins. Create your own products with simple recipes such as liquid castile soap, unrefined coconut, almond, and jojoba oils to replace moisturizing creams and lotions, and raw apple cider vinegar as an alternative to traditional conditioners.

SMART PROTOCOL

Clean Your Household Products - $0 to $$$

Opt for non-toxic cleaning products or create your own using natural ingredients like vinegar, baking soda, and essential oils. Use indoor plants, such as spider plants and peace lilies, to purify the air instead of synthetic air fresheners. Filter your drinking water and reduce plastic use by choosing glass or stainless steel containers. Avoid Teflon cookware and opt for safer materials like cast iron or ceramic. When buying furniture and mattresses, look for certifications like Oeko-Tex Standard 100 or Global Organic Textile Standard (GOTS) to ensure that harmful chemicals are not present.

Detoxification At The Cellular Level

Detoxification is a complex process that involves eliminating toxins from the body at a cellular level. The 5R protocol is a comprehensive approach employed by many functional health practitioners that helps to remove the sources of toxins, regenerate the cell membrane, restore cell energy, reduce inflammation and free radical damage, and re-establish methylation. With the guidance of a trained health professional, this strategy can help you improve cellular function, support overall health, and reduce the risk of many chronic diseases.

The 5 Rs include:

1. **Remove** sources of toxins such as pathogens, petrochemicals, toxins, and heavy metals, which can accumulate and shut down detox pathways.
2. **Regenerate** the cell membrane, which holds the intelligence of the cell and regulates hormones. Inflammation in the membrane can lead to abnormal cellular function and disease.
3. **Restore** cell energy by ensuring the proper functioning of mitochondria, which produce energy. Low ATP levels can cause fatigue, brain fog, and hormone issues.
4. **Reduce** inflammation and free radical damage caused by the detoxification process, which can change gene expression and affect cell communication.
5. **Re-establish methylation**, which repairs DNA, fights infections and gets rid of toxins. The "methylation priority principle" means the body sends methyl groups where they're most needed, based on adaptation to stress. Methyl groups turn our stress receptors on and off.

Single Nucleotide Polymorphisms (SNPs) And Detoxification

Single Nucleotide Polymorphisms (SNPs) are naturally occurring variations in a single nucleotide (A, T, C, or G) at a specific position in the DNA sequence of the human genome. SNPs can be thought of as "copying errors" that happen during the process of cell division, where an existing cell makes a copy of its DNA to create a new cell with a complete set of genetic instructions. Similar to a typo, mistakes in the copying process can lead to variations in the DNA sequence at a specific location. These variations can impact the expression of genes and affect individual traits, as well as influence susceptibility to diseases and response to treatments.

In terms of detoxification, there are several SNPs that can impact the body's ability to metabolize and eliminate toxins. One of the most well-known genes related to detoxification is the Cytochrome P450 (CYP) gene family. These genes encode enzymes that play a critical role in the metabolism of drugs, toxins, and other foreign compounds in the liver.

Certain SNPs in the CYP gene family have been associated with altered enzyme activity, which can impact an individual's ability to detoxify specific compounds.

Additional SNPs associated with detoxification include:

- **Superoxide Dismutase 2 (SOD2)**—An antioxidant enzyme that prevents the accumulation of harmful levels of superoxide.
- **NQO1**—An enzyme that detoxifies quinone breakdown products from environmental toxins such as benzene and tobacco smoke.
- **GPX1P1**—A member of the glutathione peroxidase enzyme family that detoxifies hydrogen peroxide, a reactive oxygen species formed during mitochondrial energy metabolism.
- **GSTP1**—One of many glutathione sulfotransferases (GST) enzymes that aid in the elimination of environmental toxins, including those found in tobacco smoke.
- **COMT**—Responsible for the detoxification of reactive breakdown products of estrogen, this versatile enzyme also assumes numerous roles in various other biological processes.

It's important to note that while certain SNPs may impact an individual's ability to detoxify specific compounds, the impact of these SNPs can be influenced by a range of factors, including diet, lifestyle, and environmental exposures. Additionally, not all individuals with these SNPs will necessarily experience negative health outcomes, as the impact can vary depending on a range of factors. We will discuss SNPs in more depth in Section 5—Epigenetics, Ageing & Longevity as well as resources you can use to test and analyze SNPs you may carry in your genes.

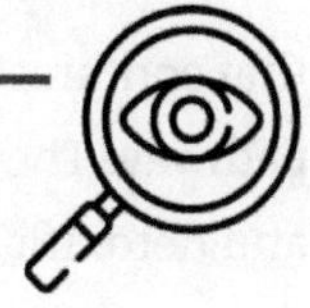

SMART CONSIDERATION

Detoxification Helpers

Detox supplements are dietary supplements designed to support the body's natural detoxification processes. They are often used to support liver function and help the body eliminate toxins and waste products:

Glutathione—Glutathione is a powerful antioxidant produced by the liver that helps neutralize harmful toxins and free radicals in the body. Liposomal glutathione is a form of glutathione that has been encapsulated in liposomes, which allows for better absorption and utilization by the body.

NAC (n-acetyl-l-cysteine)—NAC is another popular detox supplement. It is a precursor to glutathione and helps to boost glutathione levels in the body. NAC is also a potent antioxidant and has been shown to support liver function and help the body eliminate toxins. (32)

DIM (diindolylmethane)—DIM is a compound found in cruciferous vegetables such as broccoli and cauliflower. DIM has been shown to support healthy estrogen metabolism and may help to reduce the risk of certain types of cancer. (33)

Alpha Lipoic Acid (ALA)—ALA is a powerful antioxidant that helps to protect cells from damage caused by free radicals. It also helps to support liver function and has been shown to improve insulin sensitivity. (34)

Nrf2 (Nuclear factor erythroid 2-related factor 2)—Nrf2 is a supplement that contains a blend of natural ingredients that help to activate the Nrf2 pathway. The Nrf2 pathway is responsible for the activation of antioxidant and detoxification genes in the body, which helps to protect cells from damage caused by toxins and oxidative stress.

Sulphoraphane—Sulphoraphane is a compound found in cruciferous vegetables such as broccoli and kale. It has been shown to support liver function and help the body eliminate toxins. (35) Sulphoraphane also has anti-inflammatory properties and may help to reduce the risk of certain types of cancer.

Calcium-d-glucarate—Calcium-d-glucarate is a natural compound found in fruits and vegetables that has gained popularity as a supplement for its potential to promote detoxification, support hormonal balance, and reduce the risk of hormone-dependent cancers such as breast and prostate cancer. It works by inhibiting an enzyme that interferes with the body's ability to eliminate toxins and hormones and may also help lower cholesterol levels and support liver health.

Milk Thistle—Milk thistle is a plant that has been used for centuries as a natural remedy for liver issues. The active ingredient silymarin has antioxidant and anti-inflammatory properties that may reduce liver inflammation, improve function and protect it from damage caused by toxins or alcohol. It is generally considered safe for short-term use (up to six months), and there have been no reports of serious adverse effects associated with long-term use. (36)

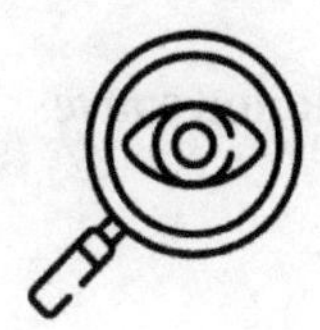

SMART CONSIDERATION

Sweat It Out

Sweating can help eliminate a range of toxins from the body, including heavy metals like lead, cadmium, and mercury, as well as environmental toxins like BPA and phthalates. In fact, studies have found that sweat can contain higher levels of some toxins than urine or blood, indicating that sweating is an important detoxification pathway that should not be overlooked. (37)

Sweat is mostly made up of water and salt but also contains metabolic waste products like urea and ammonia. When we sweat, these waste products are released from the body, which helps to reduce the overall toxin load in the body. It is vitally important to get sweaty on a regular basis, at least a few times per week.

Sauna sessions, in particular, have been found to be an effective way to induce sweating and improve detoxification. Saunas help to increase the body's core temperature, which stimulates sweat production and helps to release toxins from the body. Both traditional and infrared saunas promote sweating, detoxification, increased heart rate, and improved circulation.

Sauna blankets are a popular alternative to traditional saunas that offer similar health benefits, including detoxification. A sauna blanket is a portable, lightweight device that wraps around the body, using heat and infrared technology to create a sauna-like experience.

The benefits of sauna use extend further than detoxification, and both infrared saunas and sauna blankets are increasingly affordable and convenient options for at-home use.

SMART CONSIDERATION

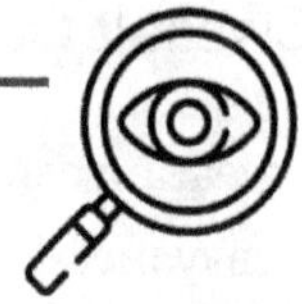

Infrared Sauna

Infrared saunas most often utilize near or far infrared wavelengths of light, rather than a combination. While both have specific benefits to the body, there are a few distinctions between them.

Far-infrared (FIR) wavelengths , typically ranging from 5,600 to 20,000 nanometers, have a longer wavelength and can penetrate deeper into the body. This deeper penetration allows FIR to generate heat within the body, leading to various benefits such as increased circulation, relaxation, pain relief, and potential detoxification effects. FIR is often associated with its ability to produce a sweat response, which can aid in eliminating toxins from the body.

Near-infrared (NIR) wavelengths range from 700 to 1,400 nanometers and are closer to the visible light spectrum. NIR is known for its photobiomodulation effects, which means it can interact with cells and tissues to stimulate beneficial processes. Near-infrared light is capable of activating the mitochondrial chelating systems in your cells. Through the stimulation of mitochondria, near-infrared light therapy promotes the release of nitric oxide and boosts ATP production, leading to healing effects like DNA repair and cellular regeneration. These effects can include improved skin health, collagen production, and wound healing. (38) NIR is also believed to have a positive impact on muscle recovery. Interestingly, only a small fraction of solar radiation consists of far-infrared wavelengths, while roughly 40% of the sunlight spectrum is near-infrared. Compared to far-infrared saunas, near-infrared saunas emit very low levels of EMFs (electromagnetic fields), as far-infrared saunas can often generate high electric fields. The majority of infrared saunas designed for at-home use far-infrared wavelengths, so be sure to research before purchasing. See Smart Resources for links to reputable sauna companies you can use as a starting point of research.

Lymphatic Points Drainage Routines

Lymphatic drainage is a therapeutic technique that aims to improve the flow of lymphatic fluid in the body. It involves a series of gentle massage movements and can be done as part of a self-care routine at home. Dr. Perry Nickelston, an expert in lymphatic drainage therapy, has developed a signature technique called the *Big 6 Tribal Lymphatic Drainage Routine.* This technique involves activating the major lymph node areas in the body to promote optimal lymphatic function. (39)

SMART PROTOCOL

Short Lymphatic Drainage Routine - $0

Follow this sequence (start with the left side):

1. Tap above the collarbones five times.
2. Tap the side of the neck/behind the angular jaw five times.
3. Tap at the pectoral area five times.
4. Tap the abdomen with both hands five times.
5. Tap the groin area five times.
6. Tap behind each knee five times.
7. Tap each arm from the shoulder down to the fingers and back up toward the armpits—front and back of the arms.
8. Tap the sides of the body to the waist.
9. Tap each leg down to the toes and back up towards the groin—front and back of the legs.
10. Finish with a full-body shake.

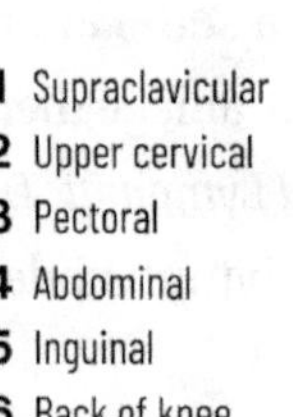

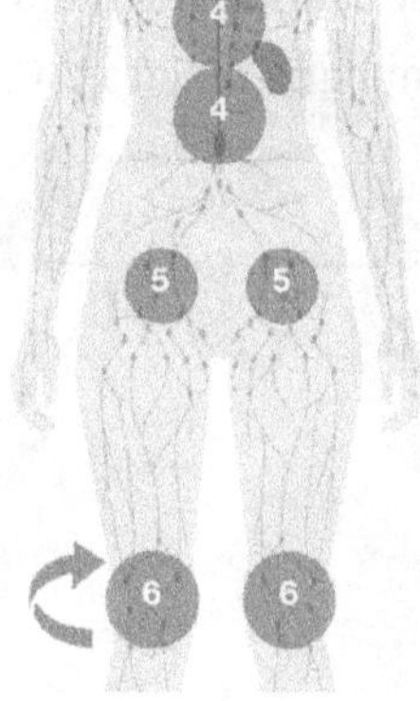

SMART PROTOCOL

Longer Lymphatic Drainage Routine - $0

Dr. Perry Nickelston also has a more extensive lymphatic routine that uses five steps for each of the lymph node points of his full lymph sequence routine. The 5 steps are:

Feather-Light Touch—The first step starts with a feather-light touch that lasts for five seconds, with the intention of stimulating enteroception. Enteroception is the awareness of the internal state of the body.

Rub Faster And Deeper—This step involves deeper pressure and faster rubbing to activate Pascinian corpuscles as these sensory receptors respond to pressure. Perform for 5 seconds.

Tap/Slap—In this step, tapping or slapping the skin activates the vibration part of the Pascinian receptors. Perform for 5 seconds.

Strokes/Pull Toward The Heart—This step involves three strokes or a gentle pulling motion toward the heart. The intention is to stimulate Ruffini receptors, which are sensitive to stretching.

Dry Brushing/Infinity Sign—The final step is to dry-brush the skin with soft, gentle bristles or make an infinity sign 3 times. This step helps to exfoliate the skin, improve circulation, and stimulate the lymphatic system.

Longer Lymphatic Drainage Routine - $0

Following the 5 steps above, work in sequence on the following lymph nodes:

Body—subclavian, pectoral, medial elbow, sternum/rib, axillary, para-aortic, mesenteric, inguinal, femoral, behind the knee, pedal.

Head—side of the neck/angle of the jaw, under the jaw, side of the jaw/masseter, nasolabial, temporal/sphenoid, occiput.

BODY

1 Subclavian
2 Pectoral
3 Medial elbow
4 Sternum/rib
5 Axillary/side of ribcage under armpit
6 Para-aortic/upper stomach under ribcage
7 Mesenteric/stomach
8 Inguinal
9 Femoral
10 Back of knees
11 Pedal/inside of ankle

HEAD

12 Side of neck/angle of jaw
13 Under the jaw
14 Masseter/side of jaw line
15 Nasolabial/side of nose
16 Temporal/sphenoid (temples)
17 Occiput/back of head-base of skull

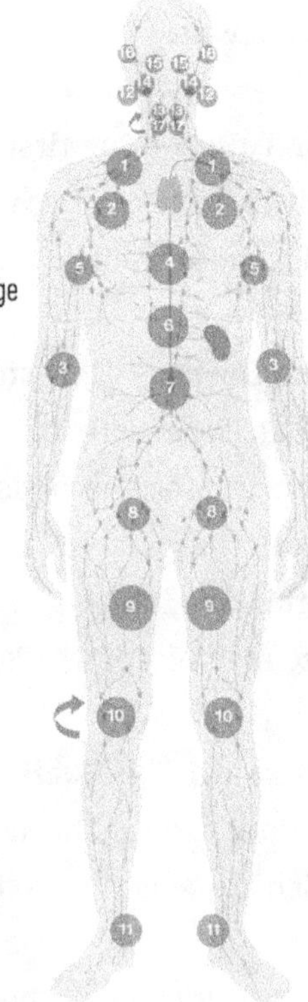

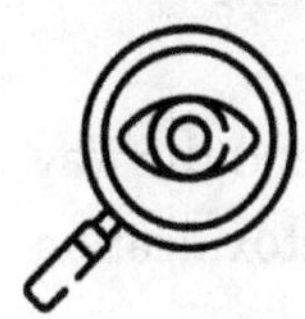

SMART CONSIDERATION

Jump Around

Rebounding involves jumping on a mini trampoline, providing a fun and low-impact way to promote lymphatic flow, detoxify the body, and boost immunity. The gentle bouncing motion stimulates lymph nodes to filter out waste and toxins, increasing circulation, reducing inflammation, and promoting efficient cell function. Rebounding also improves digestion and can be done on rebounders of varying prices, so consider your budget and choose one with features that meet your needs.

Live A Non-Toxic Lifestyle Through Consistent Detoxification Efforts

Our bodies work tirelessly to eliminate harmful substances and maintain our health, so it's important to reduce the toxic load we expose ourselves to. Detoxification should be viewed as a lifestyle choice rather than a one-time event. We can only achieve effective detoxification by consistently reducing environmental toxins from our lives and replacing them with natural, sustainable alternatives.

Although it may seem daunting to completely eliminate all sources of toxins, even small changes in the household and skin care products you use can make a significant impact. Chemicals accumulate over time, so every effort toward detoxification improves our overall health and well-being.

By adopting conscious choices about the products we use and the way we care for ourselves, we can support our body's natural detoxification processes and promote optimal health.

Section Wrap-Up

With a comprehensive approach that includes exercise, detoxification, and lymphatic support, we can enhance our overall health and vitality while reducing the risk of disease and illness for years to come. So get moving, sweat often, and work towards reducing your toxic exposure in everyday activities.

As we have explored the profound impact of exercise, movement, and detoxification on the body, we must acknowledge that our health and well-being encompass not only physicality but also the intricate connections between our body, brain, and emotions. In Section 4—Neurotransmitters, Hormones & Brain Wiring, we will examine how our brain wiring influences our thoughts, emotions, and behaviours. By uncovering the intricate workings of neurotransmitters, we will gain insights into their impact on our mental wellness and cognitive performance. Additionally, we will explore the role of hormones in regulating bodily functions and shaping our emotional states, and give practical strategies to foster a harmonious brain-body relationship.

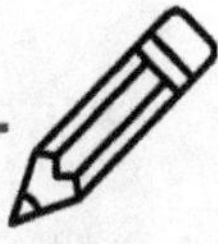

PROTOCOLS QUICK REFERENCE CHECKLIST:

PROTOCOL—Stability And Mobility Self Evaluation - $0

- [ ] *Currently doing*
- [ ] *Want to integrate*
- [ ] *Not for now*

PROTOCOL—Standing Long Jump - $0

- [ ] *Currently doing*
- [ ] *Want to integrate*
- [ ] *Not for now*

PROTOCOL—Strength Testing - $0 to $

- [ ] *Currently doing*
- [ ] *Want to integrate*
- [ ] *Not for now*

PROTOCOL—Determine FFMI - $0

- [ ] *Currently doing*
- [ ] *Want to integrate*
- [ ] *Not for now*

PROTOCOL—Muscular Endurance Test - $0 to $

- [ ] *Currently doing*
- [ ] *Want to integrate*
- [ ] *Not for now*

PROTOCOL—Assess Heart Rate Recovery - $0 to $$

- [ ] *Currently doing*
- [ ] *Want to integrate*
- [ ] *Not for now*

PROTOCOL—V02 Max Assessment - $0 to $$

☐ *Currently doing* ☐ *Want to integrate* ☐ *Not for now*

PROTOCOL—Aerobic Endurance Test - $0 to $$$

☐ *Currently doing* ☐ *Want to integrate* ☐ *Not for now*

PROTOCOL—Figure Out Fitness Priorities - $0

☐ *Currently doing* ☐ *Want to integrate* ☐ *Not for now*

PROTOCOL—Power And Speed Bias - $0 to $

☐ *Currently doing* ☐ *Want to integrate* ☐ *Not for now*

PROTOCOL—Strength Bias - $0 to $

☐ *Currently doing* ☐ *Want to integrate* ☐ *Not for now*

PROTOCOL—Build Muscle Size - $0 to $

☐ *Currently doing* ☐ *Want to integrate* ☐ *Not for now*

PROTOCOL—Building Muscular Endurance - $0

☐ *Currently doing* ☐ *Want to integrate* ☐ *Not for now*

PROTOCOL—Developing Phosphagen Energy System - $0

☐ *Currently doing* ☐ *Want to integrate* ☐ *Not for now*

PROTOCOL—Developing Fast Glycolysis Energy System - $0

☐ *Currently doing* ☐ *Want to integrate* ☐ *Not for now*

PROTOCOL—Developing Fast Glycolysis/Oxidative Energy System - $0

☐ *Currently doing* ☐ *Want to integrate* ☐ *Not for now*

PROTOCOL—Repeat Sprint Ability - $0

☐ *Currently doing* ☐ *Want to integrate* ☐ *Not for now*

PROTOCOL—Intermittent Hypoxic Hypercapnic Training - $0

☐ *Currently doing* ☐ *Want to integrate* ☐ *Not for now*

PROTOCOL—Developing VO2 Max - $0

☐ *Currently doing* ☐ *Want to integrate* ☐ *Not for now*

PROTOCOL—Developing Steady State Endurance - $0

☐ *Currently doing* ☐ *Want to integrate* ☐ *Not for now*

PROTOCOL—Post-Workout Recovery Routine - $0

☐ *Currently doing* ☐ *Want to integrate* ☐ *Not for now*

PROTOCOL—Clean Your Beauty Products - $0 to $

☐ *Currently doing* ☐ *Want to integrate* ☐ *Not for now*

PROTOCOL—Clean Your Household Products - $0 to $$$

☐ *Currently doing* ☐ *Want to integrate* ☐ *Not for now*

PROTOCOL—Short Lymphatic Drainage Routine - $0

☐ *Currently doing* ☐ *Want to integrate* ☐ *Not for now*

PROTOCOL—Longer Lymphatic Drainage Routine - $0

☐ *Currently doing* ☐ *Want to integrate* ☐ *Not for now*

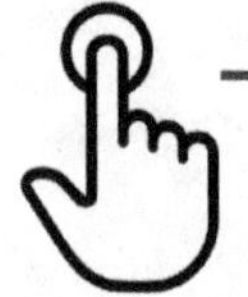

SMART RESOURCES

- FFMI Calculators—ffmicalculator.org, omnicalculator.com/health/ffmi, fitnessvolt.com/ffmi-calculator
- DEXA Scan—dexascan.com
- OxygenAdvantage®—oxygenadvantage.com
- Maximum heart rate calculator—ntnu.edu/cerg/hrmax

- Movement and exercise videos—ericcressey.com, functionalmovement.com, foundationtraining.com
- Air Purifiers—airdoctorpro.com, iqair.com, blueair.com
- Dirty Dozen—ewg.org
- Safe Drinking Water—epa.gov/waterdataepa.gov and testing—mytapscore.com
- Safe skin care—ewg.org/skindeep
- Infrared Saunas—infraredsauna.com, saunaspace.com

SMART TOOLS AT A GLANCE

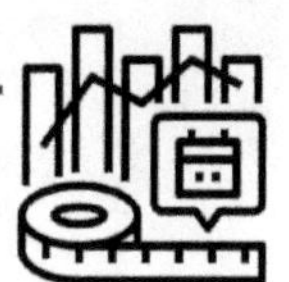

- Grip Strength Measurement—Hand Dynamometer
- Pulse Oximeter—nonin.com/technologies/pulse-oximetry
- Handheld Body Fat Monitors—Omron—omronhealthcare.com
- Tanita—tanita.com
- Withings—withings.com
- Heart Rate Monitor—Polar H10 polar.com/ca-en/sensors/h10-heart-rate-sensor
- Barefoot Shoes—vivobarefoot.com, xeroshoes.com, lemsshoes.com
- Oxygen Advantage® Sportsmask—oxygenadvantage.com/product/sports-mask

Section 4—Neurotransmitters, Hormones & Brain Wiring

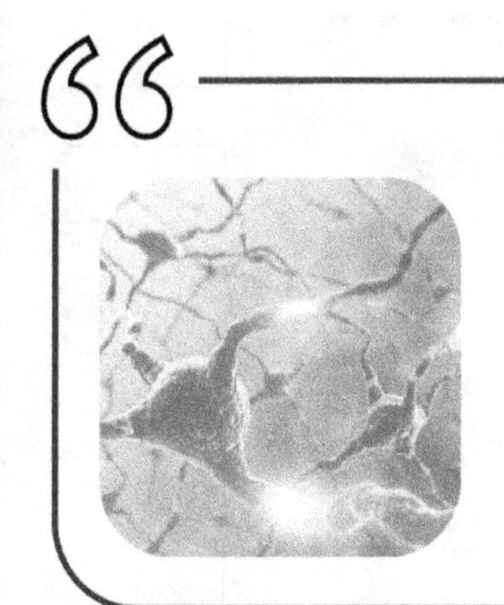

"The master control system of the body is the nerve system. The nervous system controls and coordinates every function of the body. The better your nervous system functions, the better your body functions."

—BJ Palmer

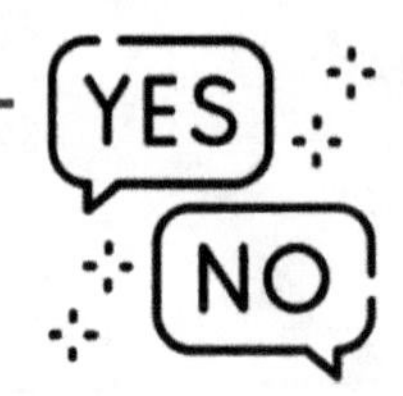

SELF EVALUATION-DISCOVERY QUESTIONS

Does stress or emotional upset cause you to feel exhausted? Y N

Do you often feel anxious, depressed, or experience mood swings?? Y N

Do you have a sensitive gag reflex or difficulty swallowing supplements? Y N

Are you able to remain calm under pressure? Y N

Do you have practical strategies to control your stress? Y N

Do you experience forgetfulness or memory loss? Y N

Is it usually easy for you to focus and stay on task? Y N

Do you have trouble retaining information or difficulty learning new skills? Y N

Do you feel mentally drained after a long day of work or activities? Y N

Do you feel energized throughout your day? Y N

Are you usually a happy person? Y N

Are you impulsive or apathetic? Y N

Do you experience addictive or pleasure-seeking behaviours? Y N

Are you motivated to complete tasks? Y N

Do you find yourself procrastinating often? Y N

Do you carry your cell phone close to your body? Y N

Have you ever had your hormone levels tested? Y N

Are you able to embrace making mistakes when learning something new? Y N

Are you able to incorporate and stick with new habits? Y N

Do you feel you are a creative person by nature? Y N

Do you meditate regularly? Y N

Do you have a regular gratitude practice? Y N

Do you use breathwork techniques to manage your state?

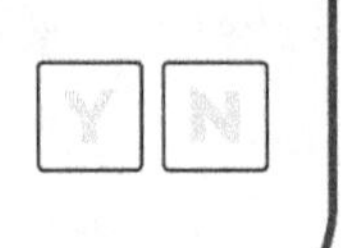

In this Section, we'll explore how neurotransmitters play a role in focus, concentration, motivation, mood, learning, and productivity, and how to optimize them for better health and a more fulfilling life. We will also talk about hormones as they are closely connected to neurotransmitters in the body's regulation of various physiological functions.

Neurotransmitters are chemicals that transmit signals between nerve cells in the brain and throughout the nervous system. Hormones are chemical messengers produced by the endocrine glands that regulate various bodily processes, including growth and development, metabolism, and reproductive functions.

The release of neurotransmitters and hormones is regulated by the nervous system and endocrine system, respectively. Neurotransmitters and hormones can affect each other's production and release, creating a delicate balance that is essential for overall health and well-being.

Brain Basics

Before we dig deeper into the topic let's go over some basic brain anatomy.

The brain is made up of billions of nerve cells called neurons, that gather and transmit electrochemical signals known as nerve impulses, across gaps called synapses. Neurons are responsible for our thoughts, emotions, actions, and sensations through these impulses. There are several different kinds of neurons, with different functions. Sensory neurons send information from sensory receptors located in the skin, eyes, nose, tongue, ears and organs to the central nervous system. Motor neurons send information from the central nervous system to muscles and glands. Interneurons transmit information between sensory and motor neurons.

The largest part of the human brain is the cerebrum, which consists of several parts. The cerebrum is divided into two hemispheres, which are connected by large fibre tracts (called the corpus callosum) that enable the left and right sides to efficiently communicate.

The outermost layer of the cerebrum is the more evolutionarily modern cerebral cortex, which consists of 4 lobes:

- **The Frontal Lobe** stretches between the temples. Much of our personality comes from this part of the brain. It is responsible for impulse control, emotion, drive, motivation, planning, and fine motor coordination.
- **The Temporal Lobes** are located to the side, just above the ears, and are responsible for hearing, speech, memory, emotional responses, and distinguishing smells. They contain the hippocampus, which is responsible for learning, memory, and the sleep-wake cycle.
- **The Parietal Lobes** lie directly behind our ears. Their primary function is to perceive sensations like touch and pressure, and to interpret these sensations, such as—judging texture, weight, size, or shape. Another function is to integrate input from the skin, muscles, joints and vision to become aware of the body in its environment.
- **The Occipital Lobe** is located in the very back of the brain and processes visual information like recognizing shapes, colours, and motions.

DIVISIONS OF THE NERVOUS SYSTEM

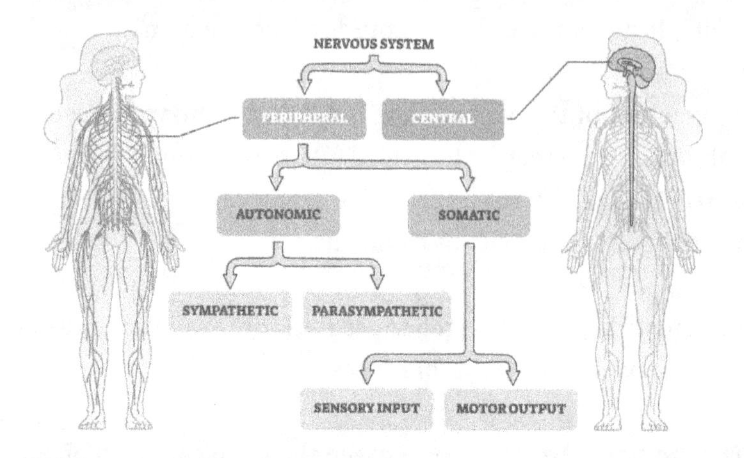

Underneath the cerebrum lies the brainstem, which consists of the more primitive medulla, pons, and midbrain. The brainstem controls the reflexes and autonomic functions (e.g. heart rate, blood pressure), limb movements, and visceral functions (e.g. digestion, urination). Behind that sits the cerebellum. The cerebellum receives input from the sensory systems, the spinal cord, and other parts of the brain and then coordinates voluntary movement.

The cerebellum communicates intimately with the cerebrum. Therefore, it is thought to be the connection between our physical environment (as it relates to movement and position of the body) and our cognition, personality, and emotions, providing the mind-body connections so to speak.

Other important parts of the brain:

- **The Basal Ganglia**, which plays an important role in planning actions that are required to achieve a particular goal, in executing well-practiced habitual actions, and in learning new actions in novel situations.

- **The Limbic System**, which is composed of the amygdala, hippocampus, thalamus, hypothalamus and cingulate gyrus. Each of these parts work together and are involved in processing the senses, emotions, memories, hormone regulation and motivation.

Neurons And Glial Cells

Neurons in the brain do not regenerate, except in one area known as the hippocampus. This means that when neurons are damaged or lost due to injury or disease, they cannot be replaced or regrown. Neurons make up roughly 10% of the brain's composition while the other 90% are glial cells, varying depending on the brain region and the individual. (1) Glial cells play an important role in supporting the function and health of neurons, including providing structural support, regulating the extracellular environment, and aiding in neuronal signalling. While neurons are responsible for processing and transmitting information in the brain, glial cells are essential for maintaining a healthy and functional nervous system.

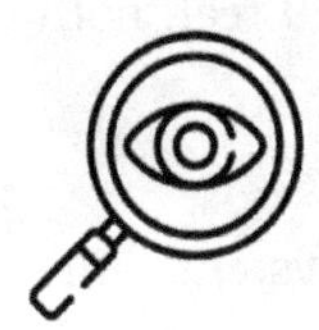

SMART CONSIDERATION

Neuronal Health—Another Good Reason To Use Heat Exposure

Science has shown that heat exposure has a positive impact on the body, specifically through the production of brain-derived neurotrophic factor (BDNF) and heat shock proteins (HSPs). (2)

BDNF is a protein that is critical for the survival of neurons and protecting them against various stresses. Heat shock proteins (HSPs) are a family of proteins that help protect cells from damage caused by stress, including heat, exercise, and exposure to toxins. They function as molecular chaperones, promoting the folding and assembly of other proteins, and helping to repair damaged proteins.

A study conducted by Dr. Rhonda Patrick, a leading expert in the field of nutritional health, genetics, and longevity, saw participants exposed to heat stress which resulted in an increase in heat shock proteins and an improvement in cognitive function. (3) Protocols and considerations for safe, deliberate heat exposure are outlined in Section 1—Sleep, Rest & Recovery for your reference.

Nervous System 101

The nervous system controls everything you do, think, and feel, both voluntary and involuntary.

The brain and spinal cord make up the central nervous system. The peripheral nervous system is made up of nerve fibres that branch off from the spinal cord and extend to all parts of the body, including the internal organs, neck, arms, torso, legs, and skeletal muscles.

The peripheral system itself is comprised of two components:

- **The Somatic Nervous System** is responsible for sending motor and sensory information to and from the central nervous system. It connects to the skin, sensory organs, and all skeletal muscles, and is responsible for many voluntary muscle movements. In addition, it is important in the sensory processing of sound, smell, touch and taste.

- **The Autonomic Nervous System** regulates certain body processes such as blood pressure, heart rate, breath rate, immune system and digestion that occur without conscious effort. The autonomic nervous system has two branches: the sympathetic nervous system and the parasympathetic nervous system. The sympathetic nervous system is often described as the "fight-or-flight" system, while the parasympathetic nervous system is often referred to as the "rest-and-digest" system.

SMART CONSIDERATION

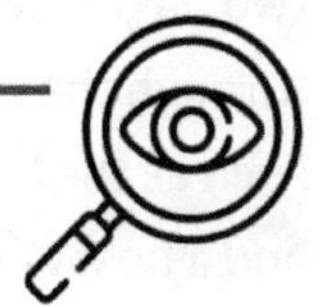

The Gut-Brain Connection

More and more research is showing the reciprocal connection between our gastrointestinal tract or "gut" and our brain. (4) The gut has its own nervous system called the enteric nervous system—the largest network of nerves in the human body, which is linked to the brain through the vagus nerve. The vagus nerve is key in balancing our autonomic nervous system, as its down-regulating effect allows for a tempered response to stress, acting as a buffer for the fight-or-flight response during stressful situations. Due to the strong connection between the brain and gut, factors such as a poor diet, stress, and the use of certain medications can affect the composition of the gut microbiome, which in turn can impact our mental health and cognitive function. In short, emerging research suggests that a healthy gut equals a healthy brain. For recommendations on promoting and sustaining a diverse and resilient microbiome, please refer to Section

2—Hydration, Fuel & Foundationals.

The Vagus Nerve

The vagus nerve (also called cranial nerve 10) is one of the largest nerve systems and is so named because it wanders like a vagabond, sending out nerve fibres from our brain to all the organs in our body. There are actually two vagus nerves—a left and a right—that start in the brainstem, exit through the jugular foramen of the skull, and branch down to vital organs such as the heart, lungs, esophagus, digestive tract, reproductive organs, and a host of others. Interestingly, 80% of information sent by the vagus nerve is afferent (meaning from the organs to the brain) whereas only 20% is efferent (meaning coming from the brain to the organs). (5)

The Polyvagal Theory, developed by Dr. Stephen Porges, provides a framework for understanding the complex interplay between our nervous system, behaviour, and emotional regulation. (6) According to the Polyvagal Theory, the vagus nerve has two branches, each with a distinct role in regulating the body's response to stress and threat. The first branch, the dorsal branch, is responsible for the "freeze-or-faint" response. This response is a form of self-protection that involves shutting down the body's systems to conserve energy and avoid detection by a potential predator or threat. In this state, the body may become immobile, appear unresponsive, or even lose consciousness.

The dorsal branch of the vagus nerve is activated in response to intense stress, trauma, or perceived threat. When this happens, the body's Sympathetic Nervous System (SNS) becomes activated, triggering the release of stress hormones like cortisol and adrenaline. These hormones can cause a range of physical symptoms, including increased heart rate, rapid breathing, and muscle tension.

On the other hand, the ventral branch of the vagus nerve is responsible for the "rest-and-digest" response, which helps the body to calm down and recover from stress. This branch of the vagus nerve affects the body functioning above the diaphragm, including the heart, lungs, and facial muscles. When the ventral vagus nerve is activated, the body's Parasympathetic Nervous System (PNS) becomes dominant, which slows down heart rate, lowers blood pressure, and promotes digestion and healing.

The ventral branch of the vagus nerve plays a critical role in social engagement and emotional regulation. When we feel safe and secure, the ventral vagus nerve helps us connect with others, communicate effectively, and experience positive emotions like joy and love. In contrast, when we feel threatened or overwhelmed, the dorsal vagus nerve may take over, leading to a freeze-or-faint response that can be immobilizing and disorienting.

Spinal health plays a significant role in directing the health of the vagus nerve. If the spine becomes compromised in its positioning or ability to move freely, the information to and from the vagus nerves becomes altered. This is why chiropractic adjustments can have such an impact on the vagus nerve.

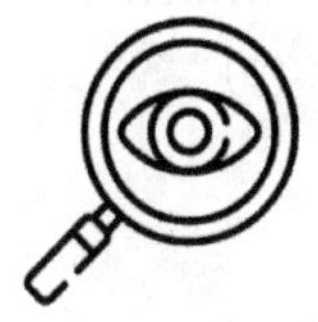

SMART CONSIDERATION

Signs Of Vagal Dysfunction

If the vagus nerve is not functioning properly, it can lead to a range of symptoms. However, it's important to note that these symptoms can vary widely depending on the specific cause and severity of the issue. Here are some signs and symptoms that may indicate a problem with the vagus nerve:

- Digestive issues (nausea, vomiting, bloating, indigestion, changes in appetite).
- Heart rate and blood pressure abnormalities (bradycardia, low blood pressure, fainting, light-headedness, irregular heart rhythms).
- Respiratory problems (shortness of breath, shallow breathing, difficulty breathing).
- Voice and swallowing difficulties (hoarseness, voice changes, difficulty swallowing, the sensation of food getting stuck).
- Gastrointestinal issues (constipation, diarrhea, decreased sensation of fullness or hunger).
- Anxiety and mood changes (anxiety, depression, mood swings).
- Dizziness and balance problems (dizziness, vertigo, balance difficulties).
- Weakness and fatigue.

Another issue linked with vagus dysfunction is chronic inflammation, as the vagus nerve releases the neurotransmitter acetylcholine—which has been shown to have an anti-inflammatory effect on the body. (7)

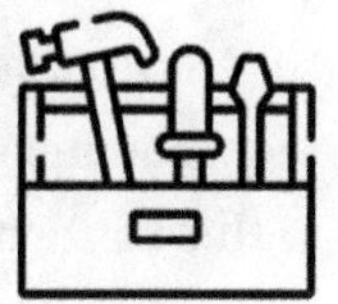

SMART TOOLS

Test Vagal Tone With Transit Time Challenge

To assess your vagus nerve health, conduct a bowel transit time test. The vagus nerve regulates digestive tract contractions and peristalsis, facilitating efficient digestion and bowel movements. To perform the test, swallow 1 tablespoon of white sesame seeds (our bodies lack the enzymes to break down their shells) with water, noting the ingestion time. Observe subsequent stools after bowel movements and record when you see the seeds until they are no longer visible. Ideally, seeds should appear 16-24 hours after ingestion. If seeds appear significantly earlier or after 24 hours, it may indicate vagal tone issues.

Heart Rate Variability, The Vagus Nerve, And Chiropractic Care

The gold standard test used to check the function and efficiency of the vagus nerve and the autonomic nervous system is Heart Rate Variability (HRV). The heart does not beat like a metronome. The SNS and PNS are constantly competing, the SNS wanting to speed up heart rate and the PNS wanting to slow it down via the vagus nerve. This even happens in one breath cycle—inhalation is SNS dominant and speeds heart rate, and exhalation is PNS dominant and slows it. This is why simply prolonging your exhale helps you to relax.

HRV devices are used to measure the variability between heartbeats. It may seem counter-intuitive to consider that heart rate should be variable, but in this context, we are referring to the periods between the PQRST beats. Greater variability during these intervals indicates higher resilience.

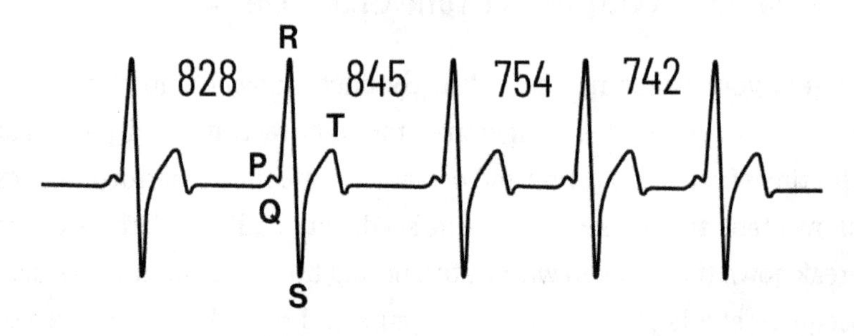

Different devices will measure different variables: the Root Mean Square of the Successive Differences (RMSSD), which is a measure of time, and the Standard Deviation of the Normal-to-Normal intervals (SDNN), which is a measure of frequency. See the following illustrations.

TIME-DOMAIN

How many heartbeats in this timeframe?

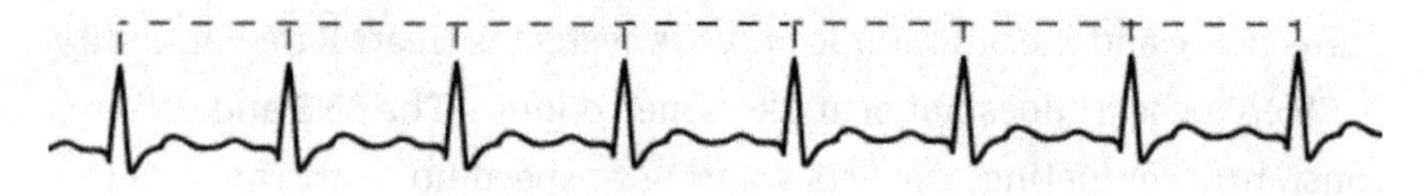

FREQUENCY-DOMAIN

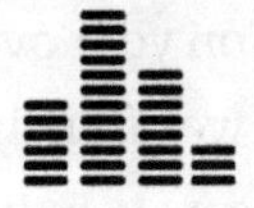

How are the RR intervals modulated?

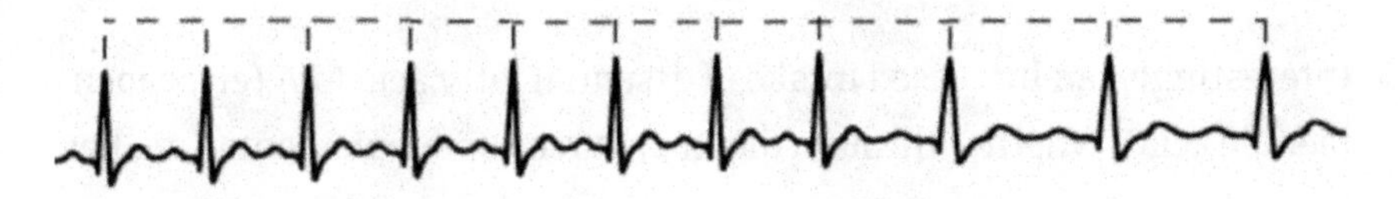

RMSSD—time-domain—is often used to measure parasympathetic nervous system activity, while SDNN—frequency-domain— can provide an overall measure of heart rate variability.

When it comes to interpreting HRV readings, it's important to understand which measurement you are looking at, and not try to compare the two. Many of the popular devices like FitBit and Oura Ring primarily measure SDNN.

HRV is a great tool to assess your nervous system adaptation, stress levels, and recovery. It's important to note that HRV is an individualized metric, so it's best to compare your HRV score to your own previous measurements rather than comparing it to others. You can establish your baseline HRV over several days to weeks, and track changes.

How much time and effort you are devoting to rest and recovery (see Section 1—Sleep, Rest & Recovery), sleep, diet and whether you may be overtraining will all be reflected in your HRV. Remember this is a metric where higher is better; a normal or increasing number indicates less stress and a greater ability to take on tasks and workouts while a lower number indicates a greater need for rest and recovery.

This is why some healthcare practitioners and strength coaches will use heart rate variability as one measure to help decide if an individual is ready to train hard on a particular day. Many chiropractors use HRV to measure the impact of chiropractic care on your overall nervous system function. In the stressful, fast-paced life we often live these days, one of the many benefits of chiropractic care appears to be its ability to increase the healing and calming side of our autonomic nervous system. (8)

Interestingly, an increased intake of essential fatty acid EPA (eicosapentaenoic acid), whether through dietary sources or supplementation, has been shown to improve symptoms of depression and boost heart rate variability. The mechanism behind this effect lies in EPA's influence on both the gut and the autonomic nervous system, particularly the connections between the heart and the brain that relay sensory information about heart rate. By elevating HRV, EPA has the ability to alleviate depression symptoms and even enhance the efficacy of low-dose antidepressant medications. This study presents a fascinating exploration of the intricate link between the brain and the body, underscoring the potential advantages of utilizing natural approaches to enhance mental well-being. (9)

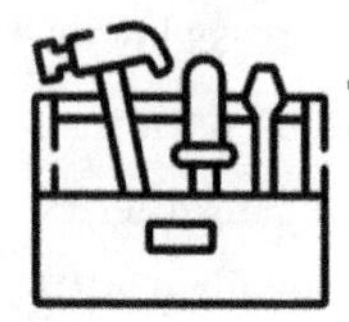

SMART TOOLS

Elite HRV

The Elite HRV App offers a convenient and user-friendly way to monitor your HRV. It is compatible with various popular wearable devices, including Garmin, Polar, and Apple Watch, or simply the Polar H10 strap paired with your smartphone. By taking just a few minutes to measure your HRV daily, the app provides valuable insights into your overall health, stress levels, and recovery status. Through HRV measurements, optional sleep quality analysis, and other factors, the app generates a daily readiness score. This score empowers you to make well-informed decisions about your training intensity, workout routines, and overall lifestyle choices, all geared toward optimizing your performance and recovery.

SMART PROTOCOL

Track HRV – $ to $$

Understand your heart rate variability with a personal HRV tracker. For the most accurate reading, track at the same time each day, ideally upon waking, and avoid physical activity or stress prior to measurement. Continue for a couple of days to determine your baseline reading. Keep a log of factors that may impact HRV, so you can identify any patterns or trends over time. If you are taking steps to better your health and fitness, you should notice an upward trend. Conversely, if you suddenly notice lower HRV readings, it could indicate illness, poor sleep quality, improper hydration, or even training too hard.

SMART PROTOCOL

HRV Biofeedback - $ to $$

One of the advantages of the Elite HRV App is its ability to provide you with real-time readings. This allows you to assess, for instance, the effect of a specific breathing practice on your HRV. Refer back to Section 1—Sleep, Rest & Recovery for the details of how to perform relaxation breathing. In the app, you have the ability to set the length of your inhale, exhale and any pauses. This means you can experiment with these variables and see the immediate effect this has. Start with a 4-second inhale and a 6-second exhale and manipulate these variables until you find the greatest effect on your HRV.

Vagus Nerve Activation

There are several easy and efficient ways to increase vagal tone at home and encourage the parasympathetic state of your nervous system.

Singing, Humming, Chanting, And Gargling—These activities all involve the muscles of the throat and vocal cords, which are innervated by the vagus nerve.

Gag Reflex—Gently tapping the soft palate on both sides of the back of the throat a few times in the morning and evening, leads to the activation of muscles at the back of the throat and the pharynx, and triggers a physical reflex in the vagus nerve.

Diaphragmatic Breathing—Also known as belly breathing, this involves breathing deeply into the diaphragm, which is the main muscle of respiration. This type of breathing is slow and rhythmic, and it helps to activate the parasympathetic nervous system, leading to a state of calm and relaxation.

Alternate Nostril Breathing—Use your right hand to block your right nostril and inhale through your left nostril for a count of 4. Then, use your ring finger to block your left nostril and exhale through your right nostril for a count of 4. Next, inhale through your right nostril for a count of 4, and then exhale through your left nostril for a count of 4. Continue this pattern, alternating nostrils with each inhale and exhale, for several minutes.

Box Breathing—Also known as square breathing, this involves inhaling, holding the breath, exhaling, and then holding again for an equal count. A common starting point is 4-4-4-4, but this can be increased or decreased for an equal number of seconds.

Vibratory Therapy—Tuning forks can be used to stimulate the vagus nerve by placing the vibrating fork on specific points on the body, such as the sternum or the mastoid process behind the ear. This is known as vibratory vagal stimulation and has been shown to have a number of therapeutic benefits, including reducing anxiety and depression, improving sleep, and reducing inflammation. (10)

SMART CONSIDERATION

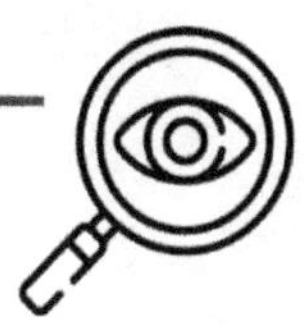

Vagal Taping

Vagal taping is a relatively new form of neuromodulation that involves the application of kinesiology tape to specific points on the neck. This technique, developed by chiropractic doctor Dr. Perry Nickelston, works by stimulating cutaneous receptors which, in turn, activate the vagus nerve. First, locate the sternocleidomastoid (SCM) muscle on one side of the neck. This is the large muscle that runs from the base of the skull down to the collarbone. Then place a strip of kinesiology tape horizontally across the SCM muscle, about one inch above the collarbone. Place another strip of tape vertically over the first strip, creating a T-shape. Repeat the process on the other side of the neck. Rub the tape gently to activate the adhesive. Typically, the tape is left in place for 3-5 days and can be removed and replaced as needed. However, the specific duration of time that the tape should be left on may vary depending on the individual and their response to the treatment. Please note that vagus taping should not be done by people with a history of carotid artery disease, stroke, or neck injury.

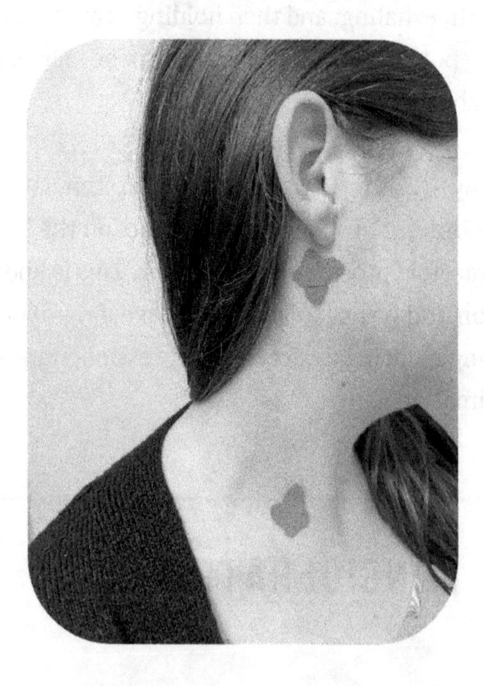

SMART PROTOCOL

Stimulate Your Vagus Nerve - $0 to $

Pick one or two of the methods of stimulating your vagus nerve from the list above, and practice daily. Keep track of how you feel, or ideally, monitor the effect on your HRV. Try different combinations of methods and see what works best for you. This could mean stimulating your gag reflex and gargling on certain days, and humming and diaphragmatic breathing on others. With practice, you will learn which methods you prefer.

SMART UPGRADES

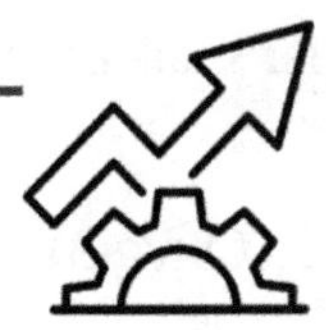

Vagal Stimulation Devices

Truvaga is a compact handheld device that stimulates the vagus nerve through the skin using energy signals. Easy to use, sessions last about 2 minutes. Results can vary; some feel immediate benefits, while others may need weeks of consistent use. The device's patented technology targets the vagus nerve, situated just 1.5cm below the skin. Users might experience a minor neck muscle contraction during use.

Another interesting device is the Sensate, a palm-sized device engineered to reduce stress and promote relaxation using sound and vibrations. Paired with its smartphone or tablet App, it offers a customizable experience. Regular use of Sensate is said to help enhance vagus nerve function, aiding in nervous system balance. Website links are provided in Smart Resources at the end of this Section.

The Three Pillars Of Brain Health

Now that we have a better understanding of the brain and nervous system, let's talk about what the brain needs to function optimally.

1. Oxygen

One of the most vital nutrients for the brain is oxygen. It is a fundamental ingredient in the creation of energy used by the body. All living creatures breathe; thus, we must have plenty of oxygen for the brain, right? Wrong! Just because we breathe to survive does not mean that we are breathing for overall health. We can change how we breathe and, to an extent, change how breathing affects our bodies. Controlled breathing—also known as "paced respiration," "diaphragmatic breathing," and "deep breathing"—have all been shown to decrease stress and anxiety, improve digestion, promote alertness and concentration, cleanse cells, improve quality of sleep and so much more. (11)

Nasal breathing results in much better oxygen uptake than mouth breathing. Nose breathing increases the arterial pressure of oxygen by 10% (12) and improves cognitive function. (13)

Vascular dementia is the second most common form of dementia after Alzheimer's disease and is due to poor blood flow to the brain. There can be many underlying reasons for poor oxygen flow to the brain. However, the most common ones tend to include systemic inflammation, smoking, low blood pressure, hypothyroidism, stress, and blood sugar dysregulation.

How can you tell if you aren't getting enough oxygen? Symptoms of poor circulation and blood flow to the brain include–low mental endurance, poor focus and concentration, poor nail health or fungal growth on toes, and cold hands, feet, or tip of the nose.

So the usual suspects apply to keeping adequate blood flow to the brain. Keep your blood pressure in check with proper diet and exercise, avoiding smoking and other toxic substances, keeping stress to a minimum, and engaging in a breathing practice including diaphragmatic breathing and most importantly nasal breathing day and night to ensure that the brain receives the appropriate amount of oxygen it needs to function optimally.

2. Proper Fuel

The human brain is an incredibly complex organ that requires a constant supply of energy to function optimally. As we mentioned in Section 2—Hydration, Fuel, & Foundationals, there are two main types of fuel that the brain can use to generate energy: glucose and ketones.

Glucose is the primary source of energy for the brain and is obtained from the breakdown of carbohydrates in the diet. When glucose levels are high, the brain uses it as its main energy source. However, when glucose levels are low, such as during periods of fasting or low carbohydrate intake, the brain may switch to using alternative sources of fuel.

Ketones are a type of molecule produced by the liver when the body is in a state of ketosis, which occurs when glucose levels are low. The brain can use ketones as an alternative energy source when glucose is not available. Studies have shown that ketones may be a more efficient source of energy for the brain compared to glucose. (14)

The brain's preference for glucose as a fuel source is well-established, but recent research has shown that ketones may offer several benefits for brain health. Ketones have been shown to improve cognitive function, enhance mood, and reduce inflammation in the brain. (15)

Adequate exercise, occasional fasting, and an overall good diet with an emphasis on healthy fats all help your body to be metabolically flexible and use ketones when necessary.

3. Stimulation

The saying "use it or you lose it" truly applies when it comes to neuroplasticity and neural generation. Just like muscles need resistance training to stay strong, the brain's neural connections do, too. The more stimulation and challenge the brain gets, the faster synapses become, the better it acquires information, and the less chance there is of memory loss and brain degeneration.

Puzzles, "brain twisters", learning (or even attempting to learn!) a musical instrument, language, or anything new helps to keep your brain young and healthy.

Neurogenesis

Neurogenesis is the process of creating new neurons. For a long time, it was believed that the adult brain was unable to generate new neurons and that our neural circuitry was fixed after a certain point in development. However, we now know that this is not the case, and that neurogenesis can occur in certain regions of the brain throughout our lives.

One of the most well-known regions of the brain, where neurogenesis occurs, is the hippocampus, a small, seahorse-shaped structure located in the medial temporal lobe of the brain. The hippocampus is involved in the formation and retrieval of memories, and neurogenesis in this region has been linked to the learning and retention of new information. Studies have shown that exercise, environmental enrichment, and other factors can stimulate neurogenesis in the hippocampus. (16) Neurogenesis also occurs in the olfactory bulb, which is involved in the sense of smell, odour discrimination, and learning.

It's worth noting that neurogenesis is a complex process, and researchers are still working to understand all of the factors that regulate it. While the hippocampus and olfactory bulb are the two main regions of the brain where neurogenesis occurs, there may be other regions where new neurons can be generated under certain conditions.

Blood-Brain Barrier

The blood-brain barrier (BBB) is a highly selective and complex barrier that separates the blood circulating in the body from the brain and the central nervous system. It is composed of specialized cells that line the blood vessels in the brain, including endothelial cells, astrocytes, and pericytes.

The blood-brain barrier plays a critical role in maintaining the proper environment for brain function by selectively allowing nutrients, oxygen, and other essential molecules to enter the brain while keeping harmful substances out. This barrier also protects the brain from toxins, pathogens, and other harmful substances that may be circulating in the bloodstream.

The blood-brain barrier is also involved in regulating the transport of molecules in and out of the brain. For example, it can prevent the entry of certain drugs into the brain, which can limit their effectiveness in treating brain diseases.

Disruption of the blood-brain barrier can occur in various neurological conditions, including stroke, traumatic brain injury, and neurodegenerative diseases such as Alzheimer's and Parkinson's disease. When the blood-brain barrier is compromised, harmful substances can enter the brain and contribute to inflammation and neuronal damage.

Neuroinflammation And Impact On The Blood-Brain Barrier

Neuroinflammation is a complex biological process that involves the activation of immune cells in the brain and central nervous system (CNS) in response to injury, infection, or disease. It is characterized by the release of various pro-inflammatory molecules, such as cytokines, chemokines, and reactive oxygen species, which can cause damage to the surrounding neurons and glial cells. The immune response in the brain is orchestrated by several types of immune cells. Microglia, which are resident immune cells of the CNS, are the first line of defence and are activated in response to any type of injury or insult. They phagocytose and eliminate debris, secrete pro-inflammatory cytokines, and initiate the recruitment of other immune cells.

While acute inflammation is a normal response to injury or infection, chronic neuroinflammation can lead to tissue damage and neuronal death and is implicated in the pathogenesis of various neurological disorders. In

Alzheimer's disease, for example, neuroinflammation has been shown to contribute to the accumulation of beta-amyloid plaques and tau tangles, which are hallmark features of the disease. (17)

Neuroinflammation can have a significant impact on the integrity of the blood-brain barrier. Inflammatory processes activate immune cells that can disrupt the tight junctions between the endothelial cells that make up the blood-brain barrier. This disruption can lead to increased permeability of the blood-brain barrier, allowing harmful substances such as pathogens, toxins, and immune cells to enter the brain.

Neuroinflammation can lead to a variety of neurological and psychiatric symptoms, including depression, anxiety, cognitive impairment, and memory loss. (18) Various lifestyle factors can contribute to neuroinflammation, including a diet high in sugar and processed foods, exposure to toxins like mold and heavy metals, and chronic stress. Addressing these factors can help reduce inflammation in the brain and promote better neurological function.

Neuroprotective Properties Of Polyphenols

Polyphenols are a class of bioactive compounds found in various plant-based foods, including fruits, vegetables, and herbs. Research suggests that polyphenols may have a range of health benefits, including anti-inflammatory effects, antioxidant properties, and potential neuroprotective effects. In particular, several polyphenols have been shown to combat neuroinflammation, which is a common factor in many neurodegenerative diseases. (19)

Resveratrol, curcumin, apigenin, luteolin, catechins, rutin, and quercetin have all been found to reduce inflammation in the brain, improve cognitive function, and protect against neurodegeneration.

It's worth noting that polyphenols only become active when they are converted to metabolites by enzymes in the microbiome. When polyphenols are consumed, they are not fully broken down and absorbed by the body. Instead, they travel to the colon, where they are metabolized by gut bacteria into smaller molecules that can be absorbed by the body. The specific gut bacteria responsible for polyphenol metabolism depend on the type of polyphenol consumed. For example, the metabolism of flavonoids, a type of polyphenol found in many fruits and vegetables, has been shown to be dependent on the presence of certain bacterial species, such as Bifidobacterium and Lactobacillus. (20) Having a diverse and healthy gut microbiome is essential for activating the beneficial effects of polyphenols.

SMART PROTOCOL

Eat More Polyphenols - $0 to $

Eat a varied diet rich in polyphenol-containing foods daily. All berries, in particular, blueberries, are one of the richest sources. Cherries, plums, pears, grapes (especially the skins), broccoli, spinach, red onions and artichokes are also good sources of polyphenols. Consume more green tea for its catechin content, and dark chocolate (70% or higher) is a rich source of polyphenols called flavanols. Consume foods that help maintain a healthy microbiome as detailed in Section 2—Hydration, Fuel & Foundationals.

Neuroplasticity

Neuroplasticity refers to the brain's ability to reorganize and adapt in response to changes in the environment, learning, and experience. It is a crucial process for the development of new skills, the recovery from injury, and the maintenance of cognitive function throughout life. Neuroplasticity is the ability of neural networks in the brain to change through growth or reorganization. These changes range from individual neuron pathways making new connections to systematic adjustments in how certain areas of the brain work—known as cortical remapping.

The brain is incredibly plastic from birth until about age 25. During this time, the brain is highly adaptable and capable of making new connections between neurons. This is because the brain is still developing and undergoing a process of pruning and refining its neural connections based on experiences and learning. As we age, the brain's ability to change and adapt gradually declines. However, this does not mean that the brain is no longer capable of neuroplasticity. The adult nervous system is still capable of a significant amount of plasticity, and research has shown that it can be improved through focused learning and other techniques that promote the growth and reorganization of neural networks. (21)

However, neuroplasticity doesn't occur instantaneously or constantly throughout the day. Instead, it occurs during specific periods of sleep and rest. This is because, during sleep, the brain is free from the constant influx of sensory input and can focus on processing and storing information acquired during wakefulness. Critical to optimizing neuroplasticity is ensuring you get adequate sleep. Sleep is necessary for the brain to consolidate and integrate new information and experiences, and it's during this process that the brain can undergo changes in neural connections and strengthen existing ones.

SMART PROTOCOL

Mindful Learning Blocks - $0

To optimize learning, consider approaching it in 90-minute blocks, as our brains alternate between periods of intense focus and restful consolidation. It may be challenging to concentrate during the first 5-10 minutes of a learning session, however, as engagement increases the brain enters a phase of heightened attention and productivity. After approximately 90 minutes, it is beneficial to take a break, allowing the brain to process and reinforce the newly acquired information. This would be an excellent time for an NSDR protocol as outlined in Section 1—Sleep, Rest & Recovery.

Testing different learning times throughout the day can help identify the most suitable moments for absorbing new knowledge, taking into account individual variations in attention and natural rhythms. Aim for a maximum of two to three such blocks per day to maintain high levels of focus and productivity.

Nootropics

Nootropics are substances or supplements that are used to enhance cognitive function, memory, creativity, and motivation. They work by increasing the levels of neurotransmitters, hormones, and other brain chemicals that are associated with cognitive performance. Some nootropics have the ability to increase blood glucose levels, which can provide the brain with an immediate source of energy. This is particularly beneficial for tasks that require sustained focus and mental effort.

Additionally, some nootropics can increase the activity of the cholinergic system, which is a network of neurons in the brain that use acetylcholine as a neurotransmitter. The cholinergic system plays a crucial role in cognitive function, including attention, memory, and learning.

There are several different types of nootropics, including:

Stimulants—These substances, such as caffeine and amphetamines, are used to increase alertness, attention, and energy.

Racetams—These substances, such as piracetam and aniracetam, are believed to enhance memory and cognitive function.

Adaptogens—These substances, such as Ashwagandha and Rhodiola, are believed to reduce stress and improve mood.

Nutraceuticals—These substances, such as omega-3 fatty acids and choline, are believed to improve brain function through nutrition.

The roles of nootropics vary depending on the specific substance and the individual using them. Some people use nootropics to improve their ability to focus on tasks or to enhance memory and learning. Others may use nootropics to reduce stress or to increase motivation and productivity. We will explore nootropics specifically for brain health further in this Section.

The Neurochemical Network—Communication Pathways Between Brain And Body

The brain and body function optimally when each neuron is properly producing, sending, and receiving biochemical messages. Your brain chemistry influences the five major areas of brain function: memory, attention, temperament, personality, and physical well-being. The biochemical messengers that enable communication between the brain and the body are called neurotransmitters. As mentioned previously, neurotransmitters are chemicals released by nerve fibres and are responsible for many processes in the body. Different neurotransmitters have different roles and carry various messages between the brain and body, from controlling alertness to assisting in digestion.

There are two types of neurotransmitters:

- **Excitatory Neurotransmitters**—These types of neurotransmitters have excitatory effects on the neurons; they increase the likelihood that the neuron will fire. Some excitatory neurotransmitters include epinephrine and norepinephrine.
- **Inhibitory Neurotransmitters**—These types of neurotransmitters have inhibitory effects on the neurons; they decrease the likelihood that the neuron will fire an action potential. Gamma-Amino Butyric Acid (GABA) is an example of an inhibitory neurotransmitter.

The number of neurotransmitters in the body is well over 100, but for the purposes of this Section, let's focus on five key neurotransmitters: acetylcholine, epinephrine/norepinephrine, dopamine, GABA, and serotonin. This sounds a bit complex but bear with us. Trying to understand your brain is a worthwhile effort and a good brain exercise in itself.

Acetylcholine

Acetylcholine is one of the most important neurotransmitters in the process of converting short-term memory to long-term, which happens in the hippocampus.

Acetylcholine tends to modify and amplify brain circuits associated with attention and focus. Poor acetylcholine activity impacts memory function and may even give symptoms of dementia and Alzheimer's. In addition, this neurotransmitter is responsible for the speed at which electrical signals are processed throughout the body.

Acetylcholine is also responsible for our intuitive, innovative, and creative nature. It creates feelings of sociability, adventurousness and enables communication.

Improve Memory And Learning With Acetylcholine—Food And Supplement Tips

Acetylcholine is a key neurotransmitter that is involved in many cognitive functions such as memory, attention, and learning. Here are some tips to optimize your acetylcholine levels for better cognitive performance.

Eat Choline-Rich Foods—Choline is a precursor to acetylcholine, so consuming choline-rich foods such as whole eggs, beef liver, chicken, fish, and mushrooms can help boost your acetylcholine levels.

Try Alpha-GPC—Alpha-GPC is a natural choline compound found in the brain that has been shown to increase acetylcholine synthesis. It also stimulates dopamine release which can enhance motivation. However, chronic use of Alpha-GPC may increase the risk of stroke and the production of TMAO, (trimethylamine N-oxide), a compound produced by gut bacteria which is associated with heart disease. To offset this, consume 600 mg of garlic along with it.

Consider Acetyl L-Carnitine (ALC)—ALC is a brain nutrient that energizes the brain, increases neurotransmitter chemicals, and repairs damage caused by stress and poor nutrition. It has also been shown to aid those with mild cognitive impairment or Alzheimer's disease. (22)

Use L-huperzine—L-huperzine inhibits the activity of an enzyme that breaks down acetylcholine, allowing more to accumulate in the synapse and improve cognitive function, particularly in memory and attention.

Manage Blood Sugar—Avoid blood sugar fluctuations as they can cause acetylcholine imbalances. Lifestyle practices such as visual meditation, reading, regular exercise, deep breathing, and taking time for yourself can help replenish this neurotransmitter.

Narrow Your Visual Field—Centering your vision on a specific target limits visual information and reduces distractions, allowing you to focus more effectively. Research shows that acetylcholine plays a key role in regulating attention and arousal, and narrowing your visual field can further enhance this effect, leading to improved cognitive performance. (23)

SMART PROTOCOL

Foods For Focus - $0 to $

Eat a diet with varied sources of choline like beef liver, wild salmon, chicken, and whole eggs. If you choose eggs, keep the yolk slightly runny to prevent oxidation of the choline. There are small amounts of choline in legumes, tofu, green vegetables, potatoes, nuts, seeds, grains, and fruit. Ensure blood sugar stability throughout the day by consuming healthy protein, fat, and carbohydrate at each meal and snack.

SMART PROTOCOL

Memory Supportive Supplementation – $ to $$

For long-term support of cognitive performance and memory retention, supplement with L-huperzine, acetyl-L-carnitine, or alpha GPC.

SMART PROTOCOL

Narrow Your Visual Field - $0

At the time of a focused task, narrow your visual field. This can be done by simply throwing on a ball cap to keep attention focused, or by entering a smaller space to complete your work.

Epinephrine And Norepinephrine AKA—Adrenaline And Noradrenaline

Epinephrine and norepinephrine are two of the three main catecholamines, which are neurotransmitters and hormones that are derived from the amino acid tyrosine. The same hormone that we refer to as adrenaline in the body is referred to as epinephrine in the brain. This discrepancy in nomenclature can be confusing, but it is important to note that both terms refer to the same hormone. Adrenaline, which is produced by the adrenal glands in the body, is released in response to stress or danger, leading to an increase in heart rate, blood pressure, and other physiological changes. Epinephrine, which is produced by the adrenal medulla and certain neurons in the brain, has a similar effect on the body but is involved in various functions in the brain, including memory consolidation and arousal.

Norepinephrine, also known as noradrenaline, is a neurotransmitter that is released by nerve cells in the sympathetic nervous system. It is also released by the adrenal glands in response to stress. Norepinephrine acts on many different parts of the body, including the heart, blood vessels, and lungs. Like epinephrine, norepinephrine increases heart rate and blood pressure, and it causes blood vessels to constrict. However, norepinephrine does not have as strong an effect on blood sugar levels as epinephrine. Norepinephrine tends to modify circuits associated with alertness and the desire to move your body.

Optimize Energy With Epinephrine

Feeling energized and focused is essential for achieving success and maintaining a healthy lifestyle. However, many of us struggle with fatigue and lack of motivation, especially as the day wears on. Luckily, there are several ways to increase energy levels naturally, including triggering the release of epinephrine in the body.

Morning Movement—Any physical activity, (swimming, walking, running, etc) particularly early in the day increases epinephrine release and helps to 'wake up' the brain. Get some exercise in the morning and reap the benefits of increased energy for the rest of your day.

Stimulating/ Energizing Breathwork—Breathwork that involves cyclic hyperventilation (deep inhales and passive exhales) such as the Wim Hof breathing technique, can increase epinephrine release through increased oxygen intake, sympathetic nervous system activation, brief changes in carbon dioxide levels in the body. Try short bursts of fast inhales and exhales for one minute, then hold your breath for about 15 seconds. Repeat as many as 25 times.

Caffeine—Regular ingestion of safe levels of caffeine (150g-400g) can optimize and increase epinephrine levels in the body. Caffeine also increases the number of dopamine receptors in the brain. Increasing dopamine receptor availability can improve cognitive performance and increase feelings of alertness and well-being. Avoid caffeine consumption after 2 pm to minimize any ill effects on sleep quality.

Voluntary Hyperventilation For A Higher Performing State

We mention several different breathing techniques throughout this book, as breathwork can have a great impact on many physiological processes and responses in the body.

Voluntary hyperventilation refers to a deliberate and conscious increase in the rate and depth of breathing.This method of breathing can increase alertness and promote a higher-performing state in the body and mind. It has gained popularity in recent years thanks to Dutch athlete, Wim Hof. His approach involves deep, rhythmic breathing exercises as well as cold exposure and meditation. This type of breathing can trigger the body's sympathetic nervous system, which activates the "fight-or-flight" response and causes the release of adrenaline and noradrenaline. You will see voluntary hyperventilation recommended several times throughout this Section; here's how to do it:

1. Begin by taking a few deep breaths to relax. Inhale deeply through your nose, filling your lungs with air, and then exhale fully through your mouth, letting go of any tension or stress.
2. When you are ready, start the breathing technique by taking a powerful breath in through your nose, filling your lungs and feeling your abdomen rise. As you reach the full inhalation, let go, relax, and exhale all the air out through your mouth.
3. Repeat this cycle of deep inhalations and relaxed exhalations for a total of 30-40 breaths. Keep a steady rhythm, but don't strain or force the breaths. It should feel invigorating but comfortable.
4. After the last exhalation, hold your breath for as long as you comfortably can. In the beginning, this may be seconds but as you get used to it it may become minutes.
5. When you feel the urge to breathe again, take a single deep breath in and hold it for 15 seconds. Then exhale fully, letting go of any tension

or stress.

6. This cycle can be repeated 3-4 times.

This technique can be practiced daily or as desired. Always listen to your body and adjust the intensity if needed. Remember to never practice the technique in water, while driving, or in any potentially dangerous situation.

Serotonin

Known as our "happy hormone," serotonin is produced in small amounts in the brain, with the remaining 80 percent to 90 percent produced in the gastrointestinal tract. (24) Serotonin provides a healing, nourishing, satisfied feeling to the brain and body. Serotonin release modifies circuits associated with bliss and remaining still.

When serotonin is secreted at optimal levels, your sleep is deep and peaceful, your mood is boosted and you think rationally. Serotonin helps to resynchronize the brain to help you feel fresh and recharged in the morning. This is because serotonin is converted into melatonin in the brain's pineal gland. Low cortisol can hinder the conversion of serotonin to melatonin and cause difficulty sleeping. If cortisol is too high, melatonin levels can drop. Therefore, it is important to keep cortisol and melatonin levels in check for proper serotonin function.

Too much serotonin can cause you to feel nervous, hesitant, distracted, vulnerable to criticism, and afraid of judgment. Meanwhile, serotonin deficiency is most associated with low mood and depression, hence why Selective Serotonin Reuptake Inhibitors (SSRIs) are commonly prescribed to help deal with the negative symptoms of depression. SSRIs ease depression by increasing levels of serotonin in the brain and blocking the reuptake of serotonin so that a good mood lasts longer.

Fortunately, there are several ways to boost serotonin production through lifestyle choices. These include balancing hormones, exercising daily, and supplementing with compounds such as 5-HTP and Tryptophan—do not take these if you are already on an antidepressant. Other nutrients and botanicals important in serotonin production are P5P (the active form of vitamin B6), niacinamide, magnesium citrate, methyl B12, and folate.

It is also very important to minimize blood sugar fluctuations in order to promote healthy levels of serotonin. Excess insulin reduces the brain's ability to clear out amyloid plaques, the plaques that are the hallmark of Alzheimer's disease. In addition, too little insulin impacts the amount of tryptophan (a precursor of serotonin) that is able to reach the brain, causing a decrease in serotonin production.

Support Mood Regulation With Serotonin

To increase the production of this 'feel good' neurotransmitter, consider the following:

Physical Touch—Physical contact, whether romantic, platonic or even cuddling with a pet, can increase serotonin levels in the body through the release of oxytocin. Oxytocin increases serotonin levels in the brain leading to a boost in mood and a reduction in stress and anxiety.

Gratitude—Observing and receiving gratitude–not giving gratitude, can impact serotonergic pathways in the brain through a complex set of interactions between different neurotransmitters and brain regions. When we observe or receive gratitude, we activate the brain's reward system, which includes the release of dopamine. Dopamine then stimulates the release of serotonin, leading to an increase in levels.

Tryptophan-Rich Foods—Tryptophan is an essential amino acid that cannot be produced by the body and must be obtained through the diet. Once consumed, tryptophan is transported to the brain where it is converted into serotonin through a series of biochemical reactions. Include foods high in tryptophan like turkey, whole milk, oats, almonds, cashews, pumpkin seeds and some cheeses to increase circulating serotonin.

Cissus Quadrangularis—Cissus quadrangularis is a plant that has been used in traditional medicine for centuries. This plant contains a number of bioactive compounds, including ketosterones, triterpenoids, and flavonoids. These compounds may have an effect on serotonin receptors in the brain, helping to regulate the production and release of serotonin. There is limited data available about the timing of cycles for taking this supplement. Some experts recommend cycling cissus quadrangularis (e.g. two days on, two days off, or two weeks on, two weeks off).

Myo-inositol—Myo-inositol is a naturally occurring substance that has been found to increase the activity of the serotonin transporter, a protein that transports serotonin into nerve cells. This increased activity, in turn, boosts the availability of serotonin in the brain and the production of serotonin by nerve cells. It can also help improve the depth and quality of sleep, curb symptoms of anxiety, and many other conditions. It is important to note that the doses of myo-inositol used in studies are typically very high, ranging from 2 to 18 grams per day. It is recommended to start with a low dose and gradually increase over time. A common starting dose is 900 mg every few days.

SMART PROTOCOL

Immediate Mood Boost - $0

Oxytocin release can occur in as little as 20 seconds. Embrace a loved one, or spend a few moments cuddling with a pet to experience a quick elevation in mood.

SMART PROTOCOL

Long-Term Mood Support - $0 to $

Keep production of serotonin stable by regularly consuming tryptophan-rich foods like turkey, chicken, parmesan cheese, eggs, and raw nuts and seeds like almonds, cashews, and pumpkin seeds. Consider supplementation of cissus quadrangularis, myo-inositol, B12 (methylcobalamin), or 5-HTP.

Dopamine

Dopamine is produced in many areas of the brain and is released by the hypothalamus (the master controller of our hormones.) Dopamine generates the signals that control voluntary movement, posture, intelligence, abstract thought, goal setting, long-term planning, and personality. It has numerous functions in the brain related to motor coordination, motivation, pleasure, and reward. Yet, having too much of this neurotransmitter can also cause impulsivity, an overly active libido, and power-seeking behaviour. It is a common phenomenon to see highly-driven and successful individuals in business or politics who, in contrast, have challenging personal lives and relationships. This can be attributed to an overemphasis on the pursuit of success and rewards, associated with the dopamine system, while neglecting emotional well-being and social connection, regulated by the serotonin system.

Dopamine is most commonly known for its association with Parkinson's disease. This is a disease brought on by the destruction of the brain's substantia nigra, one of the several places dopamine is made, and where long-term dopamine deficiency can occur.

Dopamine And Beyond—Exploring The Complexities Of The Brain's Reward System

Dopamine is a neuromodulator that plays a crucial role in our motivation and reward system. It is a chemical released by the brain that is responsible for regulating our emotions and pleasure. Dopamine is not just about pleasure, but more about the pursuit; it is also the universal currency of foraging and seeking things that will provide sustenance and pleasure in the short term and extend life in the long term. Understanding the dynamics of dopamine release can help us predict whether we will be motivated in the next hours, days, or weeks.

The dopamine system doesn't care about the specific goal or pursuit; it's about pursuing anything, healthy or not. Dopamine is not just released when we get the reward; it's also released in anticipation of getting the thing we want, which triggers action. Dopamine levels vary through baseline, peaks, and troughs. The peaks are triggered by behaviours, compounds, substances, food, etc., while the troughs are when dopamine levels go below baseline.

The peak and baseline are not independent; for every peak, there's a trough. We all have a dopamine set point, and if we continue to participate in dopamine-stimulating activities, our levels can drop in imperceptible ways until we reach a low threshold of dopamine, and eventually, we won't experience the same joy from those behaviours. The pleasure-pain balance is based on how much dopamine is there and how much is ready to be released into the system. If you do something that releases huge levels of dopamine, pleasure drops because there isn't enough dopamine to release after. This creates a cycle where the desire for something increases dopamine, but the subsequent drop in levels below baseline triggers the motivation to pursue that thing to relieve the pain of not having it.

Addiction is a progressive narrowing of things that give us pleasure. The hallmark of any addictive behaviour is that it releases dopamine at high levels. The addictive process is the same, regardless of whether a person is addicted to gambling, drugs, sex, etc. People with severe addiction suffer from a lack of homeostasis in the pleasure-pain balance.

To maintain healthy dopamine levels, it is important to avoid seeking dopamine rushes and instead focus on maintaining engagement with activities on an intermittent schedule. This means engaging in activities that provide a sense of accomplishment or pleasure, but not becoming dependent on them for a constant dopamine rush. If you regularly listen to music during exercise, try to occasionally workout without it. You can also change the background colours on your cellphone to make looking at it less appealing or pleasurable.

To promote learning, the dopamine system relies on three fundamentals: desire, motivation, and reward or lack thereof. To protect the enjoyment of an activity, it's important not to attach too many dopamine-releasing behaviours to it. This can lead to less interest and motivation over time. To overcome procrastination, try doing something that is not enjoyable (but is safe) to steepen the dopamine trough, such as a cold shower or water immersion. This can remind your brain that you are capable of doing hard things and help bring you back to baseline dopamine faster.

SMART PROTOCOL

Dopamine Detox - $0

To reset the dopamine system from unhealthy behaviour and/or addiction, it is recommended to completely abstain from the behaviour for a period of 30 days. This period of abstinence allows the brain to readjust to normal dopamine levels, and to rewire the neural pathways associated with the behaviour. During this time, the brain may experience withdrawal symptoms, which can be uncomfortable but are generally manageable. Tapering off may be required depending on the severity of the addiction, as abruptly quitting a highly addictive substance, for example, can be dangerous and even life-threatening.

Maximize Motivation And Dial In Dopamine

By leveraging certain lifestyle changes and supplements, it is possible to optimize dopamine levels and boost productivity. Here are some ways to maximize motivation and dial in dopamine:

Leverage Light—Sunlight exposure in the morning can increase dopamine receptors in the brain by stimulating the release of melanopsin, a hormone involved in regulating the circadian rhythm. To optimize dopamine levels, it is recommended to view the maximum amount of sunlight you can safely do to your eyes (do not look directly at the sun) and skin within the first hour of waking. If you wake up before the sun or in a climate where there is no morning sun, it is recommended to turn on as many bright lights overhead as you can. However, it is important to note that bright light exposure should be avoided during the late evening hours leading up to bed and throughout the night. Exposure to bright light during this time can impact the production of melatonin, a hormone that is involved in regulating sleep-wake cycles and is known to have an inhibitory effect on dopamine release. You may recall this was an important protocol in Section 1—Sleep, Rest & Recovery.

Tyrosine-Rich Foods—Tyrosine is an amino acid that is a precursor to dopamine. Consuming tyrosine-rich foods, such as meat, fish, eggs, spinach, avocados, almonds, and sesame seeds, can increase dopamine receptor availability in the brain and positively impact dopamine levels. Dopamine receptors are proteins found on the surface of brain cells that bind to dopamine molecules and help to transmit signals throughout the brain. Consuming tyrosine-rich foods may be particularly beneficial for individuals with conditions that involve low dopamine levels, such as depression and Parkinson's disease.

Mucuna pruriens—Is a natural supplement that contains L-dopa, a precursor to dopamine. However, it's important to note that mucuna pruriens is highly potent and may lead to a significant increase in dopamine levels. This sudden increase can result in a crash when the effects wear off, leading to mood swings, anxiety, and even depression. It is not recommended to use mucuna pruriens as a long-term solution to boost dopamine levels.

L-tyrosine—Is another amino acid that's used to increase dopamine levels in the brain. It's a precursor to dopamine and other neurotransmitters, including norepinephrine and epinephrine. L-tyrosine may help improve cognitive function and reduce stress, both of which are related to dopamine levels. The recommended dose of L-tyrosine is between 500mg to 1000mg per day.

Phenylethylamine (PEA)—Is a chemical that's naturally found in the brain and is believed to play a role in the release of dopamine. PEA has been shown to have mood-enhancing effects, but more research is needed to fully understand its effects on dopamine levels. (25) The recommended dose of PEA is between 300mg to 600mg per day, but as with any supplement, it's best to speak with a healthcare professional before taking it.

Cold Exposure—Cold exposure triggers the release of norepinephrine, a precursor to dopamine, and increases dopamine receptor sensitivity, leading to a stronger dopamine response overall. Deliberate cold exposure to temperatures between 45-50°F can increase dopamine levels in as little as 1 minute, and boost levels for up to 3 hours after exposure. (26) It is imperative to start slowly and gradually increase the duration and intensity of cold exposure to avoid adverse effects.

Vitamin B6—Vitamin B6, also known as pyridoxine, is involved in neurotransmitter synthesis and can increase prolactin levels, which, in turn, increases dopamine release in the brain. However, it's essential to be cautious when taking vitamin B6 supplements as too much can have adverse effects. The recommended daily intake of vitamin B6 for adults is 1.3-1.7 mg per day. High doses of vitamin B6, can lead to toxicity and may cause neurological symptoms such as numbness, tingling, and loss of sensation in the limbs and can also interfere with the absorption and metabolism of other essential nutrients such as zinc, magnesium, and vitamin B12. (27)

GABA (Gamma-Aminobutyric Acid)

GABA is made in brain cells from glutamate and functions as an inhibitory neurotransmitter. It provides calmness and even directly affects aspects of personality such as punctuality, level-headedness, confidence, practicality, objectivity, and organization. GABA is also involved in the production of endorphins, the feel-good chemicals released during exercise.

When there is an imbalance in levels of GABA, one may experience symptoms such as feelings of anxiousness, panic, overwhelm or dread, difficulty turning the mind 'off', hypertension, depression, or Obsessive Compulsive Disorder (OCD).

A GABAergic substance is any substance that enhances or inhibits the activity of the gamma-aminobutyric acid (GABA) neurotransmitter system in the brain. GABAergics can be broadly divided into two categories: GABA agonists and GABA modulators. GABA agonists directly bind to and activate the GABA receptor, while GABA modulators increase the efficacy of GABA signalling by modulating GABA receptor activity.

GABAergic substances can include both drugs and natural compounds, and they can have a variety of effects on the body and mind. Some drugs are designed to make up for GABA deficiency. However, like many other drugs, they may create side effects and other neurotransmitter imbalances. What's more, GABA medication can also lead to tolerance and addiction. Some of the most addictive medications are called benzodiazepines, which are GABA-activating drugs. These include Valium, Klonopin, and Xanax—to name just a few.

So how do we ensure that our GABA neurotransmitters are optimized? For starters, it is important that you get a proper supply of fuel to the brain (glucose or ketones—if you are keto-adapted) and of amino acids. Aerobic activity and supplementing with compounds such as L-glutamine,

L-theanine, taurine, P5P, magnesium, zinc, manganese, valerian root, lithium orotate, and passion flower extract have been shown to improve levels of GABA. (28)

It's worth considering that the benefits of GABA as a supplement are still uncertain, as there is an ongoing debate among scientists. Some experts suggest GABA may not be able to penetrate the blood-brain barrier, largely due to its large molecular size unless the barrier is compromised or "leaky." As a result, the use of GABA is frequently employed as a means of assessing whether someone has a compromised blood-brain barrier.

Modulate GABA With Natural GABAergics

Natural GABAergics are found in various plants, herbs, and foods and can have a calming effect on the central nervous system.

Kava—Kava is a plant native to the South Pacific islands, and its roots are traditionally used to make a drink that has a calming and relaxing effect. Kava contains compounds called kavalactones, which enhance the activity of GABA receptors in the brain, leading to a sense of relaxation and well-being.

Valerian Root—Valerian root is a herb that is commonly used as a natural remedy for anxiety. It contains compounds that increase GABA levels in the brain, leading to a calming effect and improved sleep quality.

Passionflower—Passionflower is a plant that has been used for centuries to treat anxiety and insomnia. It contains flavonoids and alkaloids that enhance GABA activity in the brain, provoking a sense of calmness and relaxation.

Chamomile—Chamomile is an herb that is often consumed as a tea and is known for its anxiolytic properties. It contains compounds that bind to

GABA receptors, resulting in enhanced relaxation and reduced anxiety.

Magnesium—Magnesium is a mineral that is essential for many bodily functions, including the regulation of the GABAergic system. Magnesium increases the activity of GABA receptors in the brain, leading to a calming effect and reduced anxiety.

L-theanine—L-theanine is an amino acid that is primarily found in tea leaves, especially in green tea, and it increases the activity of GABA receptors and promotes relaxation and reduced anxiety. It also increases the levels of other neurotransmitters such as dopamine and serotonin, which can contribute to its mood-enhancing effects.

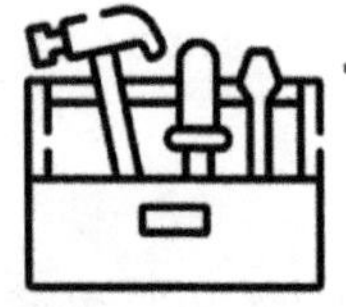

SMART TOOLS

Find Your Dominant Type

Now that you understand how certain neurotransmitters can affect behaviour, mood, cognition, and more, you may be interested in learning about your own personal dominant neurotransmitter. The following link will direct you to take *The Braverman Assessment*, created by Dr. Eric Braverman, a physician and author who is known for his work in the field of integrative medicine and neurology. He is the founder of the PATH Medical Center in New York City, which provides comprehensive medical care and specialized testing services for patients with chronic health conditions.

The Braverman Assessment is a self-administered test that consists of 110 questions and takes about 30 minutes to complete. The results of the test can help you identify your dominant neurotransmitter, which can then be used to guide you in supportive strategies for optimizing your neurotransmitter function. You can take the test at bravermantest.com or see Smart Resources at the end of this Section for the website link.

The Power Of Nitric Oxide For Cognitive Function And Brain Health

Nitric oxide (NO) is a gas that plays an important role in brain health. NO helps to regulate blood flow, neurotransmitter release, and the formation and maintenance of synaptic connections, which are essential for cognitive function.

One of the key functions of NO in the brain is its role as a neurotransmitter. NO is produced by neurons and released into the synaptic cleft, where it diffuses across the gap and activates receptors on the postsynaptic neuron. This process helps to facilitate communication between neurons and is essential for the formation and maintenance of synaptic connections.

NO is vital for regulating blood flow in the brain. It is produced by endothelial cells lining blood vessels and acts as a vasodilator, relaxing the smooth muscle cells in the vessel walls and increasing blood flow to the brain. This helps ensure the brain receives the oxygen and nutrients it needs to function properly.

Research has shown that NO may also have neuroprotective effects in the brain, protecting against oxidative stress, inflammation, and apoptosis (programmed cell death), all of which can damage brain cells and contribute to the development of neurological disorders such as Alzheimer's disease,

Parkinson's disease, and stroke. (29)

We will discuss nitric oxide more in-depth in Section 5—Epigenetics, Ageing and Longevity, as this important molecule is vital to many processes involved in ageing and longevity.

Nutrition For Brain Health—Foods And Supplements To Boost Cognitive Function

As mentioned previously, the brain requires oxygen, stimulation, and proper fuel to function optimally. Nutrition plays a critical role in brain health, affecting cognitive function, mood, and mental health. The quality of the foods we consume, particularly the types of fats and carbohydrates, can have a significant impact on brain health. Processed foods that are high in fat, sugar, and refined carbohydrates are detrimental to both metabolic and mental health, contributing to insulin resistance, obesity, and chronic mental disorders.

The ketogenic diet, which is low in carbohydrates and high in fat, has been shown to have beneficial effects on several mental disorders, including depression, PTSD, Alzheimer's, and bipolar disorder. (30) A ketogenic diet can be further enhanced by incorporating MCT (medium-chain triglyceride) oil. MCT oil can increase ketone production in the body, which provides an alternative energy source for the brain and may help improve cognitive function and protect against neurodegenerative diseases. The ketogenic diet, coupled with the potential benefits of MCT oil, induces metabolic changes in the brain and body that can improve brain health, such as lowering glucose levels, improving insulin signalling, increasing mitochondrial biogenesis, changing the gut microbiome, and repairing hormones. Together, these interventions have the potential to enhance brain function and reduce the risk of several neurological and mental disorders.

In addition to the ketogenic diet, increasing the intake of essential fatty acids, particularly omega-3s, is crucial for brain health. The brain's nerve cells and other cells are composed of structural fats that are largely derived from the foods we consume, such as essential fatty acids and phospholipids. Fat is the most crucial element for brain function. However, most people consume enough omega-6s but not enough omega-3s in their diets. Both DHA (docosahexaenoic acid) and EPA (eicosapentaenoic acid) are omega-3 fatty acids that play important roles in maintaining brain health and function, however, their effects on the brain are somewhat different.

DHA is the most abundant fatty acid in the brain, and it is particularly important for the health and function of neuronal membranes. DHA plays a crucial role in maintaining membrane fluidity and permeability, which is essential for the proper functioning of ion channels, receptors, and other membrane proteins involved in neurotransmission. Studies have also shown that DHA can reduce inflammation in the brain, protect against oxidative stress, and promote neuroplasticity, which is the brain's ability to change and adapt in response to experiences. (31)

EPA, on the other hand, is more involved in modulating inflammation and oxidative stress throughout the body, including the brain. EPA can be converted to various signalling molecules called eicosanoids, which can help to reduce inflammation and promote blood flow to the brain. Research has also suggested that EPA may have mood-regulating effects and could potentially be helpful for conditions such as depression and anxiety. (32)

To increase omega-3 intake, consume foods high in omega-3s, such as mackerel, salmon, herring, oysters, and caviar. EPA and omega-3s can also be obtained from plant-based sources like chia seeds, but the ideal source remains debatable. Adequate intake of omega-3s can improve cognitive function and mood, while deficiency has been linked to depression and other mental disorders.

Supplementing with EPA and DHA and omega-3s is advisable if one does not consume enough fish. Additionally, consuming phosphatidylserine (300mg per day) from food sources like fish and cabbage or taking a supplement can improve cognition and reduce cognitive decline. Choline (500mg-1g per day) is another nutrient that supports brain health and focus by ensuring the substrate that creates acetylcholine. The best food source of choline is egg yolks.

Recent studies have also highlighted the benefits of creatine (5g/day) for brain health- improving cognition, providing neuroprotection against age-related decline and neurological diseases, regulating mood, and potentially aiding in the treatment of depression. (33) It may also support neurological recovery after brain injuries and reduce the severity of the damage. It is believed to support brain energy metabolism by providing an additional source of adenosine triphosphate (ATP), the molecule responsible for cellular energy transfer. By increasing ATP availability, creatine may enhance brain function, particularly in tasks that require quick thinking and mental agility.

Consuming blueberries daily can enhance cognition and potentially reduce cognitive decline and oxidation of LDL. Glutamine, found in foods such as cottage cheese, meat, chicken, fish, dairy, eggs, cabbage, and spinach, is an essential amino acid needed for neurotransmitter synthesis and can be converted to glucose to be used as fuel by the brain.

SMART PROTOCOL

Exogenous Ketones For Brain Energy – $

Support brain health by incorporating exogenous ketones in the form of ketone salts or ketone esters. Ketones are specifically designed to increase blood ketone levels, which can provide a readily available source of energy for the brain.

SMART PROTOCOL

Dietary Considerations For Brain Health – $

Aim for a daily intake of 1.5-2g of healthy fats DHA and EPA through diet (salmon, sardines, anchovies) or supplementation. Consider supplementing with 300 mg of phosphatidylserine to maintain the integrity and fluidity of cell membranes. Strive to consume 500 mg-1 g of choline daily through dietary sources like egg yolks (poached or soft-boiled is better than fried to prevent oxidation of choline). You can take 5g/day of creatine monohydrate for its neuroprotective qualities. Aim to work fresh or frozen blueberries into your diet each day, and incorporate glutamine-rich foods like animal protein, beans, spinach, parsley, and cabbage. To further support glutamate production, you can take 5g of L-glutamine on an empty stomach daily to help with this important excitatory neurotransmitter. While you may recognize a few of these recommendations from earlier on in Section 2—Hydration, Fuel & Foundationals, it bears reinforcing how beneficial these nutrients are for our bodies.

Hormones 101

When discussing the factors that impact our mental and physiological states, it's essential to consider not only neurotransmitters but also hormones, which can have a significant influence. Before delving into the specific protocols for modifying our states in real time, it's important to establish some fundamental information about these biochemical messengers.

Cortisol

The adrenal glands sit just on top of the kidneys, and among the many hormones they produce is cortisol. Cortisol plays a role in regulating blood sugar levels, blood pressure, and the body's response to stress. The problem is that years of chronic stress from multiple sources (physical, emotional, nutritional, environmental) overwork and deplete our adrenals. They don't have the capacity to take on the job of the ovaries. If our adrenals are too busy making cortisol there aren't enough resources to prioritize our sex hormones: estrogen, progesterone, DHEA, and testosterone. This is why an imbalance in one hormone puts stress on all the other hormones leading to a cascading effect of symptoms and health problems.

When cortisol levels are too high, it can lead to symptoms such as weight gain, especially in the abdominal area, high blood pressure, anxiety, and irritability. High levels of cortisol can also suppress the immune system, increase inflammation, and dysregulate the insulin response.

When cortisol levels are too low, it can lead to symptoms such as fatigue, weakness, weight loss, low blood pressure, and depression. Like high cortisol, low cortisol also impacts the immune system and blood sugar regulation.

For women, it's crucial to recognize that cortisol plays a significant role in the body's stress response. (34) If the body consistently produces high levels of cortisol to manage stress, it may result in decreased levels of other essential hormones. This is because cortisol and other sex hormones are derived from the same precursor hormone called pregnenolone. Thus, if the body demands more pregnenolone to produce cortisol to cope with stress, there may be less available for hormones such as DHEA and progesterone, which can lead to insufficient hormone levels.

DHEA

Dehydroepiandrosterone (DHEA) is a hormone produced by the adrenal glands. DHEA is a precursor hormone, meaning that it can be converted into other hormones in the body such as testosterone and estrogen. DHEA is known to play a role in a variety of physiological functions, including sex hormone production, bone health, immune system function, and mood and cognition—some research suggests that DHEA may help improve mood and cognitive function, especially in individuals with depression and age-related cognitive decline. (35)

Estrogen

Estrogen is a group of hormones that are primarily produced by the ovaries in females, but they are also produced in smaller amounts by the adrenal glands in males. There are three main types of estrogen: estradiol, estriol, and estrone. Estradiol is the most potent form and is primarily responsible for the development of female secondary sexual characteristics and the regulation of the menstrual cycle. It also helps to maintain bone density, regulate cholesterol levels, and improve cognitive function. Estriol is the weakest form of estrogen and is primarily produced during pregnancy to support fetal growth and development. Estrone is the least abundant form of estrogen and is mainly produced after menopause. Estrogen receptors in breast tissue can be stimulated by estrone, which may contribute to the growth of certain types of breast cancer cells. (36)

Progesterone

Progesterone is a hormone that is primarily produced by the ovaries in females, but it is also produced in smaller amounts by the adrenal glands and in males. It is a critical hormone for female reproductive health and plays a vital role in regulating the menstrual cycle, preparing the uterus for pregnancy, and supporting fetal growth and development. Progesterone works together with estrogen to regulate the menstrual cycle and promote ovulation. After ovulation, progesterone helps to thicken the lining of the uterus, preparing it for a fertilized egg to implant and supporting early pregnancy. If pregnancy does not occur, progesterone levels drop, and the lining of the uterus is shed during menstruation. Progesterone also plays a role in maintaining bone density, regulating blood sugar levels, and promoting healthy sleep.

SMART CONSIDERATION

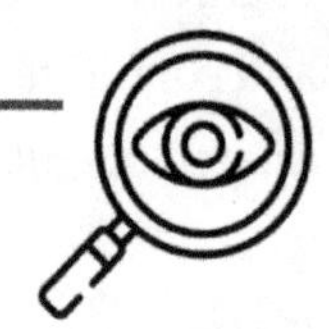

Pass On Pot

THC (tetrahydrocannabinol) is the primary psychoactive compound found in cannabis. When consumed, THC can bind to cannabinoid receptors in the brain, altering neurotransmitter release and leading to the characteristic effects of cannabis, such as euphoria, relaxation, and altered perception.

THC and other compounds found in cannabis also promote a significant increase in aromatase activity. Aromatase is the enzyme that converts testosterone to estrogen in the body. Marijuana users have a higher chance of developing gynecomastia—the development of breasts in males.

Its use has also been linked to an increase in psychosis, anxiety and depression. THC can impair cognition, including memory, attention, and executive function. Long-term use can lead to persistent deficits in these areas. THC use during adolescence can be especially risky as it has been shown to have negative effects on brain development, including a decrease in IQ and an increased risk of developing psychiatric disorders. (37)

Testosterone

Testosterone is a hormone that is primarily produced by the testes in males and in smaller amounts by the ovaries in females and the adrenal glands in both sexes. Testosterone also helps to regulate bone density, muscle mass, and fat distribution. It is involved in the development of male secondary sexual characteristics, including the growth of body hair, the deepening of the voice, reproductive health, and the growth of muscle mass. Testosterone also plays a role in red blood cell production, mood, and cognitive function. In females, testosterone helps to regulate bone density and is involved in the development of the female reproductive system. Testosterone levels naturally decline with age, and low levels of testosterone can lead to a variety of health issues, including decreased muscle mass, increased body fat, decreased bone density, and mood disorders. However, excessive levels of testosterone can also lead to negative health effects, including an increased risk of heart disease and prostate cancer.

In men, testosterone levels increase during puberty and remain relatively stable throughout adulthood, with a gradual decline after age 30. In women, testosterone levels play an important role in reproductive function and overall health. There is some research suggesting that women may have higher levels of testosterone than previously thought. One study published in 2013 in the journal *PLOS ONE* found that when testosterone levels were adjusted for body weight, women actually had significantly higher levels of the hormone than men.

The study looked at data from over 4,000 participants, both men and women and found that although men had higher absolute levels of testosterone, women had higher levels relative to their body weight. In fact, women had an average of 52% more testosterone per unit of body weight than men. (38)

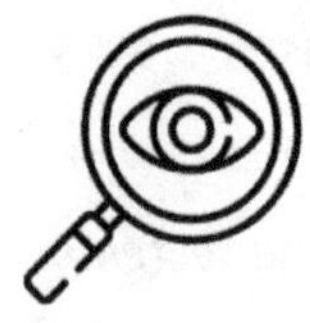

SMART CONSIDERATION

Defy Age-Related Testosterone Decline With Weightlifting

Testosterone plays a vital role in muscle growth, ligament and tendon development, and bone density, with intensity and volume being key factors in its stimulation. Heavy weight training, also known as high-intensity resistance training, is a popular type of exercise that involves lifting weights at 70-90% of your maximum effort. Research has shown that heavy weight training can increase testosterone levels in the body for up to 24 hours after the workout. (39) This effect is thought to be due to the stress that is placed on the muscles during the workout. When the muscles are stressed, they release various hormones, including testosterone, in response.

However, it's important to note that heavy-weight training should not be done to the point of failure. Going to failure, and lifting weights until you can no longer perform another rep, can actually decrease testosterone levels in the body. This is because going to failure can increase the production of cortisol, a hormone that is associated with stress and muscle breakdown.

SMART PROTOCOL

Increase Testosterone - $0 to $

If you are an experienced lifter, this protocol may be useful for you in a growth phase. To increase testosterone and growth hormone production, a 6 x 10 protocol (6 sets of 10 reps) at 80% of 1RM with a 2-minute rest between sets is recommended. It is important to adjust the load for sustainable reps over all 10 reps in each set. Testosterone is driven by intensity and volume, while growth hormone release is mainly driven by intensity, thus the prescribed work-to-rest ratio. Longer rest periods can influence the metabolic system, triggering the removal of waste products and lactates, and removing the needed stress for muscle development.

Sex Hormone-Binding Globulin

Sex hormone-binding globulin (SHBG) is a protein produced by the liver that is critical in regulating the levels of sex hormones like testosterone, estrogen, and dihydrotestosterone (DHT) in the body. SHBG binds to these hormones and transports them through the bloodstream to their target tissues. It is determined by several factors, including age, gender, and body weight. Higher levels of SHBG are associated with lower levels of free testosterone and estrogen, as these hormones are bound to the protein and unable to interact with cells.

The levels of SHBG in the body are influenced by various factors, including the three hormones that regulate its production: estradiol, insulin, and thyroxine.

SMART CONSIDERATION

Phone-Free Zones

There is increasing concern about the potential health effects of chronic exposure to the electromagnetic waves emitted by cell phones. While much of the focus has been on the potential impact on brain function and cancer risk, both males and females may be at risk of adverse effects from storing their cell phones in close proximity to their reproductive organs. For males, chronic exposure to cell phone-emitted waves on the gonads could impact sperm health by affecting swimming speed and density, as well as testosterone levels. Studies have shown that exposure to electromagnetic radiation can lead to a significant decrease in sperm motility and density, as well as reduced testosterone levels. (40) Similarly, females may experience changes in estrogen levels and menstrual cycle irregularities. Additionally, exposure to cell phone radiation has been found to lead to alterations in prolactin levels, which can impact lactation and breast development. (41)

Given the potential impact on reproductive health, it is important to be mindful of how you carry and use your cell phone. Avoid storing your phone in pockets close to the groin area, and women should never tuck the phone into a bra strap, or in the chest pocket of shirts. Instead consider carrying your phones in a bag, purse, or briefcase, or use a protective case that shields the body from electromagnetic waves.

From Cell Phones To Cellular Health—EMF Protection In The Digital Age

Electromagnetic fields (EMFs) are areas of energy produced by electrical devices and natural sources. There is research to suggest that these EMFs can activate protein structures called Voltage-Gated Calcium Channels (VGCCs) in cell membranes, leading to an increased flow of calcium into cells. This influx can prompt the production of peroxynitrite, a potent oxidant causing oxidative stress, which in turn might damage cellular components like DNA, cell membranes, and mitochondria. (42)To prevent potential harm from EMFs, it is proposed that one should either avoid them as much as possible—we know it is hard to do nowadays—or use shielding materials that block or reduce their intensity.

As studies on EMFs progress, numerous products have been developed to counteract their impacts. Among these, EMF blockers are notably effective, utilizing metallic or conductive materials to obstruct EMF transmission.

Conversely, EMF harmonizers purport to neutralize or mitigate the adverse effects of EMFs without impeding their passage. Yet, their efficacy remains under scrutiny, and the supporting science is not well-established, so caution is advised when considering their use.

Another emerging technology, EMF modulators, use microprocessors and antennas to restructure harmful EMFs. These modulators come in forms ranging from personal wearables and gadgets for electronics to larger devices safeguarding entire homes or offices from devices like routers and smart meters.

As the long-term implications of EMF exposure are still unknown, why take the risk? Not so long ago, smoking was thought to be safe too, and well, you know how that turned out. As we mentioned in Section 1—Sleep, Rest & Recovery, turning your wireless router off at night, and keeping your cell phone out of your bedroom is an important strategy for protecting your sleep, but the truth is, we are constantly exposed to these frequencies in day to day life. From our handheld devices, and Wi-Fi connections everywhere we go, to our 'smart' homes filled with appliances that can be operated remotely, we really can't escape it. While we are not endorsing any specific product or company, we have provided links on EMF protection in the Smart Resources for your consideration.

SMART PROTOCOL

Use Your Electronics Wisely - $0 to $$$

To minimize your potential exposure to EMF radiation, keep your phone away from your head and body as much as possible, and use the speaker function. Choose wired headphones over wireless options, preferably air-tube headphones which use hollow tubes to transmit sound from the device to the earpiece. Set your Wi-Fi router on a timer to turn off overnight, and consider purchasing EMF shields or modulation technology for your home and personal devices.

Supplementation For Optimal Sex Steroid Hormones

Vitamin D, zinc, and magnesium are all essential for many bodily functions, including hormone regulation. Deficiency in any of these three nutrients has been linked to low testosterone levels in both men and women. Supplementation can help to increase these levels and improve overall reproductive health.

Some lesser-known supplements can also help to optimize sex steroid hormones. Creatine, often associated with athletes and bodybuilders, has been shown to increase testosterone in some studies. Tongkat ali, also known as Eurycoma longifolia, is an herb that has been traditionally used in Southeast Asia to improve libido and sexual performance. Turkesterone is a natural plant compound that is found in certain species of plants. Some studies have suggested that turkesterone may increase testosterone levels and improve reproductive health, but more research is needed to fully understand its effects. (43) Boron is a trace mineral that is important for bone health and hormone regulation. Stinging nettle is another non-traditional supplement that has been shown to increase testosterone. While more research is needed to fully understand the effects of stinging nettle on testosterone levels, some people use it as a natural way to support reproductive health.

It is important to note to use caution when using supplements to increase hormones, as cancer cells often have a high turnover rate—they divide and grow more rapidly than normal cells. This high rate of cell turnover means that cancer cells are more likely to take up and use any hormone supplements that are introduced into the body. This can lead to a situation where hormone supplementation actually stimulates the growth and spread of cancer cells, rather than helping to control or eliminate them. These types of supplements should be used in response to tests showing low hormone levels, and under the supervision of a functional medicine practitioner who may help you cycle their use.

Human Growth Hormone (HGH)

Human growth hormone (HGH) is a peptide hormone produced by the pituitary gland that stimulates the growth of bones, muscles, and other tissues by promoting cell division and proliferation. It also has important metabolic effects, including the stimulation of protein synthesis and the breakdown of fat for energy.

HGH levels are highest during childhood and adolescence. During puberty, there is a surge in the production of HGH as the body undergoes rapid growth and development. As an individual reaches adulthood, HGH levels begin to decline gradually. In fact, research suggests that GH production decreases by about 50% every seven years after the age of 18. (44) By the time an individual reaches their 30s or 40s, GH levels may be 2-3 times lower than they were during puberty.

This decline in GH levels may lead to a decrease in muscle mass and an increase in body fat, as well as a reduction in bone density. It may also contribute to the development of age-related diseases, such as osteoporosis and cardiovascular disease. Sleep deprivation, stress, and poor nutrition can all influence HGH production and contribute to reduced levels.

Insulin-like growth factor-1 (IGF-1) is a hormone that is integral in promoting normal bone and tissue growth and development. Along with growth hormone (GH), IGF-1 helps to regulate growth and development throughout the body. IGF-1 is primarily produced in response to GH stimulation and is synthesized in various tissues such as the liver and skeletal muscles.

There are several natural ways to stimulate and support the production of human growth hormone (HGH) in the body. Here are a few strategies:

Increase (slow wave) Deep Sleep—Deep sleep is particularly important for the release of growth hormones. To increase deep sleep, aim to get 7-9 hours of sleep each night, and try to maintain a regular sleep schedule. Avoiding caffeine, alcohol, and electronic devices before bed can also improve sleep quality. Also, take note that the release of GH is maximized when we avoid eating before bedtime as insulin released in response to food intake can hinder the release of growth hormone.

Exercise—Incorporate moderate-intensity exercise for 60-75 minutes, 3 to 4 times per week. However, it's important not to work to failure, as this can increase the stress hormone cortisol, which can decrease growth hormone production.

Sauna—Heat exposure, such as in a sauna, can increase growth hormone production. Aim for a sauna temperature of 176-210F for 20-30 minutes to see an increase in growth hormone levels. Several studies have investigated the effects of saunas on growth hormone levels. One study published in *The Journal of Clinical Endocrinology and Metabolism* found that sauna use increased growth hormone levels by up to 500%. (45) The study involved

8 male subjects who sat in a sauna at 176°F for 2 sessions of 15 minutes each with a 30-minute cooling period in between. Another study published in *The Journal of Sports Medicine and Physical Fitness* found that sauna use increased growth hormone levels by as much as 1,600%. (46) The study involved 10 male subjects who sat in a sauna at 194°F for 2 sessions of 15 minutes each with a 30-minute cooling period in between. In both studies, researchers measured the subjects' growth hormone levels before and after the sauna sessions and found a significant increase in growth hormone levels after the sauna sessions.

Supplement With Arginine, Ornithine, or L-citrulline—These amino acids have demonstrated the ability to increase growth hormone production. In studies, arginine has been shown to raise growth hormone levels by 100-300% of baseline. (47) Supplementation of doses of 3-10 grams is the most effective, however, there are diminishing returns above that range—taking higher doses of arginine may not lead to further increases in growth hormone levels.

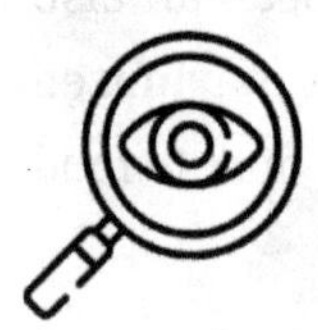

SMART CONSIDERATION

Considerations For Arginine Supplementation

It's important to note that there are some important side effects associated with arginine supplementation. Taking arginine and exercising at the same time may not be beneficial for growth hormone production, as arginine can blunt the effects of exercise. Secondly, arginine is a potent vasodilator, meaning that it can cause blood vessels to dilate and increase blood flow. While this can be beneficial for some individuals, it can be problematic for those with cardiac or blood pressure concerns, as it may lead to a drop in blood pressure.

Ornithine and L-citrulline are two other amino acids that may increase growth hormone production in the body. Ornithine is a precursor to arginine, while L-citrulline is converted to arginine in the body. Both of these amino acids have been shown to increase growth hormone levels, with doses of 2-10 grams being effective. However, as with arginine, it's important to take vasodilation concerns seriously when supplementing with these amino acids.

SMART PROTOCOL

Support Sex And Growth Hormone Production - $0 to $

To optimize the production and utilization of sex and growth hormones, the most important lifestyle factors are those that have been covered in the first three Sections of this book. Sleeping 7 quality hours per night, exercising regularly and in a variety of ways, eating a balanced, clean diet, and the intelligent use of hot and cold exposure are critical. Supplements we have covered for increasing and optimizing sex and growth hormone need to be used with careful consideration of their indications and contraindications and should be used in consultation with a functional medicine practitioner.

Thyroid Hormones

The thyroid gland is a small butterfly-shaped gland located in the front of your neck, just below your larynx. Despite its small size, this gland plays a vital role in regulating metabolism, growth, and development, and works with a whole team of glands to keep your body running smoothly. The thyroid is also involved in brain development, breathing, heart and nervous system function, body temperature, muscle strength, weight and cholesterol production.

The thyroid gland produces two main hormones, namely triiodothyronine (T3) and thyroxine (T4), which are collectively referred to as thyroid hormones. Thyroid hormone T2 (3,5,3'-triiodothyronine) is a lesser-known thyroid hormone that is structurally similar to the more well-known thyroid hormones, T3 and T4. Like T3 and T4, T2 is produced by the thyroid gland but is present in smaller quantities. While T3 and T4 have been studied extensively, research on T2 is still ongoing, and its exact role in the body is not yet fully understood.

The production of thyroid hormones is regulated by the hypothalamus and pituitary gland in the brain. The hypothalamus produces thyrotropin-releasing hormone (TRH), which stimulates the pituitary gland to release thyroid-stimulating hormone (TSH). TSH, in turn, stimulates the thyroid gland to produce T3 and T4. If this is not complex enough, there is also a hormone called reverse T3 (RT3), which decreases thyroid function. A great analogy of this is looking at T3 as the gas pedal of the thyroid and RT3 as the brakes. Elevated levels of RT3 can be a sign of toxicity from heavy metals or a sign of high stress.

A mineral called iodine is critical in the healthy functioning of the thyroid.

Historically, we would have taken iodine from the plants and vegetables we eat, as it is present in the soil. However, due to the gradual deterioration of soils, iodine is not found so easily in places where it used to be. Good sources of iodine now are fish and seaweed. Certain 'clean' diets can have negative effects on thyroid function by disrupting the body's iodine pathway. A plant-based diet, for example, can make it difficult to get enough L-tyrosine, while a carnivore diet can make it challenging to get enough iodine. While iodine is important for thyroid health, some studies have shown iodine supplementation to be contraindicated in conditions of thyroid autoimmune disease (Hashimotos).

Understanding Your Hormones and Neurotransmitters—Testing Options Explained

Hormones can be measured in different ways. Here's a brief explanation of the differences between saliva, blood, urine, and metabolite testing:

Saliva Testing—Saliva testing measures the level of free or unbound hormones in the body, which can provide a snapshot of hormone activity at a specific moment in time. This method is often used to assess hormones such as cortisol and testosterone, as well as to monitor hormone levels during hormone replacement therapy.

Blood Testing—Blood testing measures the level of hormones that are bound to carrier proteins, which transport the hormones through the bloodstream. This method can provide a more accurate measurement of the total hormone level, but it may not reflect the level of hormones that are actually active or available to the body's cells.

Urine Testing—Urine testing can measure both free and bound hormones, as well as their metabolites, or breakdown products. This can provide a more comprehensive assessment of hormone levels and activity, as well as information on how the body is metabolizing hormones.

Metabolite Testing—Metabolite testing measures the by-products of hormone metabolism, which can provide information on how the body is processing and utilizing hormones. This can help identify potential hormone imbalances and underlying health issues that may be affecting hormone metabolism.

While hormones can easily be measured, neurotransmitters are not typically tested directly. This is because neurotransmitters are produced and used within the brain and nervous system, making them difficult to measure through traditional medical testing methods. Instead, neurotransmitter activity can be indirectly assessed through techniques such as neuroimaging or neuropsychological testing. Additionally, certain metabolites of neurotransmitters can be measured in the blood or urine, but these measures are not always reliable indicators of neurotransmitter activity in the brain.

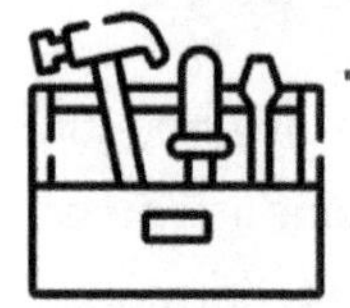

SMART TOOLS

Test, Don't Guess—Hormone Testing At Home

There are now options available to test your hormones from the comfort of your home.

ZRT saliva testing is one option. ZRT Laboratory is a company that specializes in saliva and blood hormone testing. ZRT saliva testing is often preferred over traditional blood testing by some people because it's non-invasive and easy to administer at home. This test can measure the levels of various hormones in the body, including cortisol, estrogen, progesterone, testosterone, DHEA, and melatonin.

The DUTCH test, also known as the Dried Urine Test for Comprehensive Hormones, is another non-invasive and highly accurate method of measuring hormones in the body. (48) This test uses a small sample of dried urine to analyze hormone metabolites, making it a convenient and accessible option if you are looking to monitor your levels. The DUTCH test measures various hormones, including cortisol, estrogen, testosterone, progesterone, and melatonin, among others. If you are experiencing symptoms related to hormonal imbalances, such as fatigue, weight gain, mood swings, and irregular menstrual cycles, you may want to use this test.

One of the key benefits of the DUTCH test is its ability to measure hormone metabolites, which provides insight into how hormones are being metabolized in the body. This information is crucial for identifying any hormonal imbalances and developing an effective treatment plan. The test is easy to administer. Simply collect a small sample of urine at different times of the day and mail it to the laboratory for analysis. The results are typically available within a few days, and they provide a comprehensive overview of your hormone levels and how they fluctuate throughout the day.

SMART PROTOCOL

Know Your Numbers - $0 to $

Maintain an annual blood work schedule through your primary health care provider. Depending on your location, health care system and individual practitioner, there may be limitations as to how much information can be obtained through regular blood tests. To gain deeper insights, consider consulting with a naturopathic doctor or functional medicine practitioner who can interpret the results of specialized tests like saliva or metabolites hormone tests discussed above. They can offer valuable guidance and recommend specific action steps based on your unique results.

Fundamentals Of Learning—Knowledge Acquisition And Retention

In today's fast-paced world, we often find ourselves struggling to focus and retain information. The constant barrage of information and distractions can make it challenging to concentrate on a particular task, let alone remember it later. According to Wendy Suzuki, a renowned neuroscientist, and author of the book, *Healthy Brain, Happy Life: A Personal Program to Activate Your Brain and Do Everything Better*, there are three essentials that can help us improve our learning, focus, and retention: exercise, meditation, and sleep. (49)

Exercise is not only good for our physical health, but it also has significant benefits for the brain. Exercise can offset age-related memory decline, increase focus, and reduce stress and anxiety. It can also improve mood and release dopamine, serotonin, and brain-derived neurotrophic factor (BDNF), all of which boost brain function. Cardiovascular exercise, specifically for 30-45 minutes per day, is particularly important for brain health, specifically the hippocampus and prefrontal cortex. Even just 10 minutes of walking, preferably outside, can shift mood and focus.

Meditation is another powerful tool that can help improve our learning and focus, reduce stress, and even improve memory. This is because meditation helps to calm the mind and increase our awareness of the present moment, which can help us to concentrate better on the task at hand. In her studies, Suzuki has found that guided meditation can have significant benefits for cognitive performance, stress reduction, and mood improvement. She has stated that the minimum threshold for a guided meditation to achieve these benefits is 12 minutes per day.

We've spoken about how vital sleep is for many facets of health, and brain health is no exception. Sleep is essential for consolidating memories and strengthening the connections between neurons in the brain. If you want to improve your ability to learn and retain information, make sure you're getting enough quality sleep each night. Studies have also shown that taking a nap after learning can improve memory consolidation and retention. (50) You can further enhance memory and learning by exposing yourself to specific sensory stimuli during sleep, such as particular sounds or scents that were present while actively learning. This essentially reactivates the neural networks that were engaged while learning and practicing a specific task while awake. This reactivation process strengthens the neural connections formed during wakefulness, ultimately leading to improved task performance upon repetition.

In addition to these three essentials, Suzuki identifies 4 factors that contribute to making something memorable: novelty, repetition, association, and emotional resonance. Novelty involves presenting new or unexpected information, repetition helps reinforce the information, association connects new information to existing knowledge, and emotional resonance is triggered by an emotional response. Notably, memories are formed due to the neurochemical state that occurs after an emotion, including the release of adrenaline, cortisol, epinephrine, and norepinephrine, which strengthen neural connections and enhance memory vividness.

Increase Learning Potential Through Trial And Error

To optimize our brain's potential for learning, it's important to embrace trial and error. This involves repetitions including mistakes and focusing on them for a concentrated period of up to 90 minutes. This time frame is within the ultradian cycle, which refers to the natural 90-minute cycles of heightened physiological and mental activity in the brain. By doing so, we can trigger the release of dopamine, a brain chemical that boosts motivation and aids learning.

Interestingly, the frustration that comes with making mistakes can also accelerate learning by prompting the release of these chemicals. This highlights the importance of repetition, feedback, and practice in shaping our nervous system for better performance. By strengthening and refining neural connections through repetition, we can ultimately improve our overall function. So, don't be afraid to make mistakes. They can be a powerful tool for learning and growth.

SMART PROTOCOL

Skill Acquisition - $0

To learn any skill, evidence shows certain steps are helpful. First, get into an alert state. This largely involves the release of adrenaline in the brain and body. A bout of voluntary hyperventilation that has been discussed here previously is very efficient. Next, get focused. Staring at a point or object just a few feet away for 30-60 seconds (blinking allowed) does this nicely.

Then generate as many repetitions of the skill as you safely can in 90 minutes or less, making the level of difficulty such that you make errors 15% of the time. Insert very short rest intervals, about 10 seconds every 2 minutes, but random. This allows neurons in the hippocampus and cortex involved in learning and memory to "rehearse" what you are doing at 10x speed. As much as possible use random intermittent rewards—just like casinos—to keep yourself motivated.

Studies show that learning rate and depth can be enhanced by performing a shallow nap or Non-Sleep Deep Rest (NSDR) within 1 hour of the learning bout. (51) Then get sufficient and adequate quality sleep at night. Repetitions create the stimulus but the actual rewiring of neural circuits for learning takes place during rest and sleep. Most individuals cannot do more than three 90-minute cycles of learning in a 24-hour period.

How To Leverage Adrenaline For Better Learning And Memory Consolidation

The presence of adrenaline, epinephrine, norepinephrine, and cortisol allows for the formation of memory. After a learning episode, it's recommended to create an adrenaline spike to help cement the newly learned information in your brain. Consuming caffeine can enhance memory by blocking adenosine and increasing dopamine, and epinephrine. It's best to consume caffeine immediately or 5-15 minutes after a learning episode for optimal memory enhancement and neurochemical release. Cold baths, sticking your arm in ice water, or anything that quickens breathing and widens your eyes can further stimulate adrenaline release.

After creating an adrenaline spike, it's important to take a non-sleep deep rest of at least 20 minutes to help the brain process and consolidate the newly learned information. This can be achieved through meditation, deep breathing, or simply lying down and resting your mind and body.

SMART PROTOCOL

Memory Consolidation - $0

To enhance memorization, remove and minimize distractions in your work or learning space. Turn off notifications on your devices, and ensure your space is free from physical clutter. Force an adrenaline spike with coffee, cold exposure, or breathwork after learning to solidify memory consolidation. After a focused learning bout, sit with your eyes closed for 1-10 minutes or have a short NSDR to let your brain consolidate the new information.

Binaural Beats And Brain Waves

Binaural beats are a type of auditory illusion that occurs when two slightly different frequencies are presented to each ear through headphones or earbuds. The brain processes these two frequencies and perceives a rhythmic tone that appears to be within the range of brainwaves.

Some research suggests that listening to binaural beats may have beneficial effects on health, such as reducing anxiety, improving focus and attention, and promoting relaxation. A study published in the *Journal Evidence-Based Complementary and Alternative Medicine* found that participants who listened to binaural beats experienced a significant decrease in anxiety levels compared to those who did not listen to the beats. (52) Another study published in *The Journal of Alternative and Complementary Medicine* reported that binaural beats improved participants' attention and working memory. (53)

There are several different types of brain waves, each associated with different states of consciousness and mental activity. Here are the 5 main types of brain waves and how they affect our state:

1. **Delta Waves (0.5 to 4 Hz)**—Delta waves are the slowest and have the highest amplitude of all brain waves. They are associated with deep sleep, unconsciousness, and physical healing.
2. **Theta Waves (4 to 8 Hz)**—Theta waves are associated with deep relaxation, daydreaming, and meditation. They are also present during REM sleep and may play a role in learning and memory consolidation.
3. **Alpha Waves (8 to 12 Hz)**—Alpha waves are associated with a relaxed and calm state of mind, such as when meditating or taking a break from work. They are also present during light sleep.
4. **Beta Waves (12 to 30 Hz)**—Beta waves are associated with a state of wakefulness and alertness, such as when we are actively engaged in work, conversation, or problem-solving. They can also be associated with stress and anxiety if they are too high in frequency.
5. **Gamma Waves (30 to 100 Hz)**—Gamma waves are the fastest and have the lowest amplitude of all brain waves. They are associated with high levels of cognitive processing, perception, and consciousness. Gamma

waves are also present during intense focus, peak performance, and heightened states of awareness.

Use Auditory Inputs To Augment Learning And Focus

Binaural beats are a modern approach to enhancing learning. These sounds are designed to induce an optimal state for learning, leading to benefits such as increased cognition, creativity, relaxation, pain reduction, and anxiety relief. Listening to sounds in alpha and beta waves increases alertness and recall and focus and concentration. Gamma waves also help to boost problem-solving abilities and learning.

Research has shown that playing low levels of white noise in the background can engage brain areas involved in attention, focus, cognition, and memory to a greater degree. (54) This means that incorporating white noise into your environment can have a positive impact on your ability to concentrate and retain information. White noise can affect brain activity in areas such as the dopaminergic pathway, and raising the base levels of dopamine can increase learning potential. To take advantage of this natural mechanism, try playing low levels of white noise in the background when working or studying.

Using a metronome can be a powerful tool for enhancing learning and skill acquisition. By setting a consistent and rhythmic beat, the metronome can help you stay focused on your task and remember information more easily. Matching the beat to the information you're trying to learn can further enhance memory retention. Additionally, the steady beat of the metronome can help you maintain a consistent pace and avoid distractions, ultimately improving your overall productivity. By training your brain to process information more quickly through the use of a metronome, you can accelerate your learning and acquire new skills more effectively.

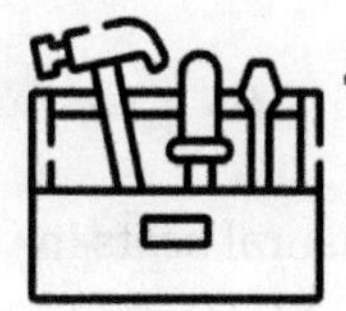

SMART TOOLS

Brain.fm

Brain.fm is a music streaming service that uses artificial intelligence (AI) to create personalized music that can enhance focus, relaxation, and sleep. The service is based on scientific research into the effects of music on the brain and has been shown to be effective at improving concentration and reducing stress. The music on Brain.fm is specifically designed to help users achieve a desired mental state. The music is created in real time and can be customized to suit individual preferences. Users can select from different genres and tempos to personalize their listening experience, and the music adapts to their changing mental state to maintain its effectiveness. In addition to its music offerings, Brain.fm also provides users with a range of guided meditations and other mindfulness exercises that can help improve focus and reduce stress.

SMART PROTOCOL

Auditory Inputs – $0 to $

For focus, concentration, and problem-solving, listen to binaural beats in the alpha, beta, and gamma wave range, or play low-level white noise in the background. For relaxation, sleep, and memory consolidation, listen to binaural beats in the delta and theta wave ranges. There are many free resources available online.

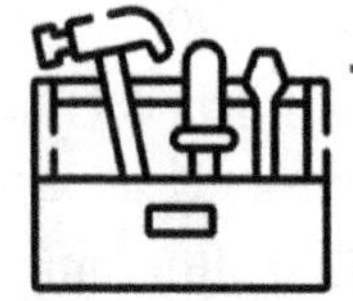

SMART TOOLS

Neuro-Training Devices

Neuro-training devices represent a new frontier in harnessing technology to optimize brain function and mental well-being. These innovative tools utilize various approaches, from biofeedback to audiovisual stimulation, aiming to enhance cognitive abilities and induce relaxation by tapping into the intricate workings of the human brain. Muse and Brain Tap are two such devices:

Muse—Muse is a brain-sensing headband that uses EEG (electroencep halography) technology to monitor brain waves and provide real-time feedback on your mental state. It comes with an App that guides users through meditation sessions and provides personalized feedback on their progress. The headband uses sensors to track the electrical activity of the brain and provides feedback on factors such as concentration, relaxation, and calmness.

BrainTap Technologies—BrainTap Technologies is a powerfully effective mind-development tool designed to help you overcome the ill effects of the fight-or-flight response while achieving physical, mental and emotional balance. Using guided imagery, vibration, binaural sounds and light frequencies to help balance the communication of the right and left brain, BrainTap helps you to relax, reboot and strengthen your busy brain.

Leverage Your Natural Brain And Body Rhythms—Understanding The Phases Of The Day

By understanding the phases of the day and how they can affect neurotransmitter levels and corresponding shifts in mood and mindset, we can create an environment that is more conducive to building and maintaining habits.

During phase one, which occurs during the first 0-8 hours after waking up, the body is in a more alert state. Elevations in norepinephrine, epinephrine, dopamine, and healthy cortisol make this an ideal time to engage in challenging activities that require overcoming a high degree of limbic friction. This can be enhanced through activities such as sunlight viewing, delaying caffeine intake, and delaying your feeding window to prolong your fasted state.

Phase two occurs during the 9-15 hours after waking up, during which levels of dopamine, epinephrine, and cortisol start to come down. Serotonin begins to rise, lending itself to a relaxed state of being that can be further enhanced with activities such as yoga nidra, warm baths, and taking an Ashwagandha supplement. It is best to taper the amount of bright light during this phase and focus on habits and activities that do not require a lot of override of limbic friction, such as journaling and music.

Phase three occurs during the 16-24 hours after waking up, and it is essential to create an environment that supports deep sleep during this phase. Keeping the environment dark and cool can help the body drop in temperature and promote restful sleep. Deep sleep is critical for wiring the neural circuits required for building and maintaining habits.

Insights Into Habit Formation And Breaking Bad Habits

According to neuroscientist Dr. Andrew Huberman, successful habit formation relies heavily on being in the right state of mind and having control over both your body and mind. (55) However, the length of time it takes to adapt to a habit can vary greatly depending on the individual and the habit itself. Some may find it takes as little as 18 days to form a habit, while others may require more than 200 days. The ultimate goal is to overcome limbic friction, the level of energy needed to engage in a habit, and achieve automaticity.

To increase the likelihood of successfully engaging in or maintaining habits, it is important to leverage the natural rhythms of brain and body hormones. During the first 0-8 hours after waking, the brain and body are more action- and focus-oriented, making it easier to overcome high limbic friction with the help of dopamine. Limbic friction describes the strain required to overcome anxiety and lack of motivation or fatigue related to building the new habit. During the 9-15 hours after waking, it is best to leverage high serotonin levels and engage in habits that do not require a lot of limbic override effort to keep stress low.

One way to determine if a habit has truly formed is if it can be performed at any point in the day without much conscious thought. For example, exercising whenever time allows is a sign of a well-formed habit. The strength of a habit is determined by the level of limbic friction and context dependence.

Breaking a bad habit is more complicated than simply rewarding or punishing oneself for engaging in the behaviour. It is important to change the neural circuitry involved. To do this, conscious awareness should be brought to the habit in question, followed by immediately engaging in a positive replacement behaviour, which does not necessarily have to be related to the habit being changed.

SMART PROTOCOL

Habit Reset - $0

Step 1—Choose six new habits to practice over the course of 21 days, with the goal of performing 4-5 of them each day. Don't punish yourself if you miss a day; simply reset and start again.

Step 2—After 21 days, stop deliberately engaging in the six habits and see which ones you naturally incorporate into your daily routine.

Step 3—Take time to assess how deeply you've rewired your nervous system for these new habits. Once you've effortlessly incorporated all six habits into your routine, you can consider starting a new 21-day program to build additional habits.

Rewiring Your Mind—Using Mind Movies For Manifestation And Motivation

Dr. Joe Dispenza is a renowned author, speaker, and researcher who has extensively studied the human mind and its potential. One of his popular concepts is that of "Mind Movies," which refers to the mental images or videos that we create in our minds, often unconsciously, and that influence our thoughts, emotions, and behaviours.

According to Dispenza, our minds are constantly creating images based on our past experiences, beliefs, and expectations, and these mental movies can either propel us toward success or hold us back from achieving our goals. (56) For example, if we constantly visualize ourselves failing or being rejected, we are more likely to experience those outcomes in real life. On the other hand, if we visualize ourselves succeeding and achieving our goals, we are more likely to take the necessary actions and make the right decisions to make that happen.

Dispenza suggests that by consciously creating and controlling our Mind Movies, we can reprogram our minds and create the reality we desire. He recommends the following steps to create effective Mind Movies:

- **Set A Clear Intention**—Start by identifying the specific goal or outcome you want to achieve and set a clear intention for it. This could be anything from starting a new business to improving your health or relationships.
- **Visualize Your Desired Outcome**—Create a mental image or video of yourself already achieving your goal. Imagine how it feels, what you see, hear, and smell, and make it as vivid and detailed as possible.
- **Add Positive Emotions**—To make your Mind Movie more powerful, add positive emotions such as joy, gratitude, and excitement. Feel as if you have already achieved your goal and let those emotions fill you up.
- **Practice Regularly**—To reprogram your mind, you need to practice

regularly. Spend a few minutes every day visualizing your Mind Movie and feeling the positive emotions associated with it. The more you practice, the more effective it will be.

- **Take Action**—Finally, take action towards your goal. Your Mind Movie is a tool to help you stay focused and motivated, but you still need to take the necessary actions to make it a reality.

If you are interested in learning more about the various courses and guided meditations Dr. Dispenza offers, see Smart Resources at the end of this Section for a link to his website.

The Role Of Dopamine And Serotonin In Time Perception And Productivity Optimization

Our perception of time is regulated by internal mechanisms controlled by dopamine and serotonin, causing us to experience events differently depending on whether we feel excited or bored. The more dopamine and epinephrine are released in the brain, the more we tend to overestimate the duration of an event, and our perception of time speeds up. Conversely, the more serotonin is released, the more we tend to underestimate how much time has passed, and our perception of time slows down. Interestingly, blinking can be leveraged for time perception. Every time we blink, our perception of time increases. If we want to speed up our perception of time, we should blink more. To slow down our perception of time, we should blink less.

Leveraging dopamine release can help build habits and segment the day into blocks of productive time. In the first half of the day, when dopamine and norepinephrine levels are higher, it is best to tackle work that involves adhering to rigid rules, such as math or tasks with a clear right or wrong answer. In the afternoon, when serotonin levels are higher, it is advisable to work on brainstorming and creative tasks that require flexibility in scheduling and completing tasks of a similar nature.

Maximize Productivity With Temperature Minimum

Did you know that your body temperature can impact your ability to perform at your best? Research has shown that your temperature minimum—the point at which your body temperature reaches its lowest point during sleep—can be a helpful indicator for scheduling your best work. (57)

Your temperature minimum generally occurs 2 hours before your average wake-up time— if you typically wake up at 7:00 AM, your temperature minimum is likely to occur around 5:00 AM.

You can be reasonably sure that your best work will be done anywhere from 4 to 6 hours after your temperature minimum. To take advantage of this natural mechanism, try scheduling your most important tasks and projects for the hours following your temperature minimum. This can help ensure that you are working at your most productive and efficient during the time when your body is naturally primed for optimal performance.

SMART PROTOCOL

Plan Projects Around Phase Of Day - $0

To maximize efficiency and productivity, schedule tasks or activities that require you to be more alert, and higher degree of limbic friction in Phase 1 (0-8 hours upon waking). Save activities that will benefit from a more relaxed state in Phase 2 (9-15 hours after waking) such as more creative projects or pursuits. Phase 3 (16-24 hours after waking) should be reserved for relaxation and deep sleep.

Creativity—Understanding The Key Elements And Practices To Enhance It

Understanding creativity and how it functions can greatly benefit productivity, habits, and mental wellness. A creative mindset can aid in developing innovative solutions, creating new habits, and refining ways of thinking. To achieve a creative mindset, both divergent and convergent thinking must be utilized. Divergent thinking is what generates new ideas and possibilities, while convergent thinking sharpens and focuses those ideas into actionable plans. Incorporating these thinking styles into daily routines can increase productivity and effectiveness in reaching goals.

Creativity is an essential aspect of life that brings a unique perspective and value to everything we do. The creative process stems from neural structures in the brain that must be accessed in a specific sequence to spark creativity in different domains of life. Creative acts are not just random combinations of things, but instead, reveal a fundamental feature of how our brains and the world work.

SMART PROTOCOL

Enhance Thinking For Creativity - $0

To enhance divergent thinking, try 5 minutes of open monitoring meditation. Close your eyes and let thoughts flow naturally without control or active engagement. Observe sensations, emotions, and experiences that arise. Maintain a relaxed and open awareness, exploring spontaneous ideas and associations. After about 5 minutes, gently bring your attention back to the present moment.

For convergent thinking, try 5 minutes of focused attention monitoring. Choose a specific sound, object, or point to focus on. Keep your attention steady and notice textures, sounds, and sensory aspects. Fully engage your senses and be present in the chosen focal point. After 5 minutes, release your focus and return to a relaxed state of awareness.

Note: Caffeine may aid convergent thinking but is not recommended for divergent thinking.

Take Movement 'Snack' Breaks

Movement snacks, also known as microbreaks or active breaks, are short bursts of physical activity that can be incorporated throughout the day to improve productivity and focus. The idea is to break up long periods of sitting and sedentary behaviour with short bouts of movement to help refresh the mind and body. Research has shown that these microbreaks can have a significant impact on productivity; that even brief periods of exercise can increase blood flow to the brain, improve mood, and enhance cognitive performance. (58)

Incorporate movement snacks into your day with the following:

Stretch Breaks—Take a few minutes to stretch your arms, legs, and back to release tension and increase blood flow.

Desk Exercises—Perform simple exercises like calf raises, squats, or leg lifts while sitting at your desk.

Walk Breaks—Take a short walk around the office or outside to get some fresh air and stretch your legs.

Stair Breaks—Take a few flights of stairs up and down to get your heart rate up and increase blood flow.

Yoga Breaks—Do a few yoga poses like downward dog or child's pose to stretch and relax your muscles.

Dance Breaks—Put on your favourite song and dance around for a few minutes to get your heart rate up and release tension.

Ultradian Rhythm

During the day, our bodies go through periods of high and low energy, with each cycle lasting about 90 minutes. This is known as the ultradian rhythm. During these cycles, our brain shifts between high-frequency beta waves, associated with alertness and concentration, and low-frequency alpha waves, associated with relaxation and daydreaming. These cycles have a significant impact on our learning and productivity as our ability to concentrate and focus typically declines after 90 minutes of continuous work. It will typically take between 5 to 10 minutes to ease in and ramp up. Taking 10-30 minute breaks every 90 minutes can help maintain energy and productivity levels. The following technique further breaks down these 90-minute cycles to help maximize productivity in alignment with our natural rhythms.

Pomodoro Technique

The Pomodoro Technique is a simple but effective time management method that can help increase productivity, improve focus, and reduce stress and burnout. (59) Developed by Francesco Cirillo in the late 1980s, the technique is based on the idea of breaking work down into shorter, focused intervals, or "pomodoros," each lasting around 25 minutes. One of the benefits of the Pomodoro Technique is that by focusing on just one task at a time, it's easier to stay motivated and avoid getting overwhelmed by the bigger picture.

To use the Pomodoro Technique, start by choosing a task that you need to complete. Set a timer for 25 minutes and work on the task until the timer goes off. Once the timer rings, take a 5-minute break. This break is a chance to stretch, get up and move around, or do something else that's unrelated to work. After the break, start another 25-minute pomodoro and repeat the cycle until you've completed three pomodoros. At this point, take a longer break of 15-30 minutes to rest and recharge. This would be a great time to take a power nap or implement an NSDR.

The key to the Pomodoro Technique is to stay focused and avoid distractions during each 25-minute interval. Turn off your phone, close your email, and focus solely on the task at hand. By taking the breaks, you're giving your brain and body a chance to rest and recharge, which can help you stay focused and productive for longer periods. These intervals are a great time to incorporate the movement snacks mentioned above.

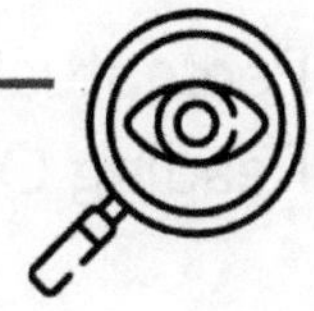

SMART CONSIDERATION

Concentration Technique For Progressive Focus Training

We mentioned that narrowing your visual field can help to increase acetylcholine and enhance memory and learning, but learning to leverage your visual field can also help to improve focus and concentration. To implement this strategy, set a timer for a short amount of time, approximately 30 seconds, and focus your gaze on one object during that time. The object can be anything in your visual field, such as a spot on the wall or a pencil on your desk. The goal is to maintain your focus solely on that object during the allotted time, without allowing your mind to wander or become distracted.

Once you have successfully completed 30 seconds of focused attention on the object, you can gradually increase the time by 5 seconds each day. For example, on day 2, you would focus on the object for 35 seconds, and on day 3, you would focus on the object for 40 seconds. This gradual increase helps to build up your ability to maintain focus for longer periods of time. It is important to remember to blink during these focused bouts, as staring at an object for extended periods of time without blinking can cause eye strain and discomfort. Using this technique can be a helpful onramp to longer periods of focused attention, like the 90-minute ultradian cycle. By practicing with shorter periods of time, you can build up your ability to stay focused for longer periods without becoming distracted or losing focus.

Perceptual Load Theory And Stimulation Control—Why Reading On A Smaller Surface Can Help You Focus

Have you ever noticed that it is often easier to hone in on information when you are reading from your cell phone or tablet as opposed to a computer screen? This is because the smaller surface area of a mobile device provides a more compact and focused area for reading, which can help reduce distractions and allow us to concentrate more deeply on the text. As a result, we may experience an increase in concentration, which can stimulate the release of neurotransmitters like epinephrine and acetylcholine in our brains. These neurotransmitters play a crucial role in our ability to focus our attention on specific tasks and retain information in our memory. While the exact mechanism behind this is still a subject of research, there are some theories that can help us understand how it may work.

One theory is related to the concept of the "perceptual load theory." This theory suggests that the amount of attentional resources required for a task depends on the perceptual demands of that task. In other words, tasks that require high perceptual demands, such as reading small text on a phone or tablet require more attentional resources than tasks that have low perceptual demands, such as reading large text on a computer or larger area. When attentional resources are focused on a task, it may lead to increased concentration and focus.

Another theory is related to the idea of "stimulation control." This theory suggests that the level of stimulation in the environment can affect cognitive performance. The higher the level of stimulation, the greater the arousal and attention, which can lead to improved cognitive performance. Reading on a phone may provide a higher level of stimulation due to the smaller screen size, which can help to enhance concentration and focus.

Support Neurotransmitters With Nootropics

As we mentioned earlier, nootropics are substances and supplements that can enhance cognitive function and support brain health. The following have all been found to be beneficial for focus and concentration.

Ginkgo Biloba is an herbal supplement derived from the leaves of the ginkgo tree. It's believed to improve blood flow to the brain and protect against cognitive decline. Some studies suggest that ginkgo biloba can improve focus, memory, and attention in healthy adults and individuals with Alzheimer's disease or vascular dementia. (60)

Bacopa Monnieri is a traditional Ayurvedic herb that has been used for centuries to enhance cognitive function and improve memory. Bacopa is believed to work by increasing the production of acetylcholine, a neurotransmitter that is essential for memory and learning. It also has antioxidant properties that can protect the brain from oxidative stress and neurodegeneration.

Rhodiola Rosea is an adaptogenic herb that has been used in traditional medicine for hundreds of years to improve mental and physical performance. Several studies have shown that Rhodiola can improve cognitive function, including attention, memory, and concentration. In one study, participants who took Rhodiola extract for 20 days showed significant improvement in their ability to concentrate and perform mental tasks. (61) Rhodiola helps to regulate levels of serotonin, dopamine, and norepinephrine. Rhodiola seems to increase aerobic capacity and decrease the perceived exertion of a workout. (62)

SMART PROTOCOL

Concentration - $0 to $

Honour your natural ultradian rhythm and phase of the day, taking advantage of your temperature minimum to concentrate when your body is at its most receptive to focused attention. Incorporate movement 'snack' micro-breaks throughout the day. Break up tasks with the Pomodoro technique and consider perceptual load theory to read on a smaller screen when intaking new information. Experiment with focus-enhancing nootropics–ginkgo biloba, bacopa monnieri, or Rhodiola Rosea if appropriate.

Increase Alertness With Body Posture And Eye Position

The relationship between body posture, eye position, and alertness is a well-researched topic in the fields of psychology, neuroscience, and ergonomics. The position of our body and eyes can greatly affect our cognitive performance.

Studies have shown that an upright posture promotes alertness and mental clarity. (63) Maintaining an upright posture with your eyes directed forward or slightly upwards encourages blood flow to the brain, which increases oxygenation and glucose supply. Additionally, an upright posture reduces muscle tension, which can improve comfort and reduce fatigue. When we look down, we are more likely to feel sleepy or fatigued. This is because looking down can cause a decrease in blood flow to the brain, leading to reduced oxygenation and glucose supply. Looking down can also cause increased muscle tension, leading to discomfort and fatigue.

In terms of eye position, when we look up or directly forward, it improves attentiveness and elevates mood. This is because looking up or directly forward stimulates the brain's reticular activating system (RAS), which is responsible for regulating our sleep-wake cycle and overall arousal level. The RAS is also involved in regulating attention and focus, so looking up or directly forward can help improve cognitive function. On the other hand, looking down can induce sleepiness because it activates the parasympathetic nervous system, which is responsible for promoting relaxation and restful sleep.

Research has shown that it is best to arrange your desk and workspace so you can sit for a period of time, and stand for a period of time. Sit-stand desks are commonly available, or they can be easily done using boxes and other common things found around the house and office. Sitting for 10-30 minutes and then standing for 10-30 minutes is best, with an overall ratio of 60% standing and 40% sitting over the course of a day. (64)

SMART PROTOCOL

Adjust Your Workstation - $0 to $$

Optimize your workstation for improved productivity by creating a setup that accommodates both sitting and standing positions. Aim to switch between these positions every 30 minutes or less. Position your screen or focal point slightly above eye level to maintain proper posture. Additionally, tailor your workspace to enhance specific types of work: a smaller space with a lower ceiling can foster concentration and focus for detailed tasks, while a larger space with a higher ceiling can stimulate abstract thinking and creativity. Consider altering your working environment or relocating to leverage the benefits of each setting, depending on the nature of your work.

The Impact Of Fasting And Feeding On Mental State

Eating and fasting can have opposite effects on the body's state, with eating shifting us toward a state of calmness and fasting shifting us toward a state of alertness.

When we eat, our body receives a steady supply of nutrients and energy, which can help to stabilize blood sugar levels and promote a feeling of calmness and relaxation. This is because our body releases insulin in response to the food we eat, which helps to transport glucose from the bloodstream into our cells, where it can be used for energy. This process can promote a feeling of satiety and relaxation, as our body is no longer in a state of hunger.

On the other hand, when we fast, our body is deprived of a steady supply of nutrients and energy, which can trigger the release of certain hormones and neurotransmitters, such as adrenaline and cortisol. These chemicals are associated with increased alertness and attention, as our body prepares to seek out food and sustain itself in the absence of regular nourishment.

Both fasted and fed states stimulate neuronal activity. You can leverage this with learning and productivity by trying one 90-minute cycle in a fasted state in the morning, and one in a fed state (being sure you haven't reached the point of a stuffed belly, as this will lead to a decrease in alertness and energy).

Neural Energy

When it comes to increasing energy levels, many people often think of food as the primary source. However, there are other ways to boost energy that don't necessarily require consuming food. One example is through the use of certain supplements or medications, such as choline, physostigmine (a prescription drug), and phosphatidylserine.

But why is it important to consider alternative ways of increasing energy? The answer lies in the fact that many of these supplements and medications, along with hormones like epinephrine and cortisol, can provide a significant boost to energy levels and immune system function without impacting blood glucose levels. In fact, these hormones play a vital role in what we could call "neural energy," which is a more powerful source of energy than that derived from food. Neural energy is fueled by neurotransmitters that create feelings of alertness, focus, and motivation, as well as the ability to move and respond to threats.

While food certainly plays a role in providing energy, it's important to recognize that there are other sources of energy that are equally important, if not more so. Hormones like cortisol and epinephrine interact with our body's various systems, including the immune system, to provide the energy and focus needed to function at our best.

SMART PROTOCOL

Increase Neural Energy And Alertness - $0

Start your day by getting early morning sunlight exposure. Delay caffeine intake for the first 90-120 minutes after waking, and instead drink water to hydrate and energize your body. Consider morning exercise or movement, as it can increase your bias toward action throughout the day. For improved alertness, try fasting and low-carb states, but make sure not to let hunger distract you. If you use time-restricted feeding, you will take advantage of this during the beginning of Phase 1 of the day. Implement voluntary hyperventilation in your day when you need an energy boost, or take a non-sleep deep rest break in the afternoon when you hit a wall. Minimize bright light exposure between 10 pm and 4 am to ensure quality sleep.

Unlocking The Benefits Of Gratitude—A Guide To Practicing Genuine Appreciation

Gratitude activates the prefrontal cortex, a region of the brain associated with executive functions such as decision-making, planning, and emotional regulation. When we approach life with a grateful mindset, we are more likely to notice and focus on the positive aspects of our experiences, even in the face of adversity or challenges. This can help us to cultivate a sense of perspective and resilience, and to maintain a more positive outlook on life.

The science of gratitude has been shown to have extraordinary positive effects on both our mental and physical health. (65) Interestingly, common practices like gratitude journaling are mostly ineffective and will not actually lead to benefits or changes in brain circuitry. (66) Gratitude is not about a 'fake it till you make it' mentality–giving and receiving thanks and gratitude must be genuine to see the benefits.

So, what does a true gratitude practice look like? It involves empathizing or sympathizing with someone who received help. This could be someone you helped, or it could be someone you heard about who received help. By connecting emotionally with the story of someone who received help, we can experience genuine gratitude and reap the benefits.

A regular gratitude practice can have a range of physiological benefits, including reducing anxiety and fear pathways, increasing motivation and pursuit pathways, and decreasing inflammatory cytokines. Unlike other practices, such as meditation or breathwork, the positive effects of gratitude practice can be felt almost instantly, making it a sustainable habit to incorporate regularly.

SMART PROTOCOL

Scientifically Grounded Gratitude Practice - $0

An ideal gratitude practice involves genuinely connecting with a story, reflecting on it for 1-5 minutes, and practicing 3 times per week.

To begin, think about a story in which someone received help or you received thanks. This story should be one that you can genuinely connect with emotionally. Next, write a few notes about the story. Consider what the struggle was, what the help was, and how it made you feel. Finally, reflect on the story for 1-5 minutes. Really connect with the emotions you experienced. This is a short and simple practice that can have powerful benefits with minimal time investment.

Mindfulness, Meditation And The Impact On Mental Wellness

Mindfulness and meditation can be powerful tools for improving brain health. Studies have shown that regular meditation can increase gray matter density in the brain, particularly in areas associated with learning, memory, and emotion regulation. Additionally, meditation has been found to reduce stress, anxiety, and depression, all of which can have negative effects on brain health. (67) Stress is one of the worst enemies of the brain and the body. Over time, chronic stress can destroy brain cells and even damage parts of the hippocampus—the region of the brain involved in the formation of new memories and the retrieval of old ones. It may be inevitable that we will experience stress at one point or another, and a certain amount of stress may even be deemed healthy (i.e. eustress: what motivates us to get work done). Incorporating meditation and mindfulness practices in your daily life can help to reduce stress levels and promote optimal brain function.

Mindfulness involves focusing on the sensations within your body, your breathing, and your thoughts in the present moment. Meditation is a practice that usually requires you to sit still and close your eyes. This has the effect of redirecting your attention from external factors (known as exteroception) to the sensations on and within your body (referred to as interoception). However, it's not always beneficial to have high levels of interoception—people with high levels of anxiety are also usually keenly aware of the bodily state in maladaptive ways. If you are prone to anxiety, walking or moving meditation may be more beneficial to avoid intrusive interoceptive thoughts.

Meditation has positive effects on mood, and being present correlates to happiness. However, be cautious with meditation time, as meditation too close to sleep may actually disrupt it since it's a practice of focus. Regular meditation may reduce sleep needs and allow people to function better cognitively and physically via cortisol management. Yoga Nidra can reduce cortisol and enhance neuromodulators as much as or more than traditional meditation. To get better at falling asleep or falling back asleep in the middle of the night, try Yoga Nidra or non-sleep deep rest. These practices have been previously outlined in this book. If your goal is to increase focus, and mood, and deliberately manage interoception/exteroception, traditional meditation is beneficial and will require some help and guidance.

SMART TOOLS

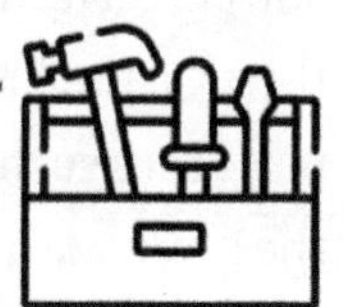

Waking Up App

This mindfulness and meditation App was created by Sam Harris, a neuroscientist, philosopher, and author. It is designed to be accessible to both beginners and experienced meditators, offering a secular and practical approach. It includes a structured introductory course that helps users develop a foundation in mindfulness. The course provides step-by-step guidance and instruction for those new to meditation. It also features a library of guided meditation sessions that cover various meditation techniques, such as breath awareness, body scans, and loving-kindness practices. In addition to guided meditations, the App offers lessons and theoretical insights. These teachings explore the nature of consciousness, the self, and the principles behind mindfulness practice. The App encourages users to establish a daily meditation habit to help maintain consistency in their practice and experience the long-term benefits of mindfulness.

Interoceptive Vs. Exteroceptive Processing

Interoception and exteroception are two related concepts that refer to the ways in which we perceive and experience different aspects of our environment and bodily states. Interoception refers to our ability to sense and perceive our internal bodily states, including sensations such as hunger, thirst, pain, and fatigue, as well as our emotional states and physiological processes such as heart rate and breathing. This information is conveyed to the brain via a network of sensory receptors located throughout the body, which transmit signals to the brain to create a sense of bodily awareness.

Exteroception, on the other hand, refers to our ability to perceive and respond to stimuli in the external environment, including sensory information such as light, sound, touch, taste, and smell. This information is also conveyed to the brain via specialized sensory receptors located in the eyes, ears, skin, tongue, and nose.

Additionally, disruptions or alterations in interoceptive and exteroceptive processing can have significant effects on our health and well-being. For example, individuals with conditions such as chronic pain or anxiety may experience heightened sensitivity to interoceptive cues, while individuals with conditions such as autism spectrum disorder may have difficulty processing and responding to exteroceptive stimuli. Understanding these states is essential to understanding the complexities of human perception and experience.

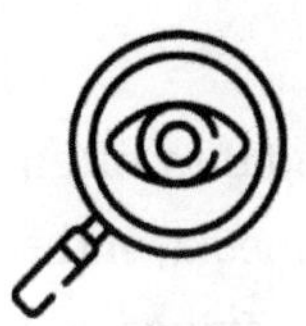

SMART CONSIDERATION

Meditate Your Opposing State

To choose the right meditation for the moment, determine whether you are in an interoceptive or exteroceptive state. Then, choose the meditation that allows you to go against the grain of your natural state to train your body, brain, and neural plasticity. One of the most important aspects of meditation is your ability to refocus when your attention wanders. That is where the magic happens in training your focus and attention. Breathwork is an important component of meditation practice, and, in fact, focusing on the breath can be a meditation in and of itself. One of the key questions to ask yourself in a meditation practice is whether you want to be more or less alert. To increase heart rate and alertness, inhale longer and/or more vigorously than exhale. To slow the heart rate down and relax, exhale longer and/or more vigorously than inhale.

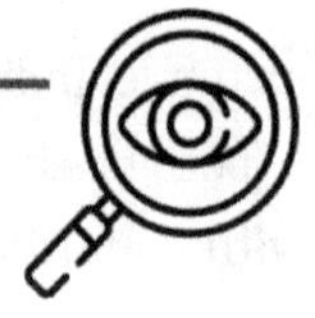

SMART CONSIDERATION

Control Cravings With Your Mind

Cravings are powerful urges that can be difficult to resist, and they often arise in response to external stimuli such as advertising, social media, or the presence of certain foods or substances. When we experience cravings, our prefrontal cortex—the part of the brain responsible for decision-making, impulse control, and planning—can be "hijacked" by the intensity of the urge. This can make it difficult to make rational choices and can lead to impulsive behaviour.

A body scan is a mindfulness practice that involves paying close attention to physical sensations throughout the body, from the head to the toes. This practice helps to draw attention inward and away from external stimuli, including cravings. When we practice a body scan, we can become more aware of our physical sensations, including any discomfort or tension in the body that may be contributing to our cravings. By bringing our attention to these sensations, we can develop a greater understanding of our internal state and gain more control over our impulses.

Physiological Sighs And Panoramic Vision—Help To Calm And Focus The Mind

Physiological sighs are deep, spontaneous breaths that occur naturally in humans and many other animals. These breaths serve an important function in regulating our respiratory and cardiovascular systems, and can also play a role in emotional regulation. You've heard the phrase 'breathed a sigh of relief' after someone experiences a stressful or tense situation. When we are feeling too alert or anxious, our sympathetic nervous system becomes activated, which can lead to a number of physical symptoms such as increased heart rate, rapid breathing, and tunnel vision. These symptoms can make it difficult to focus or concentrate and may exacerbate feelings of stress or anxiety.

Physiological sighs are thought to be generated by specialized neurons located in a small region of the brainstem called the pre-Bötzinger complex. (68) These neurons act as a central rhythm generator, coordinating the rhythmic contraction of the diaphragm and other respiratory muscles that are necessary for breathing. When we take a deep breath or sigh, we activate these neurons, which, in turn, can help to reset our breathing patterns and promote feelings of relaxation and calmness.

In addition to the physiological benefits of deep sighs, there is also evidence to suggest that looking to the horizon for panoramic vision can help to reduce feelings of tunnel vision or hyper-focus. This is because when we are hyper-focused on a task or situation, we tend to narrow our attention and become less aware of our surroundings. By looking to the horizon, we can expand our field of vision and become more aware of our surroundings, which can help to reduce feelings of stress and anxiety.

When we focus on something, we engage a part of our visual system called the fovea, which is responsible for sharp, detailed vision. This type of vision is associated with focused attention and can contribute to feelings of stress and anxiety. In contrast, when we look at a panoramic view, we engage a different part of our visual system called the peripheral vision, which is responsible for detecting movement and changes in the environment. This type of vision is associated with a more relaxed and alert state, which can promote feelings of calmness and reduce anxiety.

SMART PROTOCOL

Sigh For Serenity – $0

Perform 2-3 physiological sighs in a row. Take a deep breath in through the nose, followed by another short inhale. Hold for a few seconds and then exhale through the mouth, adding an audible 'sighing' sound. Additionally, when experiencing anxiety, expand your view by shifting your focus to a distant, panoramic point. These simple acts can help calm your mind and reduce feelings of anxiety.

SMART CONSIDERATION

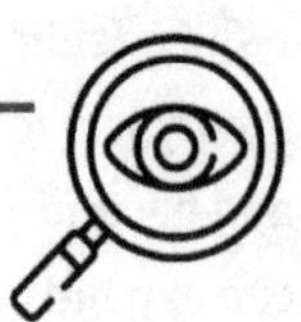

Reduce Stress With Optic Flow—Go For A Walk

When we walk forward through our environment, we generate eye movements that result in optic flow and reduce activation in the amygdala, the brain's centre for emotional processing. This means that taking a walk outside can have a positive impact on your mental well-being by reducing stress levels.

Mental Health And Self-Hypnosis

What comes to mind when you hear the word 'hypnosis'? It's likely you may envision someone on a stage being put into a hypnotic state and being coerced into clucking like a chicken or barking like a dog in front of an audience just to garner some laughs. In fact, self-hypnosis is a powerful therapeutic technique that has been shown to have a wide range of benefits for mental health and wellness. Dr. David Spiegel, a renowned psychiatrist and expert in the field of hypnosis, has conducted extensive research on the use of self-hypnosis for mental health enhancement. Dr. Spiegel's research has demonstrated that self-hypnosis is an effective tool for reducing stress and anxiety, managing chronic pain, improving sleep quality, and managing a range of mental health conditions such as depression, phobias, and addiction. (69) Self-hypnosis is vastly different from "stage hypnosis," which is often performed for entertainment purposes.

One of the primary ways to induce self-hypnosis is through progressive relaxation, a technique that involves tensing and then relaxing various muscle groups in the body. During a self-hypnotic state, individuals may experience changes in brain wave activity, such as a decrease in beta waves and an increase in alpha and theta waves. These changes in brain wave activity suggest that self-hypnosis can activate certain neural pathways in the brain, such as the anterior cingulate cortex, which is involved in regulating emotional responses. By activating these pathways, self-hypnosis can help people gain greater control over their emotions and behaviour, leading to improved mental health and well-being.

SMART TOOLS

Reveri App

To make self-hypnosis more accessible, Dr. Spiegel has developed an App called Reveri, which guides users through the process of self-hypnosis using pre-recorded audio tracks. The App has been shown to be effective in reducing anxiety and improving sleep quality in clinical trials.

Reduce Negative 'Noise'—Take A Media Break

We are constantly surrounded by information and it can be hard to tune it out and escape it. Consider taking periodic breaks from social platforms, watching the news, or consuming negative media. This can look like setting daily limits or turning off all notifications and uninstalling apps on your phone over the weekend, for example.

The news is often filled with stories of tragedy, conflict, and crisis. Constant exposure to negative news can lead to feelings of anxiety, sadness, and despair. By taking a break from consuming media, you can limit your exposure to such news, create a more positive outlook, and reduce your stress levels.

Frequent screen use can be stressful on its own. We often aimlessly scroll our phones in any spare moment of downtime, or out of boredom. Taking a break from media consumption can help give your eyes a break and provide you with some much-needed relaxation time, not to mention the fact that we can get caught up in comparison scenarios and negative comment threads on social media that can affect our mood, blood pressure, and stress levels.

When you're constantly consuming media, it can be challenging to find time for other activities that help reduce stress, such as exercise, meditation, or spending time with loved ones. Taking a break can provide you with the time and space to engage in these activities.

SMART PROTOCOL

Calming Down – $0

Exercise your empathetic and sympathetic muscles with a proper gratitude practice grounded in science. Incorporate a regular meditation practice of a minimum of 12 minutes per day and be sure to mediate against your current state, whether it is interoceptive or exteroceptive. Consider a media fast and self-hypnosis to reduce mental noise and stress.

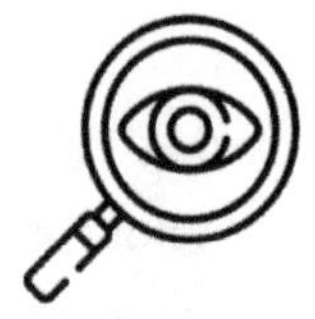

SMART CONSIDERATION

Try Focused Formulations

Throughout this Section, we have highlighted various foods, supplements, and nootropics you can incorporate into your daily routine to improve brain health, memory, focus, and cognition. However, taking multiple supplements individually can sometimes be overwhelming. Fortunately, several reputable nutraceutical companies offer proprietary formulations of brain-enhancing supplements that cater to specific results. These formulations can help you achieve greater focus, clarity, creativity, or motivation, and there are resources available to help you find the right product. For instance, mynoots.com and takethesis.com offer product lines and even personalized quiz results to help identify the ideal supplement for your needs. By leveraging these resources, you can streamline your supplement intake while optimizing your brain function and neuronal health.

Chiropractic Adjustments And Effects On The Brain

As both authors of this book are Doctors of Chiropractic, with a combined clinical experience spanning over 5 decades, we certainly would be remiss if we did not share our experience and expertise in the area of brain health. During our extensive practice, we have supported patients in improving their well-being by optimizing the function of their nervous systems. A key objective of chiropractic adjustment is to reinstate balance within the body, thereby fostering the healing process.

How does this occur? It's fascinating to discover that chiropractic adjustments can impact the functioning of the prefrontal cortex. This remarkable brain region is responsible for crucial executive functions such as planning, decision-making, memory, problem-solving, and behaviour control. Additionally, it plays a pivotal role in pain processing. Research indicates that the prefrontal cortex activates during pain experiences and has the ability to regulate pain perception by modulating other areas of the brain. (70)

Additionally, the prefrontal cortex regulates the autonomic nervous system, which controls various bodily functions such as heart rate and digestion. It also oversees the endocrine system, influencing body chemistry and hormone regulation. Moreover, the prefrontal cortex is essential for proper immune system function, enabling the body to defend against foreign invaders and infections. (71)

Chiropractic adjustments can also impact the cerebellum, often referred to as the "brain within the brain." This structure, located at the back of the brain, plays a crucial role in everyday movements, balance, and coordination. By integrating sensory inputs and fine-tuning movements, the cerebellum ensures precise and coordinated actions, as well as cognitive tasks like attention, language, and emotional responses.

Neuroscientific research has explored the effects of chiropractic care on brain function, particularly cerebellar function. Studies using advanced techniques such as electroencephalography and transcranial magnetic stimulation have demonstrated that spinal adjustments can alter how the cerebellum processes sensory information and communicates with other brain regions. (72) (73)

These findings, along with a body of research, indicate that even without pain, impaired spinal function can affect how the brain perceives body position, coordination, and movement accuracy. (74)

SMART PROTOCOL

Chiropractic Consultation And Evaluation - $ to $$

For a comprehensive understanding of your nervous system's functionality, consider scheduling an appointment with a local Doctor of Chiropractic. These healthcare professionals possess a wide range of diagnostic tools and tests, such as HRV testing, thermal and sEMG scans as well as the clinical skills to help identify and address spinal dysfunction. Correcting dysfunction and improving brain-body communication can assist in optimizing nervous system performance.

Section Wrap-Up

You now have a greater understanding of the fascinating complexities of the brain where intricate neural networks shape our cognition and behaviour. You've learned about the vital role of neurotransmitters in facilitating communication between brain cells, which allows for the transmission of signals that govern our thoughts, emotions, and actions. We have also covered the role of hormones and their profound influence on various bodily functions. Armed with this knowledge, you can enhance your concentration and focus, boost your energy levels and productivity, and achieve optimal brain health.

In Section 5—Epigenetics, Ageing and Longevity, we will venture further into the realm of human health, exploring the science of epigenetics, ageing, and longevity. Just as our brain wiring and biochemical balance shape our well-being, understanding the impact of epigenetic factors on our genetic expression and the ageing process is crucial for unlocking the secrets to extended vitality and longevity.

PROTOCOLS QUICK REFERENCE CHECKLIST:

PROTOCOL—Track HRV - $0 to $$

☐ *Currently doing* ☐ *Want to integrate* ☐ *Not for now*

PROTOCOL—HRV Biofeedback - $0 to $$

☐ *Currently doing* ☐ *Want to integrate* ☐ *Not for now*

PROTOCOL—Stimulate Your Vagus Nerve - $0 to $

☐ *Currently doing* ☐ *Want to integrate* ☐ *Not for now*

PROTOCOL—Eat More Polyphenols - $0 to $

☐ *Currently doing* ☐ *Want to integrate* ☐ *Not for now*

PROTOCOL—Mindful Learning Blocks - $0

☐ *Currently doing* ☐ *Want to integrate* ☐ *Not for now*

PROTOCOL—Foods For Focus - $0 to $

☐ *Currently doing* ☐ *Want to integrate* ☐ *Not for now*

PROTOCOL—Memory Supportive Supplementation - $0 to $$

☐ *Currently doing* ☐ *Want to integrate* ☐ *Not for now*

PROTOCOL—Narrow Visual Field - $0

☐ *Currently doing* ☐ *Want to integrate* ☐ *Not for now*

PROTOCOL—Elevate Energy Levels All Day - $0 to $

☐ *Currently doing* ☐ *Want to integrate* ☐ *Not for now*

PROTOCOL—Quick Energy Boost - $0

☐ *Currently doing* ☐ *Want to integrate* ☐ *Not for now*

PROTOCOL—Immediate Mood Boost - $0

☐ *Currently doing* ☐ *Want to integrate* ☐ *Not for now*

PROTOCOL—Long-Term Mood Support - $0 to $

☐ *Currently doing* ☐ *Want to integrate* ☐ *Not for now*

PROTOCOL—Dopamine Detox - $0

☐ *Currently doing* ☐ *Want to integrate* ☐ *Not for now*

PROTOCOL—Exogenous Ketones For Brain Energy - $

☐ *Currently doing* ☐ *Want to integrate* ☐ *Not for now*

PROTOCOL—Dietary Considerations For Brain Health - $

☐ *Currently doing* ☐ *Want to integrate* ☐ *Not for now*

PROTOCOL—Increase Testosterone - $0 to $

☐ *Currently doing* ☐ *Want to integrate* ☐ *Not for now*

PROTOCOL—Use Your Electronics Wisely - $0 to $$$

☐ *Currently doing* ☐ *Want to integrate* ☐ *Not for now*

PROTOCOL—Support Sex And Growth Hormone Production - $0 to $

☐ *Currently doing* ☐ *Want to integrate* ☐ *Not for now*

PROTOCOL—Know Your Numbers - $ to $$

☐ *Currently doing* ☐ *Want to integrate* ☐ *Not for now*

PROTOCOL—Skill Acquisition - $0

☐ *Currently doing* ☐ *Want to integrate* ☐ *Not for now*

PROTOCOL—Memory Consolidation - $0 to $

☐ *Currently doing* ☐ *Want to integrate* ☐ *Not for now*

PROTOCOL—Auditory Inputs - $0 to $

☐ *Currently doing* ☐ *Want to integrate* ☐ *Not for now*

PROTOCOL—Habit Reset - $0

☐ *Currently doing* ☐ *Want to integrate* ☐ *Not for now*

PROTOCOL—Plan Projects Around Phase Of Day - $0

☐ *Currently doing* ☐ *Want to integrate* ☐ *Not for now*

PROTOCOL—Enhance Thinking For Creativity - $0

☐ *Currently doing* ☐ *Want to integrate* ☐ *Not for now*

PROTOCOL—Concentration - $0 to $

☐ *Currently doing* ☐ *Want to integrate* ☐ *Not for now*

PROTOCOL—Adjust Your Workstation - $0 to $$

☐ *Currently doing* ☐ *Want to integrate* ☐ *Not for now*

PROTOCOL—Increase Neural Energy And Alertness - $0

☐ *Currently doing* ☐ *Want to integrate* ☐ *Not for now*

PROTOCOL—Scientifically Grounded Gratitude Practice - $0

☐ *Currently doing* ☐ *Want to integrate* ☐ *Not for now*

PROTOCOL—Sigh For Serenity - $0

☐ *Currently doing* ☐ *Want to integrate* ☐ *Not for now*

PROTOCOL—Calming Down - $0

☐ *Currently doing* ☐ *Want to integrate* ☐ *Not for now*

PROTOCOL—Chiropractic Consultation And Evaluation - $ to $$

☐ *Currently doing* ☐ *Want to integrate* ☐ *Not for now*

SMART RESOURCES

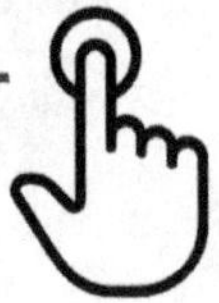

- Vagus Nerve Stimulator—truvaga.com and getsensate.com
- Mind Movies—drjoedispenza.com

- Nootropics—mynoots.com and takethesis.com
- EMF Protection—emfessentials.com, smartmeterguard.com, shieldyourbody.com, shieldedhealing.com, airestech.com

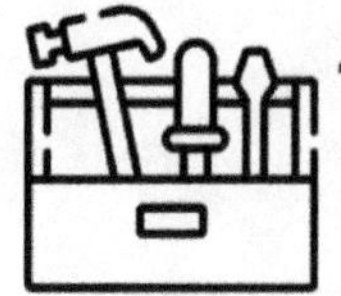

SMART TOOLS

- Elite HRV App—elitehrv.com
- Find dominant neurotransmitter—bravermantest.net
- ZRT Saliva Test—zrtlab.com/sample-types/saliva
- DUTCH Test—dutchtest.com
- Brain.fm—brain.fm
- Neuro Training Devices—Muse choosemuse.com BrainTap braintap.com
- Mindfulness/Meditation App—wakingup.com
- Self Hypnosis App—reveri.com

Section 5—Epigenetics, Ageing & Healthspan

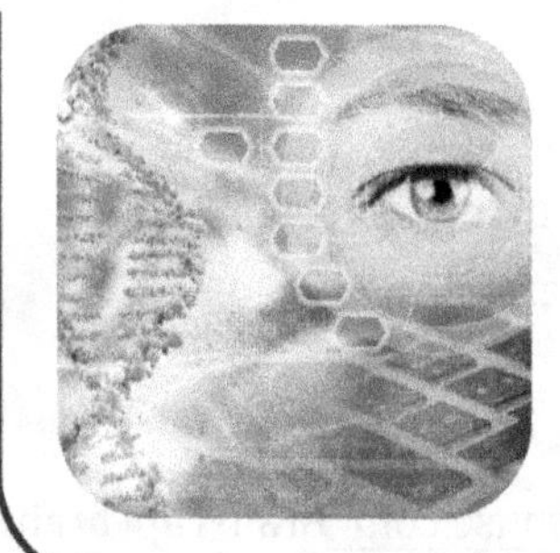

"Epigenetics is the bridge between nature and nurture, highlighting that our experiences and choices can leave a lasting impact on our genetic expression."

— Sharon Moalem

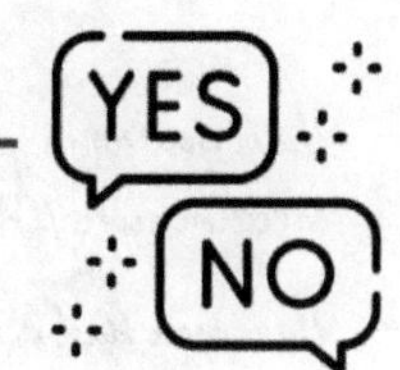

SELF EVALUATION-DISCOVERY QUESTIONS

Do you have a set of strategies to "slow down" your ageing process? Y N

Do you have health protocols that focus on the 12 hallmarks of ageing? Y N

Do you use any red light therapy devices to enhance your mitochondrial health? Y N

Do you know your level of resiliency in these categories: psychological performance & cognitive resiliency, stress response & sleep resiliency, toxicity & temperature resiliency, dietary & microbiome resiliency, inflammation and physical resiliency, pathogens & immune resiliency? Y N

Have you done any cognitive health-validated questionnaires to test your cognition? Y N

Do you know your resting heart rate, blood pressure, and radial/brachial index? Y N

Have you had an ECG and spirometry test done to know your heart and lung health? Y N

Have you done blood panels to evaluate your general health profile, cardiac profile, hormone profile and immune profile? Y N

Have you done specialty tests such as a Dexa, Fecal Immunochemical Test (FIT) for colon health or a Grail multi-cancer detection test? Y N

Have you done specialty imaging studies like CT coronary artery calcium score (CAC) or NeuroQuant MRI?	Y	N
Have you had a methylation test to test your biological age?	Y	N
Have you done genetics testing to evaluate your Single Nucleotide Polymorphisms (SNPs) to help manage your epigenetics?	Y	N
Do you use validated nutraceuticals as part of your longevity protocols?	Y	N
Do you use senolytics or calorie restriction protocols as part of your longevity protocols?	Y	N

Living longer has become an increasingly important topic in today's society due to the significant increase in human life expectancy. According to research, the human potential lifespan based on known biology is 120-150 years. (1) However, living longer has also come with a price. The risk of chronic diseases, disability, dementia, and advanced ageing prior to death has also increased. The paper 'Living Too Long' by Guy C. Brown discusses the challenges that come with living longer, as life expectancy is now up to an average of 73 years—six years longer than it was in 2000. (2) Multiple chronic conditions and preventable diseases are also becoming more common, and nearly 4 out of 5 Americans are living with them, according to a study published in Medical Care. (3)

As we grow older, we all want to maintain our vitality and live a fulfilling life. While the term "anti-ageing" may not be appealing, and can seem negative and even daunting, the idea of ageing well is one that we can all embrace. Everyone aspires to be healthy, both physically and mentally, and enjoy their lives until the end. This is where the concepts of healthspan and lifespan come into play. Although the terms are often used interchangeably, they have distinct meanings.

While the medical definition of healthspan refers to the period of time during which a person is free from disease and disability, many people may feel that this definition falls short of what they aspire to. After all, who wants to simply be free from disease and disability? We want to be able to continue to enjoy the things we love, maintain our independence, and engage with the world around us in a meaningful way.

Therefore, when we talk about healthspan, we are not just talking about avoiding illness or disability. Instead, we are talking about the period of time in which we are able to lead fulfilling lives, both physically and mentally. This includes not only being free from disease and disability, but also being able to maintain our cognitive abilities, emotional well-being, and social connections. The concept of healthspan recognizes that quality of life is just as important as the length of life.

But how do we ensure that we age well and maintain our healthspan? According to Dr. Peter Attia, it's all about backcasting. This means thinking about what we want to be doing at 70, 80, or 90 years old, and working backward from there. By measuring relevant biomarkers and taking proactive steps to set ourselves up for that life, we can increase our chances of ageing well.

In his book *Outlive: The Science and Art of Longevity,* Dr. Attia emphasizes that ageing can bring about a host of health challenges. (4) He identifies these challenges as The Four Horsemen of Death, which include diseases such as atherosclerotic cardiovascular disease (ASCVD), cancer, neurodegenerative diseases like Alzheimer's and dementia, and metabolic disease such as type 2 diabetes. These big four conditions are known to be major causes of morbidity and mortality in older adults. However, by gaining a deeper understanding of these challenges and adopting preventative measures to manage them, we can significantly improve our chances of ageing well and leading fulfilling and vibrant lives.

The Salutogenic Approach To Health

For years, the focus on health has predominantly revolved around the study of diseases rather than the study of health itself. However, the idea of salutogenesis in health promotion brings a refreshing perspective by directing our attention toward the factors that contribute to the creation and sustenance of health, instead of solely concentrating on disease prevention. The term 'salutogenesis'—derived from the Latin word for health, 'salus' and the Greek word for creation, 'genesis', was coined in the 1970s by medical sociologist Aaron Antonovsky. (5)

The salutogenic model of health emphasizes the importance of focusing on positive health outcomes, rather than simply trying to avoid negative outcomes. This model suggests that health is a dynamic process that can be influenced by a variety of factors and that we can take an active role in promoting our own health and well-being.

In this Section, we will focus exactly on this concept—what we can do to create health. Now, let us be blunt and say that you can't hack your way out of a poor diet, little sleep and no exercise. You have to do the work. You have to put in the effort, and implementing some of the key protocols outlined in the previous four Sections will help you to achieve optimal health and longevity.

Navigating The World Of Nutraceuticals—A Cautionary Tale

As we explore the realm of health and longevity optimization, it's important to exercise caution. While we'll be examining some of the latest biohacking tools and tests, we must be mindful not to rely solely on a "pill for every ill" approach commonly used in allopathic medicine. This caution extends to nutraceuticals as well, which can offer a plethora of benefits, but must not be seen as a substitute for crucial behavioural changes. We should prioritize fundamental lifestyle practices and use supplements only as a complement to our healthy habits.

We must also avoid the temptation of using supplements to address every symptom we encounter. Instead, we should use nutraceuticals in a targeted and strategic manner, with a clear understanding of how they fit into our overall approach to health. In other words, we should always strive for a balanced and integrated approach to optimizing our health, taking into account all factors that influence our well-being.

When it comes to longevity nutraceuticals, the market is flooded with supplements that claim to help us look and feel younger. While some of these supplements have a solid scientific foundation, others do not. At least not yet. Additionally, these supplements can quickly add up in cost, especially if they are taken over an extended period. Relying solely on supplements for longevity is not a sustainable solution. You don't want to end up starving yourself and living on supplements in the hope of living longer while being miserable doing it.

From DNA To Phenotype—The Intersection Of Genetics And Epigenetics

Genetics is the study of genes and their functions, including how genes are inherited from our parents and how they are expressed in an organism. Genes are the basic units of heredity, and they contain the instructions for making proteins, which are the building blocks of life. The DNA sequence of a gene determines the sequence of amino acids that make up a protein, and variations in the DNA sequence can result in changes to the protein's function.

Epigenetics, on the other hand, refers to changes in gene expression that are not caused by changes in the DNA sequence itself. Instead, epigenetic changes are modifications to the DNA molecule or to the proteins that package the DNA in the nucleus, which can affect the way genes are expressed. Epigenetic modifications can be inherited from one generation to the next and can be influenced by environmental factors such as diet, stress, and exposure to toxins.

Phenotype is the term used to describe an individual's physical appearance and behavioural characteristics, which are determined by a combination of genetics and the environment. The study of the way your environment and behaviours affect the way genes work and express themselves is called epigenetics.

Without getting too complex in explanation, epigenetic modifications encompass a range of processes that can affect gene expression without altering the underlying DNA sequence. These modifications can be grouped into several categories, including DNA methylation, histone modification, and RNA interference.

DNA methylation involves the addition of a methyl group to the DNA molecule, which can alter gene expression by inhibiting the binding of transcription factors or other regulatory proteins to the DNA. Histone modification refers to changes in the proteins that package the DNA in the nucleus, which can influence the accessibility of the DNA to the cellular machinery responsible for reading and transcribing the genetic information. Finally, RNA interference involves the regulation of gene expression by small RNA molecules that can bind to messenger RNA and inhibit translation, thereby reducing the production of specific proteins.

The Power Of Belief On Gene Expression

Dr. Bruce Lipton is a stem cell biologist and researcher who is known for his work in the field of epigenetics. He is best known for his book, *The Biology of Belief,* in which he presents his theories on the role of epigenetics in shaping human health and behaviour. (6)

According to Dr. Lipton, the environment, including the social and physical environment, plays a critical role in gene expression. He believes that our beliefs and attitudes can influence our health outcomes by altering our gene expression through epigenetic mechanisms. For example, he argues that negative beliefs and attitudes can activate stress responses in the body, which can lead to changes in gene expression that can ultimately result in disease.

Dr. Lipton's approach to genetics and epigenetics is based on the idea that our genes are not fixed, but rather can be influenced by environmental factors. He believes that we have much more control over our health outcomes than we might think and that by changing our beliefs and attitudes, we can influence our gene expression in positive ways.

While some of Dr. Lipton's ideas have been met with skepticism from some members of the scientific community; his work has undoubtedly contributed to a growing understanding of the complex interplay between genes, the environment, and human health. Hence it is essential to take responsibility for our daily habits instead of solely blaming our genes for poor health outcomes, and Dr. Lipton's work reminds us of the power of our thoughts and beliefs on our health.

Principles Of Longevity Medicine Simplified

Longevity medicine is a relatively new field that focuses on preventing or delaying age-related diseases and promoting healthy ageing. The principles of longevity medicine are grounded in the idea that there are several key factors that contribute to healthy ageing, and by focusing on these factors, we can increase our chances of living a longer, healthier life. Let's take a look into the four main categories:

Activate Hormesis—Hormesis is a term used to describe the beneficial effects that occur in response to stressors, such as exercise, caloric restriction, thermal therapy, and cognitive challenges. By subjecting the body to mild stressors, we can activate our body's natural defence mechanisms and promote cellular repair and regeneration. Some examples of hormetic activities include cardiovascular exercise, resistance training, sauna therapy, cold exposure, and mental challenges, such as learning a new language or playing a musical instrument.

Recovery And Sleep—Sleep is essential for healthy ageing. Deep, restful REM sleep and recovery from exercise are critical for repairing and rebuilding tissues, regulating hormones, and boosting immune function. Chronic sleep deprivation can lead to a host of health problems, including cognitive decline, obesity, diabetes, and cardiovascular disease. As discussed in Section 1—Sleep, Rest & Recovery, it is important to prioritize good sleep hygiene habits, such as sticking to a regular sleep schedule, creating a relaxing bedtime routine, and minimizing screen time before bed.

Protect DNA—DNA damage and oxidative stress are two of the leading causes of ageing and age-related diseases. To protect our DNA, we need to reduce our toxic load and free radicals, optimize liver and microbiome biotransformation, and optimize the ratio of antioxidants and free radicals. Some ways to reduce our toxic load and free radicals include eating a nutrient-dense diet, avoiding exposure to environmental toxins, and supplementing with antioxidants, such as vitamin C, vitamin E, and glutathione.

Find A Sense Of Purpose In Life—Having a sense of purpose in life has been linked to improved mental and physical health, as well as increased longevity. Finding purpose can involve family, work, personal goals, or relationships with friends. It is essential to identify what brings us joy and fulfilment and to pursue those activities or relationships regularly. A sense of purpose can help us maintain a positive outlook on life and give us a reason to get up in the morning.

Longevity medicine revolves around actively embracing measures to enhance healthy ageing. Although these principles may appear straightforward, they demand persistent effort and unwavering commitment to attain enduring outcomes. It becomes evident to the reader that the protocols outlined in the initial four chapters of this book embody each of these four principles.

Hormesis And Building Better Resilience

It's no secret that life can be challenging at times, and we all face obstacles that can leave us feeling drained and depleted. From environmental stressors to personal struggles, it is easy to become overwhelmed. But what if there was a way to not only overcome these challenges but actually grow stronger as a result?

As mentioned earlier, hormesis is a powerful concept that is all about using small, strategic doses of stress to stimulate growth and adaptation in the body and mind. Whether it's through targeted exercise routines, dietary changes, or other intentional practices, hormesis has the potential to transform our lives and help us thrive in the face of adversity. In other words, hormesis is the idea that what doesn't kill you makes you stronger. Furthermore, it can also be viewed as a mechanism that triggers healing and repair processes.

By intentionally pushing ourselves slightly beyond our comfort zones, we raise our resilience and improve our ability to cope with adversity. A key factor to building resilience is to focus on small, manageable goals that can be achieved over time. This will allow us to build momentum and experience small wins that can boost our confidence and motivation to continue to pursue our goals.

All areas of health—physical, mental, and emotional—work synergistically to create a state of overall well-being. When one area of health is compromised, it can affect all other areas and ultimately impact our ability to cope with stress and adversity. Building resilience is a journey, and each step you take is an opportunity to grow and learn, knowing that the challenges you face today will only make you stronger tomorrow.

The term resilience is defined as the ability to bounce back after a stressful encounter or adversity in life. Hormesis suggests that challenges that don't result in harmful effects can actually enhance resilience. As we age, a decline in biological resilience is a common occurrence, which means that older individuals may have a slower and less complete recovery after experiencing adverse events compared to their younger selves.

Want to find out how resilient you are? Take the resilience test: smartcuts .life/resilience-assessment.

Harnessing Hormesis—Incorporating Powerful Protocols Into Your Lifestyle

Throughout this book, we have presented several strategies for integrating hormesis into your daily routine. As a brief summary, we have compiled a list of some of these hormetic challenges along with some additional ones that can not only enhance your overall well-being but also foster resilience as you age.

Time-Restricted Eating (TRE) And Fasting—TRE involves restricting the time window in which you eat each day, typically to 8-12 hours, and fasting involves abstaining from food for extended periods of time, such as 16-24 hours or longer. Both of these practices have been shown to improve cellular repair mechanisms and increase resistance to future stressors.

High-Intensity Interval Training (HIIT) And Strength Training—Both HIIT and strength training involve exposing the body to physical stress, which can lead to increased muscle growth, improved cardiovascular function, and improved insulin sensitivity.

Cold Plunges And Saunas—Exposing the body to extreme temperatures from cold plunges and saunas can stimulate the production of cold and heat shock proteins and other cellular repair mechanisms.

Breathwork And Hypoxia Training—Controlled breathing techniques and exposure to low-oxygen environments such as the simulated altitude training described in Section 3—Movement, Exercise and Detoxification, can induce a state of hormesis by stimulating the production of reactive oxygen species (ROS) and other stress-response pathways.

When the body experiences low oxygen, a process called hypoxia occurs which can have both positive and negative effects. Hypoxia-inducible factor, a transcription factor that regulates the activity of certain genes, is produced in response to hypoxia and controls over 100 genes. Short bursts of low oxygen can trigger an adaptive hormetic response, while prolonged hypoxia, such as in obstructive sleep apnea, may accelerate ageing.

Similar to other stressors, low oxygen states impact the function of sirtuins, AMPK, and mTOR (which we will explain in greater detail further on), while also reducing inflammation and improving insulin sensitivity. Furthermore, low oxygen states can increase the production of stem cells and the formation of new blood vessels, aiding the body in obtaining more oxygen.

Light Therapy—Exposure to certain wavelengths of light, such as red or near-infrared light, can stimulate the production of mitochondrial ATP and enhance cellular repair mechanisms.

Hyperbaric Oxygen Therapy (HBOT)—HBOT involves exposing the body to high levels of oxygen under pressure, which can stimulate the production of new blood vessels, reduce inflammation, and enhance cellular repair mechanisms. Research has shown that hyperbaric oxygen therapy is the most effective medical intervention for targeting senescent cells and lengthening telomeres compared to other therapies. (7) Medical clinics are usually offering these therapies but there are now home units available.

Ozone Therapy—Medical ozone therapy is a popular treatment for a range of conditions such as infections, autoimmune diseases, and arthritis. This therapy exposes the body to ozone gas, which stimulates the production of antioxidants and activates stress-response pathways. This process can impact ageing. When administered, ozone produces ozonides, a compound that can kill microbes and viruses, modulate the immune system, reduce inflammation, improve red blood cell pliability, destroy free radicals, enhance mitochondrial function, and produce stem cells among many other effects. (8) Medical oxygen-ozone therapy is a potent hormetic therapy that can be administered in various ways, such as intravenously, intramuscularly, rectally, and topically.

SMART PROTOCOL

Hormetic Stressors - $0 to $$$

Depending on what you have access to and what your budget is, try to incorporate these hormetic stressors on a regular basis: time-restricted eating and fasting, high-intensity interval training and strength training, cold plunges and saunas, breathwork and hypoxia training, light therapy, hyperbaric oxygen and ozone therapy.

Phytohormesis—Leveraging Mother Nature's Stress For Longevity

Phytohormesis is a fascinating concept in the world of nutrition and longevity. It is the idea that when plants are exposed to stress, such as exposure to toxins or extreme temperatures, they produce compounds that can confer health benefits to those who consume them. By consuming these compounds, we can activate various longevity switches in our bodies, potentially leading to a longer and healthier life.

One of the most well-known compounds associated with phytohormesis is resveratrol, found in grapes and red wine. Resveratrol has been shown to activate sirtuins, a group of proteins that regulate various cellular processes related to ageing and disease. It is important to note that resveratrol is typically effective only when consumed in concentrated forms. Consuming large amounts of grapes or wine would not provide enough resveratrol to reap the benefits, making it infeasible to achieve the desired effects solely through dietary intake. Resveratrol is a fat-soluble compound that has been found to be more efficiently absorbed in the presence of other fats, such as oleic acid in olive oil, in order to achieve optimal absorption and effectiveness.

Other compounds associated with phytohormesis include allicin from garlic, capsaicin from peppers, sulforaphane from the broccoli family, curcumin from turmeric, anthocyanin from berries, quercetin and flavonoids from Himalayan Tartary buckwheat, onions, and apples, EGCG from green tea, oleuropein from extra virgin olive oil, and phenolic acids from mushrooms including shiitake, maitake, and lion's mane.

Phytohormesis is a promising concept in the world of nutrition and longevity, suggesting that consuming stressed plants can activate various longevity switches in our bodies. While more research is needed to fully understand the mechanisms behind these compounds and their effects on human health, incorporating a variety of phytohormetic foods into our diets can potentially lead to a longer and healthier life.

SMART PROTOCOL

Phytohormetic Foods - $ to $$

To reap the potential health benefits of phytohormesis, try incorporating small amounts of these phytonutrient-rich foods into your diet: red grapes, garlic, peppers, broccoli, turmeric, berries, onions, apples, green tea, olive oil, and mushrooms like shiitake, maitake, and lion's mane.

The 12 Hallmarks Of Ageing

The process of ageing is complex and multifaceted, and it is characterized by a number of physical, biological, and psychological changes that occur over time. These changes, known as the "hallmarks of ageing," are thought to be the underlying mechanisms behind the gradual decline in function and increased susceptibility to diseases that are commonly associated with getting older.

Various models of ageing have been proposed, but for the sake of simplicity in this Section, we will concentrate on the most widely accepted and recognized framework. In 2013, a paper titled, '*The Hallmarks of Aging,*' was published by renowned researchers Dr. Lenny Guarente, Dr. Jan van Deursen, and Dr. Jan Hoeijmakers. This paper identified and described nine hallmarks of ageing, which are now widely recognized as fundamental concepts in the field of ageing research. (9)

1. **Genomic Instability**—This refers to the accumulation of DNA damage over time, which can lead to the development of mutations and chromosomal abnormalities. These changes can disrupt the normal functioning of cells and increase the risk of cancer and other age-related diseases.
2. **Telomere Attrition**—Telomeres are the protective caps on the ends of chromosomes that help to maintain genomic stability. As we age, the telomeres become shorter, leading to a decline in the stability and function of our DNA.
3. **Epigenetic Alterations**—Epigenetic changes refer to changes in the way that our genes are expressed without altering the underlying DNA sequence. These changes can occur as a result of environmental factors such as diet, stress, and exposure to toxins, and they can have a significant impact on the ageing process.
4. **Loss Of Proteostasis**—Proteostasis refers to the balance of protein synthesis, folding, and degradation in the cell. As we age, this balance becomes disrupted, leading to the accumulation of misfolded proteins and the development of protein aggregates that can contribute to age-related diseases.
5. **Deregulated Nutrient Sensing**—Nutrient sensing refers to the way that cells sense and respond to changes in the availability of nutrients in the environment. As we age, the ability of cells to accurately sense and respond to changes in nutrient availability becomes impaired, leading to changes in metabolism and energy production.
6. **Mitochondrial Dysfunction**—Mitochondria are the powerhouses of the cell, responsible for producing the energy that cells need to

function. As we age, the mitochondria become less efficient and more prone to damage, leading to a decline in energy production and an increased risk of age-related diseases.

7. **Cellular Senescence**—Cellular senescence is the process by which cells stop dividing and become unable to perform their normal functions. As we age, the number of senescent cells in our bodies increases, leading to a decline in tissue and organ function.
8. **Stem Cell Exhaustion**—Stem cells are responsible for producing new cells and repairing damaged tissue. As we age, the number and function of stem cells decline, leading to a decline in the ability of tissues and organs to regenerate and repair themselves.
9. **Altered Intercellular Communication**—Intercellular communication refers to the way that cells communicate with each other and coordinate their activities. As we age, the ability of cells to communicate with each other becomes impaired, leading to changes in tissue and organ function.

More recently, 3 additional hallmarks have been recognized for their impact on ageing. (10)

1. **Chronic Inflammation Or "Inflammaging"**—Inflammaging is a chronic, low-grade inflammation that occurs as we age, characterized by immune cell activation and the production of pro-inflammatory cytokines. It is caused by factors like damaged cells, environmental stressors, genetics, and lifestyle.
2. **Disabled Macroautophagy**—Disabled macroautophagy refers to the impairment or dysfunction of the process of autophagy, which is responsible for removing cellular waste products. While autophagy was initially considered a component of proteostasis, it is now recognized as a significant factor in its own right. The decline in effective autophagy is a major contributor to the reduced turnover of organelles and an accelerant of the ageing process.
3. **Dysbiosis**—Dysbiosis refers to the imbalance in the composition and

function of the gut microbiota. The ageing process is accompanied by alterations in the gut microbiota, characterized by a decline in microbial diversity and an imbalance between beneficial and harmful bacteria. It is associated with a higher susceptibility to infections, increased inflammation, and a decline in nutrient absorption. Disruptions in gut barrier function, immune system dysregulation, and altered microbial metabolism all contribute to the dysbiotic state.

Activating Longevity—Direct And Indirect Interventions For Ageing

Ageing is an inevitable part of life, but it doesn't have to mean a decline in health and vitality. There are lifestyle, dietary, and clinical interventions that can, directly and indirectly, impact the ageing process by either activating longevity genes or preventing the pathophysiology of ageing.

Direct Activation Of Longevity Genes With Nutrient Sensors

One of the ways we can directly impact the ageing process is by activating some of the longevity genes responsible for regulating various cellular processes that are involved in ageing. One emerging area of research that holds promise in activating these longevity genes and promoting healthy ageing is the utilization of nutrient sensors. Nutrient sensors are specialized molecular systems within our cells that detect and respond to the availability of various nutrients and energy sources. These sensors play a crucial role in regulating cellular processes and can influence the activity of longevity genes such as SIRT, mTOR, and AMPK. Through the activation of nutrient sensors, we can modulate the signalling pathways associated with these longevity genes.

SIRT—Sirtuins are a family of proteins that play a crucial role in regulating cellular metabolism and stress response. By activating SIRT genes, we can increase our cellular defences against oxidative stress and inflammation, which are two key drivers of ageing. Sirtuins can be influenced by the availability of key nutrients like NAD+ (nicotinamide adenine dinucleotide). NAD+ acts as a coenzyme in cellular reactions and is involved in various metabolic processes. (11)

mTOR—Mammalian target of rapamycin (mTOR) is a protein that regulates cellular metabolism and growth. By inhibiting mTOR activity, we can reduce the rate of cellular ageing and extend lifespan.

AMPK—AMP-activated protein kinase (AMPK) is a metabolic sensor that regulates energy metabolism and stress response. By activating AMPK, we can improve mitochondrial function and reduce the risk of age-related diseases.

Both mTOR and AMPK are nutrient-sensitive kinases that regulate cellular metabolism and energy balance. Nutrient sensors help monitor the levels of nutrients, such as amino acids and glucose and influence the activity of these kinases accordingly. Researchers are exploring strategies to target these sensors to promote healthy ageing. (12)

Modulating nutrient-sensor signalling pathways through diet, exercise, or potentially developing specific interventions can offer new avenues to activate the longevity genes and extend healthspan, reducing the risks associated with age-related diseases.

Pillars Of Longevity Through Physical Health

The importance of physical fitness and preserving muscle mass and function as we age cannot be overstated. One of the significant changes that occur is the degradation of type 2 muscle fibres, also known as fast twitch muscles. These muscles are responsible for generating quick and powerful movements, such as jumping and explosive activities. As we age, the decline in these fast twitch muscles leads to a decrease in speed, strength, and size, which can have a significant impact on our physical abilities and overall quality of life.

In Section 3—Movement, Exercise & Detoxification, we detailed methodologies to balance all aspects of physical fitness. To counteract the effects of ageing on muscle health and reduce the likelihood of falls, it becomes crucial to focus on specific aspects of physical fitness. The following pillars of longevity through physical health play a vital role in maintaining strength, stability, and aerobic efficiency:

Strength—Building and preserving muscle strength is essential for maintaining mobility and functional independence as we age. Engaging in resistance training, such as weightlifting, bodyweight exercises, or resistance band workouts, can help stimulate muscle growth and enhance overall strength. Regular strength training is especially important for perimenopausal women, as it is vital for supporting bone density and reducing the risk of osteoporosis.

Stability—Balance and stability are crucial for preventing falls and injuries, especially in older adults. Balance exercises, such as standing on one leg, yoga, or tai chi, can improve stability and proprioception, reducing the risk of falling.

Aerobic Efficiency—Aerobic exercise is essential for maintaining cardiovascular health and improving the efficiency of oxygen utilization by the body. Regular aerobic activities like brisk walking, jogging, swimming, or cycling can enhance heart and lung function, leading to increased overall endurance and better energy levels.

Aerobic Peak Output/VO2 max—VO2 max is the maximum amount of oxygen that an individual can utilize during intense exercise. As we age, our VO2 max tends to decline, affecting our capacity to perform high-intensity activities. Engaging in interval training and high-intensity interval workouts can help maintain and potentially improve VO2 max, thereby enhancing aerobic peak output.

In addition to the above pillars, it is essential to address the importance of including jumping and landing safely. Jumping and landing exercises help improve muscular power, coordination, and proprioception, which are crucial for maintaining agility and reducing the risk of injuries related to falls. When done correctly and progressively, these exercises can improve bone density and reduce the impact of age-related muscle loss.

SMART CONSIDERATION

Exercise To Reverse Ageing And Boost Health At The Cellular Level

Optimizing biological systems can be achieved through exercise by choosing the right dose, type, and frequency. This can lead to improvements in the function and health of the microbiome, immune system, mitochondria, and hormonal balance. Exercise also enhances detoxification, blood circulation, and lymphatic flow.

Furthermore, exercise has been found to impact the hallmarks of ageing, such as increasing telomere length, reducing inflammation, improving mitochondrial health, and reversing harmful epigenetic changes. For instance, exercising depletes energy in muscles and organs, activating AMPK which improves insulin sensitivity and inhibits mTOR, leading to autophagy and cellular clean-up. Additionally, exercise activates the sirtuin pathway for DNA repair and reduces inflammation. The slight bump in oxidative stress triggered by exercise leads to the activation of antioxidant enzymes. The benefits of exercise for health and longevity are well-documented in scientific research.

Indirect Activation Of Genes That Prevent The Pathophysiology Of Ageing

In addition to directly activating longevity genes, we can also indirectly prevent the pathophysiology of ageing by activating genes that regulate cellular processes that are involved in ageing. Some of the key cellular processes that we can target include mitochondrial homeostasis, DNA protection, cellular signalling, and cell responsiveness.

Mitochondria Homeostasis—Mitochondria are the powerhouses of our cells, responsible for producing energy in the form of ATP. As we age, the function of our mitochondria declines. By activating genes that regulate mitochondrial homeostasis, we can improve mitochondrial function and reduce the risk of age-related diseases. One essential coenzyme that plays a significant role in mitochondrial function and overall cellular energy metabolism is Nicotinamide adenine dinucleotide (NAD+). NAD+ is crucial for mitochondrial function and helps regulate the activity of enzymes that are involved in energy production.

DNA Protection—As mentioned earlier, DNA damage is a key driver of ageing and age-related diseases. By activating genes that protect our DNA, we can reduce the risk of mutations and cellular dysfunction that can contribute to ageing.

Cellular Signalling—Cellular signalling pathways play a critical role in regulating cellular metabolism, stress response, and ageing. By activating genes that regulate cellular signalling, we can improve cellular communication and reduce the risk of age-related diseases.

The insulin/insulin-like growth factor signalling (IIS) pathway is one of these important cellular signalling pathways that play a key role in the regulation of growth, metabolism, and ageing. It is activated by the hormones insulin and insulin-like growth factor (IGF), which bind to their respective receptors on the surface of cells. This activates a series of intracellular signalling pathways that lead to the activation of various transcription factors, which in turn regulate the expression of genes involved in a variety of biological processes. The IIS pathway plays a central role in the regulation of glucose homeostasis, and its dysregulation has been implicated in a number of diseases, including diabetes and cancer. (13)

Cell Responsiveness—Cellular responsiveness refers to the ability of our cells to respond to stressors and maintain homeostasis. By activating genes that improve cell responsiveness, we can improve our cellular defences against ageing and age-related diseases.

An important example of such cell responsiveness is Nrf2 (Nuclear factor erythroid 2-related factor 2). Nrf2 is a protein, specifically a transcription factor, that is activated by a variety of stimuli, including oxidative stress, inflammation, and certain chemicals and drugs. When activated, Nrf2 binds to specific DNA sequences called Antioxidant Response Elements (AREs) and promotes the expression of genes involved in antioxidant and detoxification pathways. Studies have suggested that activating Nrf2 may have therapeutic potential in a variety of diseases, including neurodegenerative diseases, cancer, and cardiovascular disease. (14) Activating Nrf2 has been shown to have antioxidant and anti-inflammatory effects and may help to protect against the development of these and other diseases.

Ageing is a complex process that is influenced by many different factors. By directly activating longevity genes and indirectly preventing the pathophysiology of ageing, we can slow down the ageing process and reduce the risk of age-related diseases.

Nutraceuticals That Impact Longevity Genes And Pathways

Nutraceuticals, as mentioned in previous Sections, are natural compounds found in and derived from foods that have potential health benefits, including impacting longevity genes and pathways.

Let's start with the nutraceuticals that affect the sirtuin gene, they are resveratrol, curcumin, green tea EGCG, emodin (rhubarb), NMN (nicotinamide mononucleotide) and NR (nicotinamide riboside). We will discuss NMN, and NR in more detail a bit later.

What about nutraceuticals for the other longevity pathways? The mTOR pathway can be influenced by quercetin, coffee flavonoids, magnesium, and alpha-ketoglutarate. The AMPK pathway can be affected by resveratrol, curcumin, berberine, rose hips, burdock root, alpha-lipoic acid, and EGCG. Berberine, curcumin, and resveratrol can impact the IIS gene. And finally, the Nrf2 pathway can be influenced by EGCG, sulforaphane, curcumin, black pepper, NAC, quercetin, resveratrol and pomegranate.

Again, let's reinforce that we do not want to end up taking a million supplements. Rather, we should carefully consider what we want to include in our longevity plan and prioritize lifestyle protocols whenever feasible.

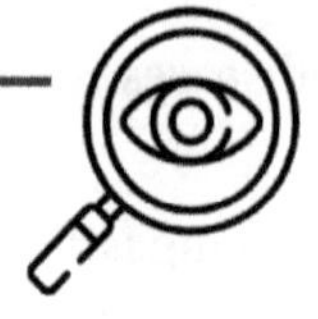

SMART CONSIDERATION

Kaufmann Anti-Ageing Protocol

Many professionals are dedicated to the study of anti-ageing medicine and longevity. Dr. Sandra Kauffmann, author of *The Kaufmann Protocol: Why We Age and How to Stop It*, is recognized for her work on the science of ageing and her efforts to educate the public about age-related cellular decay and the potential ways to slow or prevent it. Her protocol aims to slow down ageing and potentially prolong human life by targeting seven key aspects of ageing that involve cellular function. Unlike focusing on symptoms, Dr. Kaufmann's approach addresses the root causes of ageing, offering potential benefits for both lifespan and quality of life. The protocol encompasses lifestyle adjustments, dietary changes, and specific supplements. (15) For more information on more in-depth supplementation for ageing, you can explore her protocols at kaufmannprotocol.com. While Dr. Kaufmann's work is highly regarded by some, it's important to note that the field of anti-ageing medicine is still in its developmental stages. While the strategies proposed in the *Kaufmann Protocol* may show beneficial effects, ongoing research is necessary to determine the extent to which they can slow ageing or extend life.

Known Factors That Impact Longevity—Environment, Diet, And Lifestyle

Throughout this book, we have already extensively discussed several recognized factors that impact longevity. From the significance of exercise, maintaining muscle mass and strength, the crucial role of a nutrient-rich diet that minimizes inflammation, to the harmful effects of environmental toxins, and the value of social connections and a sense of purpose, there are additional factors that merit attention.

Body Composition And Mass Index (BMI)—Maintaining a healthy body weight is crucial for promoting longevity. Both high and low body mass index (BMI) values can be detrimental to overall health and increase the risk of chronic diseases like heart disease, diabetes, and certain cancers. To optimize health outcomes, it is essential to strike a healthy balance by following a nutritious diet and engaging in regular exercise. While BMI can be a useful tool for assessing body weight, it may not provide the most accurate measurement of body composition. As mentioned in Section 3—Movement, Exercise & Longevity, an alternative method for assessing body fat and muscle mass is through a DEXA scan, which is considered a more precise method for determining body composition.

Tobacco Use—Smoking and other forms of tobacco use are major risk factors for chronic diseases and premature death. Quitting smoking can be one of the most important things you can do to improve your health and extend your lifespan.

Alcohol Use—While there are studies suggesting that alcohol consumption can have some health benefits, it is crucial to be mindful of the amount and frequency of alcohol consumption. Research indicates that various aspects of alcohol use, including the volume of alcohol consumed and heavy drinking sessions are linked to an increase in chronic diseases and can have a significant impact on health. (16)

Polypharmacy—Taking multiple medications, or polypharmacy, can also impact our health and longevity. It's important to work with your healthcare provider to minimize the number of medications you take and ensure that they are all necessary and beneficial.

How Do We Test For Health In Ageing?

How can we check if we're healthy and ageing well? Sure, we can go for our regular check-ups with our family doctor, but those basic tests only tell us so much. It's important to be careful because sometimes those tests might say we have a "clean bill of health" when actually there could be some hidden issues that haven't been checked. Also, depending on where we live, those extra tests might not be so easy to get access to and can be expensive. At the end of the day, it's up to us to decide how much we're willing to spend and invest in finding out more about our health.

A comprehensive annual wellness exam should involve a detailed history and physical examination, as well as various validated questionnaires, in-office tests, and routine blood tests.

During a comprehensive annual wellness exam, several validated questionnaires are often used to evaluate a patient's cognitive abilities, functional status, and mental health. These questionnaires may include the Montreal Cognitive Assessment (MOCA), the Katz Activities of Daily Living (ADL) Index, and the Montgomery-Asberg Depression Rating Scale (MADRS). Additionally, the Adverse Childhood Experience (ACE) and Perceived Stress Scale (PSS) can be used to assess the impact of stressful experiences on an individual's mental and physical health. Together, these questionnaires provide a thorough evaluation of a patient's overall health and well-being.

In-office tests that may be conducted during a comprehensive annual wellness exam include blood pressure and resting heart rate measurements, Ankle-Brachial Index (ABI) testing, electrocardiograms (ECG), and spirometry. These tests can provide valuable information about a patient's cardiovascular and respiratory health.

Routine blood tests are an important part of a comprehensive annual wellness exam and may include a general profile, Comprehensive Metabolic Panel (CMP-14), Complete Blood Count (CBC) with differential, thyroid panel, HbA1c, 25-Hydroxy vitamin D, iron panel, and RBC magnesium. A cardiac profile may also be conducted which may include a lipid panel with risk ratio, lipid particle size, apolipoproteins— apo A, apo B, and apo E, APOE genes, oxidized LDL, C-reactive protein, homocysteine, MMP-9, fibrinogen, and TMAO. A hormone profile and immune profile could also be conducted during the exam, which may include a T- and B-cell panel and total immunoglobulins.

Specialized tests, including the Grail multi-cancer early detection test, Fecal Immunochemical Test (FIT), and FIT-fecal DNA (Cologuard), can be administered as required. Furthermore, imaging studies such as CT coronary artery calcium scoring, which assesses calcified plaques, and the Cleerly heart test, which evaluates both calcified and soft plaque in the coronary arteries, along with NeuroQuant MRI and whole-body MRI, may be performed as well. (17)

SMART PROTOCOL

Comprehensive Annual Wellness Exam - $0 to $$$

Decide on what tests you would like to add to your annual wellness routine. Cost and accessibility are the main two factors. While state/provincial healthcare systems and insured healthcare may have limitations on the tests they can provide, seeking guidance from a functional medicine practitioner and/or naturopathic doctor can help you find labs that offer the tests you need. These alternative healthcare providers can also assist you in navigating any potential insurance coverage or out-of-pocket costs associated with the tests.

SMART TOOLS

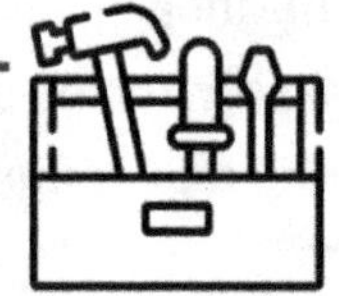

InsideTracker

InsideTracker is a personalized health and wellness platform that uses blood and DNA analysis to provide insights into a person's health and performance. The platform was founded in 2009 by a team of scientists, physicians, and nutritionists, and it has since grown to become a popular tool among athletes, health enthusiasts, and individuals who are interested in optimizing their overall health. The InsideTracker platform offers various plans that include blood tests that test up to 47 biomarkers for health, including ApoB, cholesterol, glucose, cortisol, and many more for a complete and holistic analysis of your health. The results of these tests are then used to create a personalized health and wellness plan, which includes recommendations for nutrition, exercise, and other lifestyle factors.

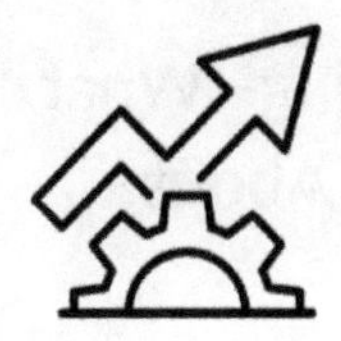

SMART UPGRADES

Brain SPECT

There are brain mapping tools that can evaluate the brain's activity and help identify areas that require attention. Brain SPECT (Single Photon Emission Computed Tomography) is a type of neuroimaging technology that uses nuclear medicine to evaluate blood flow and activity in the brain. It allows physicians to see areas of the brain that are working well, working too hard, and not working hard enough. Brain SPECT has been used to study a range of conditions including Alzheimer's disease, seizures, strokes, head trauma, chemical exposure, Lyme disease, brain inflammation, and drug toxicity. Research has shown that adding a brain SPECT scan to a psychiatric evaluation can change the diagnosis and treatment plan in many cases. (18) Dr. Daniel Amen is a physician, psychiatrist, and founder of Amen Clinics, which specializes in the treatment of brain-related disorders. Dr. Amen's work has garnered a significant following, and he continues to be a leading voice in the field of brain health and psychiatry. To learn more about his approach and use of Brain SPECT technology, please visit amenclinics.com.

Single Nucleotide Polymorphisms (SNPs) Testing—What It Is, How It Works, And What It Can Tell You About Your Health

You may be familiar with genetic testing as a means to find relatives. In fact, our DNA, which is composed of nucleotides, contains the information necessary to trace our family tree by examining the unique order of these building blocks. But genetic testing offers more than just genealogy. For instance, functional genomics is a field that explores the function and regulation of genes, providing insights into complex traits and diseases by analyzing gene expression, protein interactions, and other genomic data. Additionally, we can use genetic testing to detect single nucleotide polymorphisms (SNPs), which are variations in individual nucleotides. These SNPs, occurring about once in every 100 to 300 nucleotides, can be considered little errors or changes in our genetic code and can happen anywhere in the genome. (19)

As we mentioned in Section 3—Movement, Exercise & Detoxification, SNPs can have a wide range of effects on individual biology. Some SNPs have been linked to differences in susceptibility to certain diseases, such as cancer, heart disease, and diabetes. Other SNPs can affect an individual's response to drugs, such as altering the way a drug is metabolized or affecting how it interacts with its target in the body. Additionally, some SNPs may be associated with differences in overall health outcomes, such as lifespan, cognitive function, and immune function.

The impact of SNPs on an individual's health can be influenced by many factors, including environmental exposures, lifestyle, and other genetic variations. Additionally, just because a person has a particular SNP does not necessarily mean that they will develop a certain condition or disease. Given the widespread occurrence of SNPs in the human genome, they have become an important focus of genetic research aimed at understanding the underlying causes of various diseases and developing personalized treatments based on an individual's genetic makeup.

Here are a few SNPs that are commonly measured due to their high clinical relevance:

The MTHFR genes have been linked to an increased risk of heart disease, stroke, and certain cancers. (20) MTHFR is involved in the methylation cycle, which is a process that helps regulate the levels of certain neurotransmitters and hormones. Individuals with variations in the MTHFR gene may have a decreased ability to process folic acid, which can lead to an increased risk of certain health conditions.

The GST/GPX genes are involved in the detoxification of harmful substances in the body. Variations in these genes have been linked to an increased risk of certain cancers and neurological disorders. (21) GST/GPX is vital in protecting the body from oxidative stress, which can lead to cell damage and increased risk of disease.

The COMT gene provides instructions for making an enzyme that breaks down certain neurotransmitters, including dopamine and norepinephrine. Variations in this gene have been linked to differences in cognitive function and the risk of psychiatric disorders. (22) Individuals with variations in the COMT gene may have a decreased ability to process certain neurotransmitters, which can lead to an increased risk of certain health conditions.

The MAOA gene provides instructions for making an enzyme that breaks down certain neurotransmitters, including serotonin and norepinephrine. Variations in this gene have been linked to an increased risk of certain psychiatric disorders, including depression and anxiety. MAOA plays a critical role in regulating the levels of certain neurotransmitters and maintaining good mental health. (23)

The NOS3 gene provides instructions for making an enzyme that is involved in the regulation of blood pressure and the control of blood flow. Variations in this gene have been linked to an increased risk of cardiovascular disease, including heart attacks and stroke. (24) NOS3 is instrumental in regulating blood pressure and maintaining good cardiovascular health.

The PEMT gene provides instructions for making an enzyme that is involved in the production of phosphatidylcholine, a type of fat molecule found in cell membranes. Variations in this gene have been linked to an increased risk of certain liver diseases and fatty liver. (25) PEMT is fundamental in maintaining the health of the liver and protecting it from disease.

The DAO gene provides instructions for making an enzyme that breaks down histamine, a substance that is involved in the immune response and the regulation of blood pressure. Variations in this gene have been linked to an increased risk of certain allergies and certain autoimmune disorders. (26) DAO plays a crucial role in regulating the levels of histamine and protecting the body from disease.

The APOE gene encodes a protein involved in the metabolism of lipids (fats) in the body. This gene has three common alleles, known as ApoE2, ApoE3, and ApoE4. Each person inherits two copies of the ApoE gene, one from each parent. Studies have shown that the ApoE4 allele is associated with an increased risk of developing Alzheimer's disease and other age-related cognitive impairments. (27)

The SOD2 gene provides instructions for making an enzyme that helps protect cells from damage caused by free radicals. Variations in this gene have been linked to an increased risk of certain cancers and cardiovascular disease.

SNPs can be analyzed through various tests, including genotyping, DNA sequencing, array-based genotyping, and next-generation sequencing (NGS). There are many platforms combining educational tools, protocols and nutritional supplements designed to help easily translate, identify and address SNPs. These platforms enable you to test, translate and target SNPs you carry to allow for more precise and customized nutrition and lifestyle recommendations that are tailored to your needs.

SMART PROTOCOL

SNPs Testing - $$

There are two main ways to access your SNPs information. The first option involves using a company like 23andMe to obtain your raw data which can then be analyzed using various other platforms to gain further insights into your genetic makeup. The second option is to use companies that provide private direct-to-consumer SNP testing services. These companies offer the ability to analyze your genetic information and provide personalized genetic analysis based on your SNPs. For more information on such companies and platforms refer to the Smart Resources at the end of this Section.

The Anti-Ageing Duo—Autophagy And Senolytics

Researchers are currently exploring various methods to counteract the negative effects of ageing, such as targeting cellular processes that contribute to maintaining cell health and preventing age-related diseases. (28) Among these methods, two have gained particular attention: autophagy and senolytics. Both of these processes play crucial roles in maintaining cellular equilibrium and promoting healthy ageing. Autophagy is a natural cellular mechanism that breaks down and recycles old or damaged cellular components, while senolytics are compounds that selectively eliminate senescent cells as these cells can lead to age-related ailments. Together, these approaches may offer the potential to delay the ageing process and promote healthier ageing overall.

Autophagy is essential for maintaining cellular homeostasis, preventing the accumulation of toxic substances, and promoting cellular health. Autophagy is a highly regulated process that involves the sequestration of cellular components into double-membrane structures called autophagosomes, which then fuse with lysosomes to break down the contents into their constituent parts. You can think of autophagy as a sort of clean-up crew, working to remove damaged proteins and organelles in the body.

Senolytics, on the other hand, are compounds that selectively kill senescent cells. Senescent cells are cells that have stopped dividing and are in a state of permanent growth arrest, meaning they are no longer able to divide and replicate like normal cells. Senescence is a natural process that occurs as a response to various types of cellular stress, such as DNA damage, oxidative stress, and telomere shortening, which occurs during each round of cell division. However, when these senescent cells accumulate in the body over time, they can contribute to age-related diseases, such as osteoarthritis, atherosclerosis, and Alzheimer's disease. Senolytics work by targeting specific pathways that are activated in senescent cells, causing them to undergo cell death.

While autophagy and senolytics are both involved in the ageing process and have potential anti-ageing effects, they operate through different mechanisms. Autophagy promotes cellular health by removing damaged or unwanted components, while senolytics eliminate senescent cells that contribute to age-related diseases. Both autophagy and senolytics have been studied for their potential to promote healthy ageing and prevent age-related diseases, and ongoing research is exploring how these processes may work together to promote cellular health and longevity. (29)

Promoting autophagy can be accomplished through a range of strategies, with caloric restriction and intermittent fasting being among the most well-known. However, it's important to note that for individuals aged 50 and above who prioritize muscle mass preservation, longer fasting periods may not be advisable as they could potentially have counterproductive effects. In the case of cancer or other serious medical conditions, it is crucial to consult with a medical expert to consider the clinical goals of triggering autophagy and manage them effectively.

Other autophagy strategies include regular exercise, dietary interventions like low-carbohydrate or ketogenic diets, consuming natural compounds such as curcumin, quercetin, berberine, and spermidine, and incorporating a diet rich in phytochemicals from fruits, vegetables, and herbs. Additionally, recent research has highlighted the potential of spermidine, a lesser-known compound found in certain foods and available as a supplement, to improve lifespan and healthspan by up to 25%. (30)

SMART UPGRADES

Rejuvenate Naturally—Senolytic Supplements

Regarding senolytics, numerous reputable companies offer natural senolytic supplement regimens. Some of these supplements are designed for short-term use, taken just a few days monthly, while others suggest a daily dose in smaller quantities for consistent removal of senescent cells. As research in this field continues to unfold, the choice of senolytic supplements should be made based on your individual health goals. Here are two that we suggest:

Qualia Senolytics is a senolytic supplement protocol from the company Neurohacker Collective, which combines natural ingredients, including adaptogens like Longvida Optimized Curcumin® and piperlongumine, with herbal tonics, polyphenols, and Senactiv® to support mitochondrial health, increase endurance, and protect against oxidative stress. The supplement is designed to be taken for two days every month.

InfiniWell is another company that offers a natural senolytic supplement protocol that includes a combination of fisetin, quercetin, curcumin, and piperine, which have been shown to selectively target and eliminate senescent cells. Designed for implementation over several weeks, the protocol aims to enhance overall health and diminish the chances of age-related diseases.

How Caloric Restriction (CR) And Fasting Mimicking Diet Could Be The Key To A Longer Life

We could not talk about autophagy without mentioning caloric restriction or the fasting-mimicking diet. Calorie restriction is a dietary strategy that involves reducing the number of calories consumed while maintaining adequate nutrition. This approach has been studied extensively for its potential to extend lifespan and promote healthspan, which is the period of life free from age-related diseases.

Research has shown that CR can increase the lifespan of many species, including rodents, dogs, and primates. In humans, studies have suggested that CR may improve health outcomes such as cardiovascular health, cognitive function, and reduced inflammation, which are all important factors for healthy ageing. (31) One theory behind why CR may be effective in extending lifespan is that it reduces oxidative stress and inflammation in the body. By consuming fewer calories, the body produces less metabolic waste, which can lead to a decrease in inflammation and oxidative damage. This reduction in damage may help to slow down the ageing process and delay the onset of age-related diseases.

CR has also been shown to improve cellular health by increasing autophagy, which is the process by which cells break down and recycle damaged components. This can help reduce the accumulation of damaged molecules in the body and improve overall cellular function.

However, extreme calorie restriction can lead to malnutrition, which can have serious health consequences. While experimenting with CR can provide benefits as a preventative measure for increasing longevity, special consideration must be made for elderly individuals, especially those with frailty. Appetite naturally decreases as we age, and those of advanced years must be aware of consuming adequate high-quality protein and calories for proper body functioning.

Fasting mimicking diet (FMD) has emerged as a popular dietary regimen due to its potential health benefits. This regimen involves adhering to a low-calorie, low-protein, and low-carbohydrate diet for several days, with the goal of replicating the physiological effects of fasting without abstaining from food entirely. Valter Longo, a renowned expert in FMD, is a Professor of Gerontology and Biological Sciences at the University of Southern California, as well as the Director of the Longevity Institute. Longo's extensive research and numerous studies on FMD have cemented his authority in this field. (32)

FMD has been shown to activate the autophagy process and studies have also suggested that FMD can improve metabolic markers such as blood glucose levels, insulin sensitivity, and cholesterol levels. (33) It may also lead to weight loss, although this may vary depending on the individual's starting weight and other factors.

FMD typically involves following a specific meal plan for five consecutive days, which includes consuming low-calorie soups, broths, and energy bars designed to provide the body with the necessary nutrients while keeping calorie intake low. After the five days, individuals can return to their regular diet, although some may choose to repeat the FMD cycle periodically for ongoing health benefits. Dr. Longo has developed and patented a commercial FMD program called ProLon, which is a pre-packaged meal kit designed to make the FMD process easier and more convenient for individuals.

SMART PROTOCOL

Caloric Restriction/Fasting Mimicking Diet And Senolytics - $ to $$

Explore implementing caloric restriction or a fasting-mimicking diet on a quarterly or yearly basis. Additionally, it may be beneficial to investigate senolytic protocols and determine which approach and companies align with your specific needs and goals.

The Link Between Dietary Habits And Longevity

While we would all love to be told the magic formula to stop the ill effects of ageing in its tracks, that simply isn't possible. There is no one-size-fits-all approach to any aspect of our health, and individual healthspan and longevity are no exception. There is no one diet that has been shown to reduce ageing, but over the past decade, there have been numerous studies conducted on the diets of certain populations of people who have the highest number of centenarians per capita. Dubbed "Blue Zones", these are regions of the world where people live significantly longer and healthier lives compared to other parts of the world. These areas have been studied by researchers to understand the factors that contribute to their longevity.

The term "Blue Zones" was first coined by Dan Buettner, a National Geographic Fellow, who identified five regions of the world where people live exceptionally long lives. (34) These regions are:

1. Okinawa, Japan
2. Sardinia, Italy
3. Nicoya, Costa Rica
4. Ikaria, Greece
5. Loma Linda, California (a community of Seventh-day Adventists)

Research has shown that people in these regions have certain lifestyle factors in common that contribute to their longevity. These factors include a plant-based diet with small amounts of meat and dairy, regular physical activity through daily routines, strong social connections and community, a sense of purpose and fulfillment, and stress reduction strategies.

Studies have shown that people in Blue Zones not only live longer, but also have lower rates of chronic diseases such as heart disease, diabetes, and cancer. In addition, their mental health and cognitive function also tend to be better.

The study of longevity is a complex field where multiple factors come into play, such as the environment, stressors, and genetics. It's crucial to acknowledge that the topic is far from being black and white, as it involves intricate interactions and dependencies among these variables.

Age Gracefully—Understanding The Two Types Of Ageing And How To Slow The Clock

Intrinsic and extrinsic ageing are two different processes that contribute to the overall ageing of the human body. Intrinsic ageing, also known as chronological ageing, refers to the natural, inevitable process of ageing that occurs over time, regardless of external factors. It is largely determined by genetics and is characterized by a gradual decline in the body's ability to repair and regenerate cells, tissues, and organs. Intrinsic ageing is associated with the progressive deterioration of body systems, such as the cardiovascular, respiratory, and immune systems, and the increased risk of age-related diseases, such as cancer, Alzheimer's disease, and osteoporosis.

Extrinsic ageing, on the other hand, refers to ageing that is influenced by external factors, such as environmental exposures, lifestyle choices, and other external stressors. These factors can accelerate the ageing process by causing damage to the body's cells, tissues, and organs, and by interfering with the body's natural repair mechanisms. Extrinsic ageing is often characterized by visible signs of ageing, such as wrinkles, age spots, and sagging skin, which are largely caused by exposure to ultraviolet (UV) radiation from the sun, pollution, smoking, and other environmental factors.

While both intrinsic and extrinsic ageing contribute to the overall ageing process, the degree to which they affect our individual ageing trajectory can vary depending on a variety of factors, including genetics, lifestyle choices, and environmental exposures. As such, it is important to adopt healthy lifestyle habits, such as regular exercise, a balanced diet, and avoiding harmful environmental exposures, in order to promote healthy ageing and reduce the risk of age-related diseases.

Discover Your TruAge—Innovative Blood Test Reveals Your Biological Age

Considering the intricate interplay between intrinsic and extrinsic ageing, it's no wonder that researchers and individuals alike are increasingly seeking ways to better understand and manage the ageing process. This desire has given rise to a breakthrough in the field of ageing research: TruAge biological testing. While chronological age simply reflects the number of years since birth, biological age provides insight into how well your body is functioning and can be a more accurate indicator of overall health and vitality.

TruAge is a revolutionary blood test developed by TruDiagnostic™, a biotech company that specializes in cutting-edge diagnostic technologies. TruAge is a test that evaluates your biological age, which gives an estimate of how your body is ageing in comparison to your chronological age. The test measures specific biomarkers in the blood that have been associated with the ageing process, such as markers for inflammation, oxidative stress, telomere length, and cellular senescence. Based on the levels of these biomarkers, TruAge provides an overall score that reflects an individual's biological age.

TruAge can be utilized by healthcare providers to evaluate overall health status and risk for age-related diseases, as well as monitor the effectiveness of interventions aimed at slowing down or reversing the ageing process. Additionally, it can be used by individuals who are interested in optimizing their health and longevity.

Inside Tracker, the mobile blood testing company we previously discussed also offers an InnerAge test that gives insight into an individual's biological age. However, there are differences in their methodology and approach.

InsideTracker's age test analyzes biomarkers associated with various aspects of health and wellness, such as inflammation, glucose metabolism, and liver function. It then compares an individual's biomarker levels to a reference population to calculate a "biological age" that may be higher or lower than their chronological age. Based on the results, InsideTracker provides personalized recommendations for diet, exercise, and supplementation to optimize health and potentially reverse biological ageing.

On the other hand, the True Diagnostic TruAge test employs epigenetic analysis to measure an individual's "epigenetic age," which is based on DNA modifications influenced by environmental factors such as diet, stress, and pollution. The test analyzes DNA methylation patterns at specific sites to calculate an individual's epigenetic age, which may differ from their chronological age. The results are then utilized to provide personalized recommendations for lifestyle changes to improve health and potentially slow down epigenetic ageing.

SMART PROTOCOL

TruAge And InnerAge Tests - $ to $$

Perform a TruAge test. There are two options: TruAge Pace or TruAge Complete. TruAge Pace is a snapshot of how quickly you are ageing at this very moment. This is for those who want a brisk view of their rate of ageing and telomere length. TruAge Complete is the most comprehensive longevity-based biomarker test on the market including 10 reports. Alternatively, perform an InnerAge test from Insidetracker. For more information, see the links provided in the Smart Resources at the end of this Section.

Boosting NAD+ Levels—Exploring NMN, NR, And Niacinamide Supplements

NMN (nicotinamide mononucleotide) and NR (nicotinamide riboside) have gained popularity as dietary supplements due to their potential to increase NAD+ levels in cells. NAD+ is a coenzyme that plays a crucial role in many biological processes, including energy metabolism, DNA repair, and cellular signalling. As we age, our body's ability to produce NAD+ declines—our NAD+ levels drop by approximately 50% every 20 years, which may contribute to age-related diseases. (35) As we age, the production and recycling pathways of NAD+ are switched off, resulting in decreased levels of NAD+. Furthermore, older cells tend to consume and waste more NAD+ which leads to insufficiency in NAD+ levels crucial for optimal cellular function. NMN and NR have been shown to boost NAD+ levels, with potential health benefits such as improving cardiovascular and cognitive function and increasing lifespan in animal studies. (36)

However, the effectiveness of these supplements may be influenced by the salvage pathway, a biological pathway that recycles NAD+ from other metabolites. Additionally, the absorption of these supplements can be an issue, raising questions about which supplement is better, NMN or NR, or niacinamide, a form of vitamin B3.

SMART UPGRADES

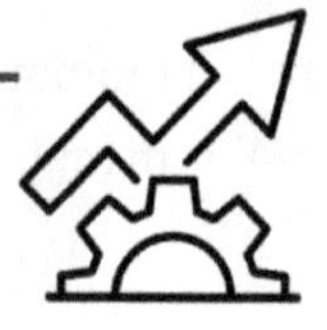

Harness The Benefits Of Next-Gen NAD+ Supplements

Among the many NAD+ supplements on the market, two recent formulations stand out with their innovative approaches to combat NAD+ decline. The first one, Nuchido TIME+ is said to activate NAMPT Nicotinamide phosphoribosyltransferase, which is an essential and rate-limiting enzyme involved in the biosynthesis of NAD+. It also contains ingredients that support NAD+ production, recycling, and reducing wastage. The second one, NAD Regen supplement by Biostack Lab, also addresses NAD+ decline by maintaining production and recycling pathways while providing precursors and reducing inflammation. It contains NAD3®, YÜTH™, resveratrol, niacinamide, and black pepper extract for efficacy. Both supplements provide a comprehensive approach to support cellular health and optimize NAD+ levels.

It is important to note that while there is some promising research on the potential benefits of various combinations of supplements aimed at increasing NAD+ levels, more studies are needed to fully understand their long-term effects and which combination of supplements may be the most effective for supporting cellular health and optimizing NAD+ levels. It is also important to note that an increase in NAD+ levels may potentially accelerate tumour growth in certain individuals, therefore it is best to exercise caution if this applies to your medical history.

Recharge Your Cells With Nitric Oxide—The Essential Molecule For Peak Performance

Nitric Oxide is a cellular signalling molecule that controls nearly every aspect of our health. Without NO, our cells are deprived of the oxygen and nutrients they need to operate at their best. NO plays a critical role in various functions, including blood flow regulation, immune response, and brain cell communication. There are two pathways to produce NO: the arginine to NO pathway and the nitrate to nitrite to NO pathway. (37)

The arginine to NO pathway involves the conversion of the amino acid arginine to nitric oxide (NO) by nitric oxide synthase (NOS) enzymes. There are 3 types of NOS enzymes in humans: endothelial NOS (eNOS), neuronal NOS (nNOS), and inducible NOS (iNOS). eNOS is present in blood vessel cells and regulates blood flow, nNOS is found in neurons and skeletal muscle cells and regulates neurotransmission, and iNOS is produced in response to inflammation and bacterial infections and has a role in host defence but can be harmful in certain pathological conditions. Dysregulation of NOS activity is linked to various diseases, including cardiovascular disease and cancer. The arginine to NO pathway is mainly responsible for producing NO in endothelial cells lining blood vessels, which is important for regulating vascular tone and blood flow. Research has shown that by the time we reach age 40, we produce half or less of the nitric oxide we did at age 20, and it continues to decline the older we get. One study found there was a loss of up to 75% of endothelium-derived NO in 70 to 80-year-old patients compared to that of healthy 20-year-olds. (38)

The nitrate to nitrite to NO pathway, on the other hand, involves the conversion of dietary nitrates to nitrites by bacteria in the mouth and then to NO in the stomach and circulation. This pathway is important for maintaining NO production in situations where the arginine to NO pathway is compromised, such as in individuals with endothelial dysfunction or low arginine levels. It is also crucial to note that stomach acid is necessary to produce NO, and we need iodine to make stomach acid.

The nitrate to nitrite to NO pathway occurs when we consume nitrate-rich foods such as leafy green vegetables, beets, and pomegranates. The bacteria in our mouths reduce nitrate to nitrite, which then decomposes to form NO in our acidic stomach. It's worth noting that using mouthwash or fluoride can negatively affect our mouth bacteria, which can impact the nitrate to nitrite to NO pathway. Therefore, it's crucial to be mindful of our oral hygiene practices. It's also worth noting that while cured meats are high in nitrates, they are not beneficial for our health. Despite containing nitrates, these meats have been linked to several health issues, and it's recommended to limit or avoid their consumption.

Due to the standard American diet, which only provides approximately 100-150 milligrams of nitrate per day, many people suffer from nitrate deficiency. This deficiency in the essential molecule can result in various health issues. (39) However, consuming nitrate-rich foods and taking appropriate supplements, such as those offered by Berkeley Life or Bryan Nitriceuticals, can help address this issue. Both of these supplements are specifically designed to enhance nitric oxide production via the pathways mentioned above and help promote cardiovascular health, exercise performance, and blood flow.

Nitric oxide plays a critical role in various bodily functions, and understanding the pathways to produce it and taking appropriate measures can support the body's nitric oxide production and reduce the risk of health issues associated with nitric oxide deficiency. Vinpocetine and hawthorn extract are other nutraceuticals that have been shown to increase nitric oxide and improve physical performance and resiliency.

It's worth noting that exercise and exposure to UVA radiation from the sun can also help increase nitric oxide production. Research has shown that one hour of daily aerobic exercise for a month can increase nitric oxide levels, reduce blood pressure, and increase antioxidants in the body. (40) Exposure to UVA radiation from the sun can also help release nitric oxide into the skin, and the effects can last for days. (41)

There are saliva test strips available to test NO levels. This is recommended in order to assess your NO level and decide which approach you should take to increase it.

SMART PROTOCOL

Nitric Oxide - $ to $$

To improve NO levels, monitor them using NO strips and consider supplements from reputable companies like Berkeley Life and Bryan Nitriceuticals. Eat nitrate-rich foods and ensure adequate HCL and iodine levels. Avoid mouthwash to help maintain the nitrate to nitrite to NO pathway and practice nasal breathing.

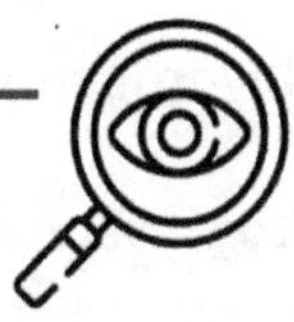

SMART CONSIDERATION

Supercharge Your Antioxidant Defence With Molecular Hydrogen

Molecular hydrogen is a remarkable supplement that helps counteract the harmful effects of excessive free radicals caused by radiation exposure, chemical exposure from household cleaning items, beauty products, processed foods, intense exercise, or air travel. This innovative supplement is highly effective in reducing oxidative stress and providing highly bioavailable magnesium for a healthy brain, muscles, cells, kidneys, and heart.

The science behind molecular hydrogen is fascinating. It activates intracellular antioxidants, which effectively reduce inflammation and enhances mitochondrial functions, leading to better cellular energy. (42) For optimal results, it is recommended to take molecular hydrogen 1-2 times a day to combat oxidative stress effectively.

SMART PROTOCOL

Hydrogen Water - $

To prepare, simply dissolve one or two tablets of molecular hydrogen in 12 oz of room-temperature water. It's essential to note that the cooler the water, the longer it takes for the tablets to dissolve, so it's best to use a timer set to 90 seconds or 1 ½ minutes. Avoid exceeding the time limit, as the hydrogen gas will dissipate, and the supplement will lose its effectiveness.

It's also recommended to drink the solution in one go, so bottoms up!

Revitalize Your Cells With Mitochondrial Boosting Urolithin A

Urolithin A is a gut metabolite derived from the breakdown of polyphenolic compounds. When you consume these compounds, your gut microflora digests them, converting them into smaller molecules that are more easily absorbed. This process categorizes Urolithin A (UA) as a postbiotic—essential nourishment for the gut microbiome.

The ability to produce Urolithin A varies among individuals, based on the unique composition of their gut microbiome. Having a complex and diverse population of gut microbiota increases your capacity to produce it. Tests using advanced mass spectrometry can determine whether you are an efficient producer of Urolithin A through a simple blood spot test.

Central to UA's health benefits is its ability to rejuvenate mitochondrial health. Mitochondria, our cellular energy factories, diminish in function as we age. UA reinvigorates them by promoting mitophagy, the purging of damaged mitochondria, leading to heightened cellular energy and health.

Beyond mitochondrial boost, UA has demonstrated anti-inflammatory properties, countering chronic inflammation tied to diseases like heart ailments, cancer, and Alzheimer's. (43) It's also an antioxidant powerhouse, guarding against oxidative stress, which can instigate age-related conditions and cognitive decline. (44) Plus, it's been linked to enhanced muscle function and metabolism, offering potential benefits against age-driven muscle deterioration.

SMART CONSIDERATION

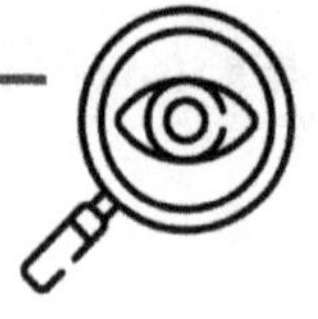

Elevate Your Cellular Energy With Ultra-Concentrated Urolithin A (UA)

Mitopure is a brand that has developed a highly concentrated form of UA using a patented process. Their UA supplement contains 10 times the concentration of UA found in traditional sources of ellagitannins, such as pomegranates. A link to their website is provided in the resources listed at the end of this Section.

Peptides—The Power Of The Body's Mini-Proteins

Peptides, which are composed of amino acids, are often referred to as the "building blocks of life" and are typically obtained through food sources. When two amino acids join together, they form a dipeptide, and as the length of the amino acid chains increases, the names of the resulting compounds change. Amino acid chains that contain 3 to 6 amino acids are known as short-chain peptides or bioregulators, while longer chains of amino acids are called proteins and then hormones.

Research spanning over 40 years has revealed that short-chain peptides, or bioregulators, have the potential to act as gene switches. This discovery has significant implications for precision medicine and its management. (45)

Research has also shown that certain peptides can also exhibit potent healing properties, making them attractive candidates for therapeutic use. For instance, some peptides have been found to stimulate the production of collagen, a protein that is crucial for skin health and elasticity. Other peptides have been shown to promote wound healing and tissue repair, making them promising options for treating injuries or accelerating recovery after surgery. (46)

Some peptides are believed to have anti-ageing effects by boosting cellular repair mechanisms, enhancing cognitive function, and promoting longevity. These properties have made them a topic of great interest in the field of anti-ageing medicine, with some researchers exploring their potential use as supplements or therapies to enhance healthspan.

Peptide delivery methods vary based on the peptide and its purpose. Some are oral, but stomach acids and enzymes can degrade many peptides. Injection into the bloodstream is a common delivery method with subcutaneous and intramuscular injections offering precise dosing. Other delivery methods include transdermal patches, nasal sprays, and topical creams for peptides that aren't suitable for oral or injection delivery.

The field of peptides is rapidly growing as researchers continue to explore their potential applications in medicine, but it is important to note that many of these peptide-based treatments are not yet approved by the U.S. Food and Drug Administration (FDA). The approval process can be lengthy and expensive, involving multiple stages of clinical trials and regulatory reviews.

Here are several examples of commonly used regenerative peptides. It's important to note that in many countries, these substances are primarily available through a prescription from a practitioner specializing in functional medicine:

1. **Thymosin Alpha-1**—This peptide is a synthetic version of a naturally occurring thymic peptide that has been shown to have immunomodulatory effects. It is being studied for its potential to treat viral infections, cancer, and autoimmune disorders.
2. **BPC-157**— This peptide is a synthetic version of a naturally occurring peptide found in gastric juice. It has been shown to have regenerative effects on various tissues and is being studied for its potential to treat musculoskeletal injuries and inflammatory bowel disease.
3. **Sermorelin**—This peptide is a synthetic version of a naturally occurring growth hormone-releasing hormone (GHRH) and is used to stimulate the release of growth hormone in the body. It is being studied for its potential to treat growth hormone deficiency and age-related decline in growth hormone levels.
4. **MOTS-c And SS 31**—These are mitochondria-targeted peptides that have been shown to have anti-ageing effects by improving mitochondrial function. They are being studied for their potential to treat age-related diseases and conditions.
5. **GHK-Cu And GHK**—These peptides are synthetic versions of a naturally occurring peptide found in human plasma. They have been shown to have regenerative effects on various tissues and are being studied for their potential to treat skin ageing, wound healing, and other conditions.
6. **Epitalon**—Epitalon is a synthetic peptide comprising 4 amino acids (alanine, glutamic acid, aspartic acid, and glycine) that is being researched for its potential anti-ageing properties. Its mechanism of action is thought to involve the activation of telomerase, an enzyme that helps preserve the length of telomeres, which are protective caps located at the ends of chromosomes.

The Potential Of Stem Cells In Regenerative Medicine

Stem cells are unique cells that have the ability to develop into many different types of cells in the body, making them incredibly versatile and valuable for medical research and therapy. There are two main types of stem cells: embryonic stem cells and adult stem cells.

Embryonic stem cells are derived from embryos and have the potential to develop into any type of cell in the body. However, their use in research and therapy is controversial due to ethical concerns surrounding the use of embryos.

Adult stem cells, on the other hand, are found in various tissues throughout the body, including bone marrow, fat, and blood vessels. They are more limited in their ability to differentiate into different cell types than embryonic stem cells, but they still have the potential to be used in medical therapies.

One of the most promising areas of research involving stem cells is regenerative medicine. This field explores the potential of stem cells to regenerate damaged or diseased tissues and organs, including those affected by conditions such as heart disease, Parkinson's disease, and diabetes.

Stem cell therapy involves the transplantation of stem cells into a patient's body to replace or repair damaged or diseased cells. The hope is that the transplanted stem cells will differentiate into the appropriate type of cell and integrate into the tissue, leading to improved function and potentially even a cure.

Stem cell therapy is still in its early stages, and much research is needed to fully understand its potential benefits and risks. Despite the challenges, stem cells hold enormous promise for the treatment of a wide range of diseases and conditions. Ongoing research and development in this field may lead to groundbreaking new therapies and cures that could transform the future of medicine.

Dr. Christian Drapeau, a renowned author and speaker in the realm of stem cells and regenerative medicine, has made significant strides in discovering natural ingredients that can stimulate stem cells. Having penned several influential books such as *The Stem Cell Theory of Renewal* and *Cracking the Stem Cell Code,* he has helped to shed light on the complexities of stem cell science and its implications for regenerative medicine. (47)(48) His works thoroughly discuss cutting-edge stem cell research and their potential applications. Furthermore, he introduces natural stimulants that could revolutionize treatment for a variety of health conditions, including ageing, arthritis, diabetes, and heart disease.

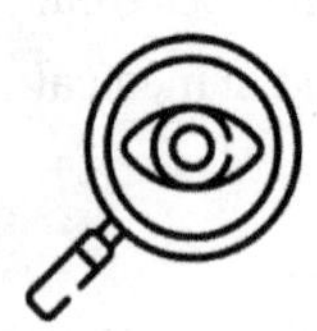

SMART CONSIDERATION

Natural Supplement For Enhanced Stem Cell Health And Regeneration

You may choose to consider supplementation to improve stem cell health and regeneration. STEMREGEN® is a dietary supplement that aims to enhance stem cell health and regeneration using a blend of natural ingredients. STEMREGEN® is a blend of plant extracts that have been documented to support the release of stem cells from the bone marrow, thereby increasing the number of circulating stem cells, as well as the migration of stem cells into tissues. It includes StemBerry™ sea buckthorn berry extract, Aphanizomenon flos-aquae, seaweed extract, notoginseng extract, and 1-3 beta-glucan. This supplement, available at kalyagen.com/product/stemregen, can be a valuable addition to your longevity regimen.

Strategic Supplementation—The Power of Cycling and Pulsing

It can be overwhelming to think of taking ALL the supplements we talk about in this book, but just like you would not eat EVERY healthful food in one day, pulsing or cycling your supplement intake can be a valuable practice.

Supplement cycling refers to the use of dietary supplements in a planned and systematic manner with specific periods of usage and discontinuation. This approach is commonly employed by athletes, bodybuilders, and fitness enthusiasts to enhance performance, support recovery, and optimize overall health.

Typically, cycles range from a few weeks to a few months. During the "on" phase of a cycle, individuals take the supplement as directed, usually following recommended dosages. The "off" phase follows, during which the supplement is discontinued for a specific period.

Supplement cycling helps to maintain the effectiveness of the supplements taken. While certain supplements (multivitamins, magnesium, fish oil etc), are typically designed for daily use to ensure a consistent intake of essential nutrients, others, such as Tongkat Ali, an herbal supplement often used to support hormonal balance, may be cycled intermittently. This can help you continue to experience the desired benefits without needing to continuously increase dosages. Cycling can also allow the body to reset and regulate its natural processes. You may decide to try a few 'new to you' supplements outlined in this book, experimenting with them for a couple of months, and then decide to try a few others. Rather than continuously adding more capsules to take, you can alternate instead. Cycling can help to prevent overwhelm, and you still reap the benefits.

Pulsing supplements is very similar, but is often done on a daily or weekly schedule. Some are taken in a day-on, day-off pattern, or are taken a few times per week. An example of this is resveratrol. According to Dr. David Sinclair, a renowned Harvard Medical School professor, who has been at the forefront of longevity research for decades, taking resveratrol every other day instead of daily is recommended based on his research. (49) By intermittently exposing the body to resveratrol, you activate hormetic pathways and promote longevity and healthspan.

Methyl-folate is another supplement that may be best to pulse. This is where SNPs testing we mentioned can give you vital information, as it allows you to tailor your supplementation based on your specific genetic variations. Some individuals with certain genetic variants may be more susceptible to over-methylation. Over-methylation can result in imbalances in neurotransmitters like serotonin, dopamine, and norepinephrine, potentially leading to mood disorders or anxiety. Pulsing methyl-folate can help control methylation levels and minimize symptoms of over-methylation in this instance.

You certainly don't need to have genetic testing done to practice cycling or pulsing, however, as stated above, it is unrealistic to take every supplement all the time. Experiment to find out what works best for you.

The Significance Of A Robust Social Network And Its Influence On Lifespan

Social connections play a vital role in providing a sense of belonging and support. When we have strong social connections, we feel less isolated and more connected to the world around us. These connections serve as a valuable source of emotional support, particularly during challenging times. It's important to recognize that social connections go beyond mere enjoyment with friends and family; they are crucial for our overall health and longevity. Numerous studies have demonstrated that individuals with robust social connections tend to lead longer and healthier lives compared to those who lack such connections. (50) This phenomenon is even observed in the Blue Zones we previously mentioned, where strong social connection is a common trait.

For older adults, active involvement in the community and nurturing social ties becomes increasingly significant as they may be vulnerable to isolation and loneliness. Maintaining social connections has been linked to various cognitive benefits, including improved memory, faster processing speed, and enhanced problem-solving abilities. Research has also revealed that socially active individuals have a reduced risk of cognitive impairment and dementia, and for those already diagnosed, social engagement can help slow down the progression of these conditions. (51)

Adopting the right mindset and developing positive habits are key factors in achieving success and happiness in life. A positive mindset empowers us to overcome challenges, stay motivated, and reach our goals. This applies not only to ourselves but also to the company we keep. The people we surround ourselves with significantly influence our mindset, attitude, and overall well-being. It is essential to surround ourselves with individuals who inspire us, challenge us, and provide support. Quality should always be prioritized over quantity when it comes to our friendships and connections.

It is crucial to invest time in nurturing our social connections, pursuing our passions, and living authentically. Our health and longevity are contingent upon these factors, and we all deserve to lead meaningful and fulfilling lives.

SMART PROTOCOL

Sustain Social Connection - $0 to $

Try joining a club or group that aligns with your interests, volunteering in your community, attending community events, and making time to prioritize connections with friends and family. Staying socially engaged doesn't need to be complicated or time-consuming. Simple activities like going for a walk with your friend, or chatting with a neighbour can all contribute to better brain health.

Section Wrap-Up

The study of epigenetics has revolutionized our understanding of ageing and longevity, revealing a remarkable interplay between gene expression and environmental factors. Epigenetic modifications, which dynamically regulate gene activity, exert a profound impact on the ageing process. They act as a crucial bridge connecting our genetic blueprint to the influences of our surroundings, ultimately shaping our well-being and lifespan. This dynamic nature of ageing has led us to recognize that it is not solely dictated by our genetic code but also strongly influenced by our lifestyle choices, environment, and personal experiences. These groundbreaking discoveries have shattered the belief that ageing follows a predetermined path, igniting excitement and hope for interventions that can decelerate ageing and foster extended health and vitality. In fact, we stand at the brink of a promising new era, where healthy ageing and an elongated healthspan may soon become a tangible reality.

PROTOCOLS QUICK REFERENCE CHECKLIST:

PROTOCOL—Hormetic Stressors - $0 to $$$

☐ *Currently doing* ☐ *Want to integrate* ☐ *Not for now*

PROTOCOL—Phytohormetic Foods - $0 to $$

☐ *Currently doing* ☐ *Want to integrate* ☐ *Not for now*

PROTOCOL—Comprehensive Annual Wellness Exam - $0 to $$$

☐ *Currently doing* ☐ *Want to integrate* ☐ *Not for now*

PROTOCOL—SNPs Testing - $0 to $$

☐ *Currently doing* ☐ *Want to integrate* ☐ *Not for now*

PROTOCOL—Caloric Restriction/Fasting Mimicking Diet And Senolytics - $ to $$

☐ *Currently doing* ☐ *Want to integrate* ☐ *Not for now*

PROTOCOL—Nitric Oxide - $0 to $$

☐ *Currently doing* ☐ *Want to integrate* ☐ *Not for now*

PROTOCOL—Hydrogen Water - $

☐ *Currently doing* ☐ *Want to integrate* ☐ *Not for now*

PROTOCOL—Sustain Social Connection - $0 to $$

☐ *Currently doing* ☐ *Want to integrate* ☐ *Not for now*

SMART RESOURCES

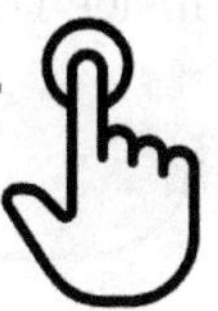

- Resilience Assessment—smartcuts.life/resilience-assessment
- Kaufmann Longevity Protocol—kaufmannprotocol.com
- Brain SPECT—amenclinics.com/services/brain-spect
- SNPs Testing and Analysis—seekinghealth.com, functionalgenomicanalysis.com, selfdecode.com, drnathaliepuregenomics.com
- Senolytic Supplements—InfiniWell infiniwell.com, Neurohacker Collective neurohacker.com/shop/qualia-senolytic
- TruAge Test—trudiagnostic.com/products/truage-complete-epigenetic-collection
- NAD Supplements—nuchido.com, biostacklabs.com/products/nadregen
- Nitric Oxide Supplements—berkeleylife.com , Bryan Nitriceuticals no2u.com
- Molecular Hydrogen Tablets—shop.drinkhrw.ca
- Urolithin A—mitopure.com

- STEMREGEN®—kalyagen.com/product/stemregen

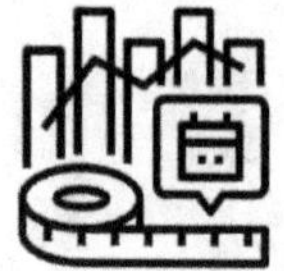

SMART TOOLS AT A GLANCE

Inside Tracker—insidetracker.com

Conclusion

Take Action—Integrating The SmartCuts Protocols Into Your Life

At the beginning of this book, you were encouraged to download the complimentary PDF—**Summary of SmartCuts Protocols**, which contains all the protocols outlined in SmartCuts. You were asked to make note of the protocols you are currently following, the ones you would like to integrate, and those that are not quite a perfect fit for you at this present time. Now, let's start by focusing on identifying your non-negotiables—the habits that you are committed to practicing consistently, regardless of the circumstances. These non-negotiables are the foundation you will build upon, providing stability and ensuring that you always prioritize your well-being in specific areas.

Step 1—With the SmartCuts Protocols Summary in hand, make sure it is fully completed with the protocols you are currently doing, those you intend to integrate, and any that are not for this time and confirm that you understand the protocols.

Step 2—Go to smartcuts.life/integration-worksheets or scan the following QR code to download the **SmartCuts Integration Worksheets:**

Step 3—Use page 1 and 2 of the SmartCuts Integration Worksheets to list the protocols you already identified as "currently doing" from the **Summary of SmartCuts Protocols,** by using the space provided in the first column. Indicate your protocol frequency (daily, weekly, monthly, quarterly) by checking the appropriate boxes. Are there other health habits or protocols you are currently doing that you could also add to the list? This could include supplements you take, specific workouts or training routines, meditation and breathwork practices, dietary habits for different time frames (daily, weekly, monthly), and even periodic full detoxes as an example of a non-negotiable you do quarterly. Take your time and be thorough in documenting these habits.

Step 4—Next, go through your list and honestly assess whether you are consistently practicing these habits. If you find that you sometimes or rarely follow them, use the Notes space provided to jot down the reasons why. It could be that your priorities have shifted, there may be certain barriers that are preventing you from being consistent, or you simply just forgot about it. Life happens, and we understand that. This exercise is not about strict regimentation, but rather about striving for consistency. Missing a workout occasionally is normal, but if you find yourself skipping them regularly, it may be time to refocus. Be kind, but firm with yourself.

Step 5—Once you have completed your inventory, it's time to review the protocols you identified earlier that you would like to integrate into your routine. Use pages 3 and 4 of the SmartCuts Integration Worksheets to write down these protocols in the first column and indicate the frequency at which you aspire to consistently practice them. To hold yourself accountable, there is a "date" column. Look at your calendar and commit to a starting date for each protocol. In the "Action To Take" section, note down any preparations that need to be made to ensure your success. For instance, if you plan to purchase an at-home sauna, you might need time to research different models that suit your needs and budget accordingly. It could also be something as simple as ordering a supplement or buying a specific item from the grocery store. Putting your plan on paper will help you stay focused and on track.

Remember, when it comes to developing healthy habits, there is no one-size-fits-all solution. What works for one person may not work for another. Therefore, it's crucial to take some time to reflect on your own health goals and needs in order to determine which habits will become non-negotiables in your health journey.

The advantage of having access to these PDFs is that you can revisit and reassess your non-negotiable habits as you make progress. In six months, practices like mouth taping and nasal breathing may have become second nature in your routine, indicating that it's time to introduce more advanced protocols. Alternatively, if you initially started with beginner protocols outlined in Section 3—Movement, Exercise, & Detoxification, you might feel ready to level up and incorporate intermediate or advanced protocols in that specific area. This flexibility allows you to continuously evolve and tailor your health journey to match your growth and capabilities. Regularly evaluating and updating your protocols, helps you ensure that your habits remain aligned with your goals and keep pushing you forward.

Living the Journey—Dr. Sly and Dr. Beauchamp's Daily, Weekly, and Monthly Routines for Optimal Wellness

One of the most frequently asked questions that we get is "how do you integrate this into your life?" or "what does a typical day look like for you?". Just like you, we are also on a continuous, ever-evolving journey when it comes to our own health. What we prioritize and practice may be vastly different from one another, and that's completely natural. Due to this fact, we have purposefully not included our current non-negotiables in the text of this book, but rather have listed our routines on our website, where we can update it as we add and remove specific habits in real time. Each of us is biologically unique, and our personal protocols reflect that individuality. Embracing and celebrating our differences allows us to embrace a holistic approach to health, recognizing that what works for one person may not work for another. Each of us has non-negotiable routines that happen daily, weekly, monthly, quarterly and yearly.

However, it's important to note that these routines are not set in stone. We view our health journey as an ongoing experiment, constantly exploring and fine-tuning what works best for us at different points in time. The routines we share on the website provide a snapshot of how we approach our health and wellness at a given moment.

At smartcuts.life, you can find detailed insights into what a typical day or week looks like for each of us. From morning rituals and dietary habits to exercise routines and stress management techniques, we aim to provide a comprehensive overview of our current practices. By sharing our routines with you, we hope to encourage you to embrace flexibility and experimentation in your own health journey. It's natural for priorities and circumstances to change over time, and it's essential to be open to modifying your habits to align with your changing needs.

So we invite you to go to smartcuts.life, and discover how we approach our daily lives in pursuit of optimal well-being. We hope that you too, will be inspired and motivated to take charge of your own health destiny.

Note From the Authors

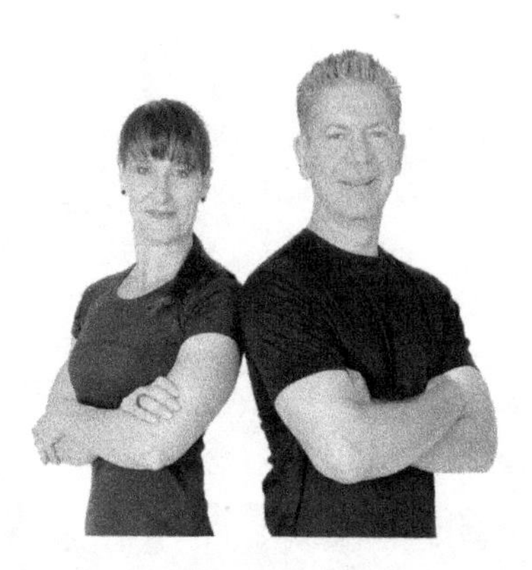

Dear Readers,

As we come to the conclusion of our book, *SmartCuts—Biohack Your Healthspan: Cutting-Edge Protocols For Greater Energy and Performance*, we want to express our heartfelt appreciation for joining us on this extraordinary journey. Throughout these pages, we have explored the boundless potential of optimal health protocols and "biohacking" to elevate your healthspan and supercharge your energy and performance.

However, this is just the beginning of your transformative experience. To continue your pursuit of optimal health and well-being, we warmly invite you to explore our website. There, you will discover a wealth of resources, personalized health programs, and coaching precisely tailored to meet your unique needs. Embark on a transformative journey with us, whether as an individual reaching for your full potential or an organization seeking enhanced vitality and productivity. Let biohacking be your path of self-discovery, guided by our expertise. Embrace its power and experience the profound impact it can bring to your life.

We invite you to visit our website at smartcuts.life and take the next step on this extraordinary adventure.

With deepest gratitude and excitement,
Dr. Paul Sly & Dr. Nathalie Beauchamp

About the Authors

Dr. Paul Sly

Dr. Paul Sly, B.Sc. (Hons.), DC is a chiropractor in private practice in Arnprior, Ontario. He works with a diverse and active population of clients of all ages, including professional strength and powerlifting athletes and hockey players.

Dr. Sly has always focused not only on the treatment and rehabilitation of injuries and pain, but on prevention, health and longevity, and ultimately performance enhancement.

Beyond chiropractic techniques which form the foundation of his practice, Dr. Sly uses acupuncture and dry needling, various soft tissue therapies, and exercise prescription with his clients. He is certified in Functional Movement Systems® and is a Master Instructor for Oxygen Advantage®. The addition of functional breathing and simulated altitude techniques not only for overall health but maximizing athletic performance has been transformational to his work.

Dr. Sly loves to research current evidence based techniques and practices. He believes modern information technology makes it possible to translate this data, which previously took a decade or more to make its way into clinical practice, and communicate it to clients in an individualized way.

When Dr. Sly is not in his clinic or consulting with clients, he can be found at home on his farm with his family, working out at the gym, or enjoying a variety of sports and activities on land and water.

To connect with Dr. Sly:

- Website: drpaulsly.com
- Email: paul@achc.ca
- LinkedIn: linkedin.com/in/dr-paul-sly-corporate-wellness-trainer-oxygen-advantage-master-instructor/

* * *

Dr. Nathalie Beauchamp

Dr. Nathalie Beauchamp, B.Sc., D.C., IFMCP is a well-known chiropractor, wellness consultant, radio and TV personality, former professional bodybuilder, and the author of the books *Hack Your Health Habits*, *Fired Up & Feeling Great*, and *Wellness On The Go*.

After overcoming her own health issues as a young adult, Dr. Beauchamp embarked on a mission to empower people all over the world to take control of their health to lead happier and more fulfilling lives. For over 25 years she has developed health programs and solutions that place an emphasis on the prevention of common lifestyle-related diseases. She focuses on longevity, bio-hacking, and natural health solutions that address root-cause issues, rather than patching symptoms.

Dr. Beauchamp believes that there is no one-size-fits-all solution to health and therefore holds bio-individuality as the foundation of her approach. Her care is specifically tailored toward her patients' individual needs, while her writing seeks to provide all the health information her readers require to make the best decisions for their own well-being.

Dr. Beauchamp is based in Ottawa, Ontario, Canada, but extends her reach across the globe. With "Dr. Nat" what you see is what you get as she practices what she preaches. In her downtime, you will find her at the gym, enjoying the great outdoors, or researching the latest advancements in natural health science.

Her ultimate goal is to help as many people as possible achieve better health and well-being in a way that works for them, leaving them with more energy, vitality, longevity, and life satisfaction.

To connect with Dr. Nathalie:

- Website: drnathaliebeauchamp.com
- Email: drnathalie@drnathaliebeauchamp.com
- LinkedIn: linkedin.com/in/drnathaliebeauchamp/

References

Introduction

In-Text References:

1. Statistics Canada. (2013). Directly measured physical activity of Canadian adults, 2007 to 2011. Retrieved August 2, 2022, from https://www150.statcan.gc.ca/n1/pub/82-625-x/2013001/article/11807-eng.htm
2. Statistics Canada. (2021, September 1). Canadian Health Measures Survey: Activity monitor data, 2018-2019. Retrieved August 11, 2022, from https://www150.statcan.gc.ca/n1/daily-quotidien/210901/dq210901c-eng.htm
3. Yang L, Cao C, Kantor ED, et al. Trends in Sedentary Behavior Among the US Population, 2001-2016. JAMA. 2019;321(16):1587–1597. doi:10.1001/jama.2019.3636
4. National Institute of Diabetes and Digestive and Kidney Diseases. (n.d.). Diabetes statistics. Retrieved August 11, 2022, from https://www.niddk.nih.gov/health-information/health-statistics/diabetes-statistics

Section 1 - Sleep, Rest & Recovery

In-Text References:

1. Rachel Leproult, P. D. (2011, June 1). *Effect of 1 week of sleep restriction on testosterone levels in young healthy men*. JAMA. Retrieved August 18, 2022, from https://jamanetwork.com/journals/jama/fullarticle/1029127
2. Huberman, A. (2022, August 8). *Sleep toolkit: Tools for optimizing sleep & sleep-wake timing*. Huberman Lab. Retrieved August 18, 2022, from https://hubermanlab.com/sleep-toolkit-tools-for-optimizing-sleep-and-sleep-wake-timing/
3. Zhang J, Jin X, Li R, Gao Y, Li J, Wang G. Influence of rapid eye movement sleep on all-cause mortality: a community-based cohort study. Aging (Albany NY). 2019 Mar 13;11(5):1580-1588. doi: 10.18632/aging.101858. PMID: 30867337; PMCID: PMC6428105.
4. Iliff, J. et al. (2014) Impairment of Glymphatic Pathway Function Promotes Tau Pathology after Traumatic Brain Injury. *Journal of Neuroscience*, 34(49) p.

16180–16193. Retrieved April 16, 2021, from
https://pubmed.ncbi.nlm.nih.gov/25471560/

5. Benveniste, H. (2016) Glymphatic System May Play Key Role in Removing Brain Waste. *Neurology Reviews*, 24(10) p. 13.
6. Lee, H., Xie, L., Yu, M., Kang, H., Feng, T., Deane, R., Logan, J., Nedergaard, M., & Benveniste, H. (2015). The Effect of Body Posture on Brain Glymphatic Transport. *Journal of Neuroscience*, 35(31), 11034–11044. https://doi.org/10.1523/jneurosci.1625-15.2015
7. Svensson S, Olin AC, Hellgren J. Increased net water loss by oral compared to nasal expiration in healthy subjects. Rhinology. 2006 Mar;44(1):74-7. PMID: 16550955.
8. Huberman, A. (2022, August 8). *Sleep toolkit: Tools for optimizing sleep & sleep-wake timing*. Huberman Lab. Retrieved August 18, 2022, from https://hubermanlab.com/sleep-toolkit-tools-for-optimizing-sleep-and-sleep-wake-timing/
9. Tsai, H. J., Kuo, T. B., Lee, G.-S., & Yang, C. C. (2014). Efficacy of paced breathing for insomnia: Enhances vagal activity and improves sleep quality. *Psychophysiology*, 52(3), 388–396. https://doi.org/10.1111/psyp.12333
10. J Stem Cells. 2015;10(4):287-94. Effect of Mobile Phone-Induced Electromagnetic Field on Brain Hemodynamics and Human Stem Cell Functioning: Possible Mechanistic Link to Cancer Risk and Early Diagnostic Value of Electronphotonic Imaging
11. Huberman, A. (2022, July 17). *Using light (sunlight, Blue Light & Red Light) to optimize health*. Huberman Lab. Retrieved August 18, 2022, from https://hubermanlab.com/using-light-sunlight-blue-light-and-red-light-to-optimize-health/
12. Brian Hoyer: *The dangers of EMF exposure and how to make your bedroom a safe haven* - get over yourself podcast with Brad Kearns. (2021, June 7). Retrieved August 18, 2022, from https://bradkearns.com/2020/03/17/brian-hoyer/
13. Huberman, A. (2022, August 8). *Sleep toolkit: Tools for optimizing sleep & sleep-wake timing*. Huberman Lab. Retrieved August 18, 2022, from https://hubermanlab.com/sleep-toolkit-tools-for-optimizing-sleep-and-sleep-wake-timing/
14. Team, F.H. (2021, December 20). *The best temperature for sleep*. Cleveland Clinic. Retrieved August 18, 2022, from https://health.clevelandclinic.org/what-is-the-ideal-sleeping-temperature-for-my-bedroom/
15. McKeown, P. (2021). *The breathing cure: Exercises to develop new breathing habits for a healthier, Happier and longer life*. OxyAt Books.
16. McKeown, P. (2021). *The breathing cure: Exercises to develop new breathing habits for a healthier, Happier and longer life*. OxyAt Books.
17. Purohit, D. (2022, April 28). *Try this: A practice to feel refreshed, revived, and refocused!* Dhru Purohit - Exploring the Inner Workings of the Brain and the Body. Retrieved August 18, 2022, from https://dhrupurohit.com/try-this-yoga-nidra/
18. Chen, Hsin-Yung & Yang, Hsiang & Chi, H.-J & Chen, H.-M. (2013). Physiological Effects of Deep Touch Pressure on Anxiety Alleviation: The Weighted Blanket Approach. Journal of Medical and Biological Engineering. 33. 463-470. 10.5405/jmbe.1043
19. Reynolds, S., Lane, S. J., & Mullen, B. (2015, April 8). *Effects of deep pressure stimulation on physiological arousal*. American Occupational Therapy Association.

Retrieved August 18, 2022, from https://research.aota.org/ajot/article-abstract/69/3/6903350010p1/5994/Effects-of-Deep-Pressure-Stimulation-on?redirectedFrom=fulltext

20. Kayla Barnes: *Brain Health + biohacking*. Karla Barnes | Brain Health + Biohacking. (n.d.). Retrieved August 24, 2022, from https://www.kaylabarnes.com/
21. Laukkanen T, Khan H, Zaccardi F, Laukkanen JA. Association Between Sauna Bathing and Fatal Cardiovascular and All-Cause Mortality Events. JAMA Intern Med. 2015;175(4):542–548. doi:10.1001/jamainternmed.2014.818
22. Šrámek, P., Šimečková, M., Janský, L., Šavlíková, J., & Vybíral, S. (n.d.). *Human physiological responses to immersion into water of different temperatures - European journal of applied physiology*. SpringerLink. Retrieved August 22, 2022, from https://link.springer.com/article/10.1007/s004210050065
23. Soberg S;Löfgren J;Philipsen FE;Jensen M;Hansen AE;Ahrens E;Nystrup KB;Nielsen RD;Solling C;Wedell-Neergaard AS;Berntsen M;Loft A;Kjær A;Gerhart-Hines Z;Johannesen HH;Pedersen BK;Karstoft K;Scheele C; (n.d.). *Altered brown fat thermoregulation and enhanced cold-induced thermogenesis in young, healthy, winter-swimming men*. Cell reports. Medicine. Retrieved August 22, 2022, from https://pubmed.ncbi.nlm.nih.gov/34755128/
24. Soberg S;Löfgren J;Philipsen FE;Jensen M;Hansen AE;Ahrens E;Nystrup KB;Nielsen RD;Solling C;Wedell-Neergaard AS;Berntsen M;Loft A;Kjær A;Gerhart-Hines Z;Johannesen HH;Pedersen BK;Karstoft K;Scheele C; (n.d.). *Altered brown fat thermoregulation and enhanced cold-induced thermogenesis in young, healthy, winter-swimming men*. Cell reports. Medicine. Retrieved August 22, 2022, from https://pubmed.ncbi.nlm.nih.gov/34755128/
25. Søberg, P., Rasmussen, R., & Pedersen, P. K. (2015). Effects of long-term whole-body cold exposures on plasma concentrations of ACTH, beta-endorphin, cortisol, catecholamines and cytokines in healthy females. Cryobiology, 71(3), 448-455. Retrieved February 23, 2023, from doi: 10.1016/j.cryobiol.2015.10.128
26. Huberman, A. (2022, August 8). *Sleep toolkit: Tools for optimizing sleep & sleep-wake timing*. Huberman Lab. Retrieved August 18, 2022, from https://hubermanlab.com/sleep-toolkit-tools-for-optimizing-sleep-and-sleep-wake-timing/
27. Examine.com. (2023, February 1). *Inositol health benefits, dosage, safety, side-effects, and more: Supplements*. Examine. Retrieved February 21, 2023, from https://examine.com/supplements/inositol/
28. DiNicolantonio, J., Land, S., Kennedy, T., & Greenfield, B. (2021). *Win: Achieve peak athletic performance, optimize recovery and become a champion: Strength, speed, endurance, recovery*.
29. Bannai M;Kawai N;Ono K;Nakahara K;Murakami N; (n.d.). *The effects of glycine on subjective daytime performance in partially sleep-restricted healthy volunteers*. Frontiers in neurology. Retrieved February 23, 2023, from https://pubmed.ncbi.nlm.nih.gov/22529837/
30. Ramar K;Dort LC;Katz SG;Lettieri CJ;Harrod CG;Thomas SM;Chervin RD; (n.d.). *Clinical practice guideline for the treatment of obstructive sleep apnea and snoring with Oral Appliance therapy: An update for 2015*. Journal of clinical sleep medicine: JCSM: official publication of the American Academy of Sleep Medicine. Retrieved February 23, 2023, from https://pubmed.ncbi.nlm.nih.gov/26094920/
31. Rivera-Oliver, M., & Díaz-Ríos, M. (2014, February 13). *Using caffeine and other adenosine receptor antagonists and agonists as therapeutic tools against*

Neurodegenerative Diseases: A Review. Life Sciences. Retrieved August 29, 2022, from https://www.sciencedirect.com/science/article/abs/pii/S0024320514002215?via%3Dihub

32. Rodriguez, J. (2016, December 9). *When should you drink your morning coffee?* Advanced Sleep Medicine Services, Inc. Retrieved August 29, 2022, from https://www.sleepdr.com/the-sleep-blog/when-should-you-drink-your-morning-coffee/
33. Maryann. (2022, August 18). *Episode 84 – sleep toolkit: Tools for optimizing sleep & sleep-wake timing: Huberman Lab • Podcast notes*. Podcast Notes. Retrieved August 29, 2022, from https://podcastnotes.org/huberman-lab/episode-84-sleep-toolkit-tools-for-optimizing-sleep-sleep-wake-timing-huberman-lab/
34. https://www.healthline.com/health/5-tibetan-rites
35. Varani, K., Gessi, S., Merighi, S., Iannotta, V., Cattabriga, E., Spisani, S., ... & Borea, P. A. (2010). Effect of low-frequency electromagnetic fields on A2A adenosine receptors in human neutrophils. British journal of pharmacology, 161(4), 883-895. doi: 10.1111/j.1476-5381.2010.00900.x
36. Tucker, J. (2021, April 20). *The science behind percussion massage*. Chiropractic Economics. Retrieved September 6, 2022, from https://www.chiroeco.com/percussion-massage/
37. Null. (2021, March 15). *Rest easy: How percussive therapy can improve your sleep: On The move: Therabody wellness blog*. Therabody. Retrieved February 21, 2023, from https://www.therabody.com/ca/en-ca/blog/home/therabody-x-biostrap-sleep-study

General References:

- Shielded Healing. (n.d.). *Podcasts & interviews*. Shielded Healing. Retrieved August 18, 2022, from https://shieldedhealing.com/pages/media
- *Asprey, D. (2021, August 3). Inclined bed therapy: Sleep on an incline for a better night's sleep. Bulletproof.* Retrieved September 6, 2022, from https://www.bulletproof.com/sleep/sleep-hacks/inclined-bed-therapy-sleep/
- Jessen, N. A., Munk, A. S. F., Lundgaard, I., & Nedergaard, M. (2015, December). *The Glymphatic System: A beginner's guide*. Neurochemical research. Retrieved September 6, 2022, from https://www.ncbi.nlm.nih.gov/pmc/articles/PMC4636982/

Section 2 - Hydration, Fuel and Foundations

In-text References:

1. Huberman, A. (2023, February 22). *Guest series: Dr. Andy Galpin: Optimal Nutrition & Supplementation for Fitness*. Huberman Lab. Retrieved February 27, 2023, from https://hubermanlab.com/dr-andy-galpin-optimal-nutrition-and-supplementation-for-fitness/
2. Adan, A. (2012). Cognitive performance and dehydration. *Journal of the American College of Nutrition*, 31(2), 71–78. https://doi.org/10.1080/07315724.2012.10720011

3. Sawka, M. N., Cheuvront, S. N., & Carter, R. (2005). Human water needs. *Nutrition Reviews, 63*. https://doi.org/10.1111/j.1753-4887.2005.tb00152.x
4. *Facts on fluids - how to stay hydrated.* Facts on Fluids - How to Stay Hydrated - Unlock Food. (n.d.). Retrieved February 28, 2023, from https://www.unlockfood.ca/en/Articles/Water/Facts-on-Fluids-How-to-Stay-Hydrated.aspx
5. National Academies of Sciences, Engineering, and Medicine. (2004). Dietary Reference Intakes for Water, Potassium, Sodium, Chloride, and Sulfate. Washington, DC: The National Academies Press.
6. DiNicolantonio, J. (2017). The Salt Fix: Why the Experts Got It All Wrong—and How Eating More Might Save Your Life. Harmony.
7. YouTube. (2022, March 14). *Using salt to optimize mental & physical performance Huberman lab podcast #63*. YouTube. Retrieved February 25, 2023, from https://www.youtube.com/watch?v=azb3Ih68awQ
8. [Svensson, S et al. Increased Net Water Loss By Oral Compared to Nasal Expiration in Healthy Subjects. Rhinology 44, no.1 (2006):74.
9. Pollack, G. H. (2013). The Fourth Phase of Water: Beyond Solid, Liquid, and Vapor. Seattle, WA: Ebner & Sons.
10. Phillips, S. M., Chevalier, S., & Leidy, H. J. (2016, February 9). *Protein "requirements" Beyond the rda: Implications for optimizing health.* Applied Physiology, Nutrition, and Metabolism. Retrieved February 2, 2023, from https://cdnsciencepub.com/doi/full/10.1139/apnm-2015-0550
11. Stokes T;Hector AJ;Morton RW;McGlory C;Phillips SM; (n.d.). *Recent perspectives regarding the role of dietary protein for the promotion of muscle hypertrophy with resistance exercise training.* Nutrients. Retrieved February 15, 2023, from https://pubmed.ncbi.nlm.nih.gov/29414855/
12. *Saturated fat.* www.heart.org. (2023, January 24). Retrieved March 1, 2023, from https://www.heart.org/en/healthy-living/healthy-eating/eat-smart/fats/saturated-fats
13. News, I. (2015, June 17). *FDA takes step to remove artificial trans fats in Processed Foods.* The National Provisioner RSS. Retrieved February 23, 2023, from https://www.provisioneronline.com/articles/102050-fda-takes-step-to-remove-artificial-trans-fats-in-processed-foods
14. Simopoulos, A. P. (2002). Omega-3 fatty acids in inflammation and autoimmune diseases. *Journal of the American College of Nutrition*, *21*(6), 495–505. https://doi.org/10.1080/07315724.2002.10719248
15. Vahdat, M., Hosseini, S.A., Khalatbari Mohseni, G. et al. Effects of resistant starch interventions on circulating inflammatory biomarkers: a systematic review and meta-analysis of randomized controlled trials. Nutr J 19, 33 (2020). https://doi.org/10.1186/s12937-020-00548-6
16. https://journals.physiology.org/doi/full/10.1152/ajpendo.00093.2009
17. YouTube. (2022, February 28). *How to enhance your gut microbiome for Brain & Overall Health | Huberman Lab Podcast #61*. YouTube. Retrieved March 1, 2023, from https://www.youtube.com/watch?v=15R2pMqU2ok
18. Sgritta, M., Dooling, S. W., Buffington, S. A., Momin, E. N., Francis, M. B., Britton, R. A., & Costa-Mattioli, M. (2019). Mechanisms underlying microbial-mediated changes in social behavior in mouse models of autism spectrum disorder. *Neuron*, *101*(2), 246-259.e6. https://doi.org/10.1016/j.neuron.2018.11.018

19. Wastyk, H. C., Fragiadakis, G. K., Perelman, D., Dahan, D., Merrill, B. D., Yu, F. B., Topf, M., Gonzalez, C. G., Van Treuren, W., Han, S., Robinson, J. L., Elias, J. E., Sonnenburg, E. D., Gardner, C. D., & Sonnenburg, J. L. (2021). Gut-microbiota-targeted diets modulate human immune status. *Cell*, *184*(16), 4137–4153. https://doi.org/10.1016/j.cell.2021.06.019
20. Vighi, G., Marcucci, F., Sensi, L., di Cara, G., & Frati, F. (2008). Allergy and the gastrointestinal system. *Clinical & Experimental Immunology*, *153*, 3–6. R
21. Camilleri, M. (2009). Serotonin in the gastrointestinal tract. *Current Opinion in Endocrinology, Diabetes and Obesity*, *16*(1), 53–59.
22. M. B. Distrutti, G. Gargiulo, F. Romeo, M. Vincenzo, and E. Cipriani."Dietary fiber and butyrate improve intestinal homeostasis and neuroprotective signaling in aged mice." Nutritional Neuroscience 21, no. 10 (2018): 715-725.
23. Ríos-Covián, D., Ruas-Madiedo, P., Margolles, A., Gueimonde, M., de los Reyes-Gavilán, C. G., & Salazar, N. (2016). Intestinal short chain fatty acids and their link with diet and human health. *Frontiers in Microbiology*, 7.
24. Katz, S. E., & Pollan, M. (2012). *The art of fermentation: An in-depth exploration of essential concepts and processes from around the world.* Chelsea Green Pub.
25. Ferriss, T. (2019). *The 4-hour chef: The simple path to cooking like a pro, learning anything, and living the good life.* Houghton Mifflin Harcourt.
26. Davis, W. (2022). *Super gut: Reprogram your microbiome to restore health, lose weight, and turn back the clock.* Collins.
27. Marsh, P. D. (2016). The human oral microbiome. Journal of Oral Microbiology, 8, 32112. https://doi.org/10.3402/jom.v8.32112
28. Peedikayil FC, Sreenivasan P, Narayanan A. Effect of coconut oil in plaque related gingivitis - A preliminary report. Niger Med J. 2015;56(2):143-147. doi:10.4103/0300-1652.153406.
29. Shanbhag VK. Oil pulling for maintaining oral hygiene - A review. J Tradit Complement Med. 2016 Jun 6;7(1):106-109. doi: 10.1016/j.jtcme.2016.05.004. PMID: 28053895; PMCID: PMC5198813.
30. *News.* Canadian Centre on Substance Use and Addiction. (n.d.). Retrieved Feb 14, 2023, from https://www.ccsa.ca/more-6-drinks-week-puts-your-health-risk-new-canadas-guidance-alcohol-and-health
31. Heather J Leidy, Rebecca J Lepping, Joanne M Savage, and Wayne W Campbell. International Journal of Obesity. Volume 32, pages 881–888 (2008). "Higher protein intake preserves lean mass and satiety with weight loss in pre-obese and obese women."
32. Leidy, H. J., & Racki, E. M. (2010, July). *The addition of a protein-rich breakfast and its effects on acute appetite control and food intake in 'breakfast-skipping' adolescents.* International journal of obesity (2005). Retrieved March 3, 2023, from https://www.ncbi.nlm.nih.gov/pmc/articles/PMC4263815/
33. YouTube. (2022, March 21). *Controlling sugar cravings & metabolism with science-based tools | huberman lab podcast #64.* YouTube. Retrieved March 1, 2023, from https://www.youtube.com/watch?v=VAEzZeaV5zM
34. Del Pozo S, Gómez-Martínez S, Díaz LE, Nova E, Urrialde R, Marcos A. Potential Effects of Sucralose and Saccharin on Gut Microbiota: A Review. Nutrients. 2022 Apr 18;14(8):1682. doi: 10.3390/nu14081682. PMID: 35458244; PMCID: PMC9029443.

35. YouTube. (2022, July 18). *Dr. Charles Zuker: The Biology of Taste Perception & Sugar Craving | Huberman Lab Podcast #81*. YouTube. Retrieved Feb 15, 2023, from https://www.youtube.com/watch?v=UChhXiFPRgg
36. Östman, E., Granfeldt, Y., Persson, L., & Björck, I. (2005). Vinegar supplementation lowers glucose and insulin responses and increases satiety after a bread meal in healthy subjects. *European Journal of Clinical Nutrition*, 59(9), 983–988. https://doi.org/10.1038/sj.ejcn.1602197
37. Seidita A, Soresi M, Giannitrapani L, Di Stefano V, Citarrella R, Mirarchi L, Cusimano A, Augello G, Carroccio A, Iovanna JL, Cervello M. The clinical impact of an extra virgin olive oil enriched mediterranean diet on metabolic syndrome: Lights and shadows of a nutraceutical approach. Front Nutr. 2022 Aug 4;9:980429. doi: 10.3389/fnut.2022.980429. PMID: 35990331; PMCID: PMC9386289.
38. Carnevale R, Silvestri R, Loffredo L, Novo M, Cammisotto V, Castellani V, Bartimoccia S, Nocella C, Violi F. Oleuropein, a component of extra virgin olive oil, lowers postprandial glycaemia in healthy subjects. Br J Clin Pharmacol. 2018 Jul;84(7):1566-1574. doi: 10.1111/bcp.13589. Epub 2018 May 2. PMID: 29577365; PMCID: PMC6005585.
39. American Heart Association. (n.d.). Suggested Servings from Each Food Group. Retrieved fromhttps://www.heart.org/en/healthy-living/healthy-eating/eat-smart/nutrition-basics/suggested-servings-from-each-food-group
40. Kong, W.-J., Zhang, H., Song, D.-Q., Xue, R., Zhao, W., Wei, J., Wang, Y.-M., Shan, N., Zhou, Z.-X., Yang, P., You, X.-F., Li, Z.-R., Si, S.-Y., Zhao, L.-X., Pan, H.-N., & Jiang, J.-D. (2009). Berberine reduces insulin resistance through protein kinase C–dependent up-regulation of insulin receptor expression. *Metabolism*, *58*(1), 109–119. https://doi.org/10.1016/j.metabol.2008.08.013
41. YouTube. (2021, April 19). *How our hormones control our hunger, eating & satiety | Huberman lab podcast #16*. YouTube. Retrieved March 12, 2023, from https://www.youtube.com/watch?v=17O5mgXZ9ZU
42. YouTube. (2021, October 18). *Nutrients for Brain Health & Performance | Huberman Lab Podcast #42*. YouTube. Retrieved March 1, 2023, from https://www.youtube.com/watch?v=E7W4OQfJWdw
43. Braverman, E. R., & Pfeiffer, C. C. (1987). *The healing nutrients within: Facts, findings, and new research on amino acids*. Keats Pub.
44. de Cabo, R., & Mattson, M. P. (n.d.). *Effects of intermittent fasting on health, aging, and disease | nejm*. New England Journal of Medicine. Retrieved February 8, 2023, from https://www.nejm.org/doi/full/10.1056/NEJMra1905136
45. Gabel, K., Hoddy, K. K., Haggerty, N., Song, J., Kroeger, C. M., Trepanowski, J. F., Panda, S., & Varady, K. A. (2018). Effects of 8-hour time restricted feeding on body weight and metabolic disease risk factors in obese adults: A pilot study. *Nutrition and Healthy Aging*, 4(4), 345–353. https://doi.org/10.3233/nha-170036
46. Mattson MP, Longo VD, Harvie M. Impact of intermittent fasting on health and disease processes. Ageing Res Rev. 2017 Oct;39:46-58. doi: 10.1016/j.arr.2016.10.005. Epub 2016 Oct 22. PMID: 27770653.
47. Panda, S. (2018). *The circadian code: Lose weight, supercharge your energy, and transform your health from morning to midnight.* Rodale, an imprint of the Crown Publishing Group.

48. Pelz, M. (2023). *Fast like a girl: A woman's guide to using the healing power of fasting to burn fat, boost energy, and balance hormones*. Hay House.
49. Catherine Greene and Carolyn Dimitry (n.d.). Recent growth patterns in the U.S. Organic Foods Market. USDA ERS. Retrieve March 2, 2023, from https://www.ers.usda.gov/publications/pub-details/?pubid=42456
50. NSF International. (n.d.). NSF International dietary supplement certification. Retrieved February 12, 2023, from https://www.nsf.org/services/by-industry/dietary-supplements/dietary-supplement-certification
51. *Nutreval: Genova diagnostics*. NutrEval | Genova Diagnostics. (n.d.). Retrieved March 2, 2023, from https://www.gdx.net/products/nutreval
52. Calder, P. C., Carr, A. C., Gombart, A. F., & Eggersdorfer, M. (2020, April 23). *Optimal nutritional status for a well-functioning immune system is an important factor to protect against viral infections*. MDPI. https://doi.org/10.3390/nu12041181
53. Simopoulos, A. P. (2008). The importance of the omega-6/omega-3 fatty acid ratio in cardiovascular disease and other chronic diseases. *Experimental Biology and Medicine*, 233(6), 674–688. https://doi.org/10.3181/0711-mr-311
54. Simopoulos, A. (2002). The importance of the ratio of omega-6/omega-3 essential fatty acids. *Biomedicine & Pharmacotherapy*, 56(8), 365–379. https://doi.org/10.1016/s0753-3322(02)00253-6
55. Kubala, Jillian, M.S., R.D. (2022,February 9). *What Is Collagen and What Is It Good For?* Healthline. Retrieved February 23, 2022, from https://www.healthline.com/nutrition/collagen#what-it-does
56. Bantilan Ms, R. C. D. (2019, November 7). *What Is Bovine Collagen, and Does It Have Benefits?* Healthline. https://www.healthline.com/nutrition/bovine-collagen#what-it-is
57. DiNicolantonio, J. (2016). The collagen supplement: Alternative medicine for a healthy body. Healthy Living Publishing.
58. Swaminathan, R. (2003, May). *Magnesium metabolism and its disorders*. The Clinical biochemist. Reviews. Retrieved February 2, 2023, from https://www.ncbi.nlm.nih.gov/pmc/articles/PMC1855626/.
59. Gröber U, Werner T, Vormann J, Kisters K. Myth or Reality-Transdermal Magnesium? Nutrients. 2017 Jul 28;9(8):813. doi: 10.3390/nu9080813. PMID: 28788060; PMCID: PMC5579607.https://doi.org/10.1111/j.1365-2249.2008.03713.x
60. Roschel, H., Gualano, B., Ostojic, S. M., & Rawson, E. S. (2021, February 10). *Creatine supplementation and Brain Health*. MDPI. Retrieved March 2, 2023, from https://www.mdpi.com/2072-6643/13/2/586
61. Chevalier, G., Sinatra, S. T., Oschman, J. L., Sokal, K., & Sokal, P. (2012). Earthing: Health implications of reconnecting the human body to the Earth's surface electrons. *Journal of Environmental and Public Health*, 2012, 1–8. https://doi.org/10.1155/2012/291541
62. Ober, C., Sinatra, S. T., & Zucker, M. (2010). *Earthing: The Most Important Health Discovery Ever?* Basic Health Publications.

General References:

- Greenfield, B. (2022, June 8). *Best creatine for Muscle Repair, cognition, endurance, and more!* Ben Greenfield Life - Fitness, Diet, Fat Loss and Performance Advice.

Retrieved March 2, 2023, from
https://bengreenfieldlife.com/article/supplements-articles/best-creatine/

Section 3—Movement, Exercise & Detoxification

In-text References:

1. Volpi, E., Nazemi, R., & Fujita, S. (2004). Muscle tissue changes with aging. *Current Opinion in Clinical Nutrition and Metabolic Care*, 7(4), 405–410. https://doi.org/10.1097/01.mco.0000134362.76653.b2
2. Nazri NSM, Vanoh D, Soo KL. Natural Food for Sarcopenia: A Narrative Review. Malays J Med Sci. 2022 Aug;29(4):28-42. doi: 10.21315/mjms2022.29.4.4. Epub 2022 Aug 29. PMID: 36101538; PMCID: PMC9438863.
3. Virginia A. Hughes and others, Longitudinal Muscle Strength Changes in Older Adults: Influence of Muscle Mass, Physical Activity, and Health, The Journals of Gerontology: Series A, Volume 56, Issue 5, 1 May 2001, Pages B209–B217, https://doi.org/10.1093/gerona/56.5.B209
4. Donato AJ, Tench K, Glueck DH, Seals DR, Eskurza I, Tanaka H. Declines in physiological functional capacity with age: a longitudinal study in peak swimming performance. J Appl Physiol (1985). 2003 Feb;94(2):764-9. doi: 10.1152/japplphysiol.00438.2002. Epub 2002 Oct 18. PMID: 12391125; PMCID: PMC5063028.
5. YouTube (January 26, 2023) Dr. Andy Galpin: How To Assess & Improve All Aspects of Your Fitness | Huberman Lab Guest Series. YouTube. Retrieved May 24, 2023, from https://hubermanlab.com/dr-andy-galpin-how-to-assess-improve-all-aspects-of-your-fitness/
6. Dercon, Q., Nicholas, J. M., James, S.-N., Schott, J. M., & Richards, M. (2021, September 29). *Grip strength from midlife as an indicator of later-life brain health and cognition: Evidence from a British birth cohort - BMC geriatrics*. BioMed Central. Retrieved May 12, 2023, from https://bmcgeriatr.biomedcentral.com/articles/10.1186/s12877-021-02411-7
7. Jiang, R., Westwater, M. L., Noble, S., Rosenblatt, M., Dai, W., Qi, S., Sui, J., Calhoun, V. D., & Scheinost, D. (2022a, September 9). *Associations between grip strength, brain structure, and mental health in > 40,000 participants from the UK Biobank - BMC Medicine*. BioMed Central. Retrieved May 17, 2023, from https://bmcmedicine.biomedcentral.com/articles/10.1186/s12916-022-02490-2
8. Genton, L., Hans, D., Kyle, U. G., & Pichard, C. (2002). Dual-Energy X-ray absorptiometry and body composition: Differences between devices and comparison with reference methods. *Nutrition*, *18*(1), 66–70. https://doi.org/10.1016/s0899-9007(01)00700-6
9. Vicente-Campos, D., López, A. M., Nuñez, M. J., & Chicharro, J. L. (2014). Heart rate recovery normality data recorded in response to a maximal exercise test in physically active men. *European Journal of Applied Physiology*, *114*(6), 1123–1128. https://doi.org/10.1007/s00421-014-2847-4
10. Suzic Lazic, J., Dekleva, M., Soldatovic, I., Leischik, R., Suzic, S., Radovanovic, D., Djuric, B., Nesic, D., Lazic, M., & Mazic, S. (2017). Heart rate recovery in elite

athletes: The impact of age and exercise capacity. *Clinical Physiology and Functional Imaging*, 37(2), 117–123. https://doi.org/10.1111/cpf.12271

11. Kline, G.M., Porcari, J.P., Hintermeister, R., et al. (1987). Estimation of VO2 Max from a one-mile track walk, gender, age, and body weight. Medicine and Science in Sports and Exercise, 19(3), 253-259.
12. Cooper, K. H. (1968). A means of assessing maximal oxygen intake. *JAMA*, *203*(3), 201. https://doi.org/10.1001/jama.1968.03140030033008
13. YouTube. (2022, March 28). *201 - deep dive back into zone 2 training | iñigo san-millán, Ph.D. & Peter Attia, M.D.* YouTube. https://www.youtube.com/watch?v=-6PDBVRkCKc
14. O'Keefe, J. H., O'Keefe, E. L., & Lavie, C. J. (2018). The Goldilocks zone for exercise: Not too little, not too much. Missouri medicine. Retrieved August 17, 2021, from https://www.ncbi.nlm.nih.gov/pmc/articles/PMC6139866/
15. Penfield, W., & Boldrey, E. (1937). Somatic motor and sensory representation in the cerebral cortex of man as studied by electrical stimulation. Brain, 60(4), 389-443.
16. Episode 65: Dr. Andy Galpin: How to build strength, Muscle Size & Endurance: Huberman lab · podcast notes. Podcast Notes. (2022, March 31). Retrieved June 24, 2022, from https://podcastnotes.org/huberman-lab/episode-65-dr-andy-galpin-how-to-build-strength-muscle-size-endurance-huberman-lab/.
17. Isner-Horobeti ME, Rasseneur L, Lonsdorfer-Wolf E, Dufour SP, Doutreleau S, Bouitbir J, Zoll J, Kapchinsky S, Geny B, Daussin FN, Burelle Y, Richard R. Effect of eccentric versus concentric exercise training on mitochondrial function. Muscle Nerve. 2014 Nov;50(5):803-11. doi: 10.1002/mus.24215. Epub 2014 Aug 30. PMID: 24639213.
18. Heller, H. C., & Grahn, D. A. (2012, May 14). Enhancing Thermal Exchange in Humans and Practical Applications. Temperature. https://doi.org/10.1089/dst.2012.0004
19. Shift Adapt. (n.d.). Art of Breath. Retrieved May 25, 2023, from https://shiftadapt.com
20. Cintineo, H. P., Arent, M. A., Antonio, J., & Arent, S. M. (2018). Effects of protein supplementation on performance and recovery in resistance and endurance training. *Frontiers in Nutrition*, *5*. https://doi.org/10.3389/fnut.2018.00083
21. Woorons, X., Mucci, P., Aucouturier, J., Anthierens, A., & Millet, G. P. (2017). Acute effects of repeated cycling sprints in hypoxia induced by voluntary hypoventilation. *European Journal of Applied Physiology*, 117(12), 2433–2443. https://doi.org/10.1007/s00421-017-3729-3
22. McKeown, P. (2015). *The oxygen advantage: Simple, scientifically proven breathing technique to help you become healthier, slimmer, faster, and Fitter*. William Morrow & Company.
23. ScienceDaily. (2022, March 3). *Meta-analysis of 15 studies reports new findings on how many daily walking steps needed for longevity benefit*. ScienceDaily. Retrieved April 18, 2023, from https://www.sciencedaily.com/releases/2022/03/220303112207.html
24. Stanley, J., Peake, J. M., & Buchheit, M. (2013). Cardiac parasympathetic reactivation following exercise: Implications for training prescription. *Sports Medicine*, 43(12), 1259–1277. https://doi.org/10.1007/s40279-013-0083-4

25. *Dr. Timothy R. Morris, Functional Naturopathic Doctor*. Retrieved May 25, 2023, from https://www.trmorrisnd.com/.
26. Wolverton, B. C., Bounds, K., & Johnson, A. (1989). *Interior landscape plants for indoor air pollution abatement - Final Report*. NASA. Retrieved May 15, 2023, from https://ntrs.nasa.gov/citations/19930073077
27. Sajid, M., & Ilyas, M. (2017). PTFE-coated non-stick cookware and toxicity concerns: A perspective. *Environmental Science and Pollution Research*, 24(30), 23436–23440. https://doi.org/10.1007/s11356-017-0095-y
28. Stapleton, H. M., Eagle, S., Anthopolos, R., Wolkin, A., & Miranda, M. L. (2011). Associations between polybrominated diphenyl ether (PBDE) flame retardants, phenolic metabolites, and thyroid hormones during pregnancy. *Environmental Health Perspectives*, *119*(10), 1454–1459. https://doi.org/10.1289/ehp.1003235
29. Thrasher, J. D., & Kilburn, K. H. (2001). Embryotoxicity and teratogenicity of formaldehyde. *Archives of Environmental Health: An International Journal*, 56(4), 300–311. https://doi.org/10.1080/00039890109604460
30. Barry, V., Winquist, A., & Steenland, K. (2013). Perfluorooctanoic acid (PFOA) exposures and incident cancers among adults living near a chemical plant. *Environmental Health Perspectives*, *121*(11–12), 1313–1318. https://doi.org/10.1289/ehp.1306615
31. U.S. Environmental Protection Agency. (2017). *Volatile Organic Compounds' Impact on Indoor Air Quality*. EPA. Retrieved May 5, 2023, from https://www.epa.gov/indoor-air-quality-iaq/volatile-organic-compounds-impact-indoor-air-quality
32. Mokhtari, V., Moini , A., Kalantar , S. M., Shahhoseini , M., & Afsharian , P. (2017). *A review on various uses of N-acetyl cysteine*. Cell Journal (Yakhteh). 19(1), 11-17. Retrieve May 2, 2023, from https://www.celljournal.org/article_250409.html
33. Thomson, C. A., Ho, E., & Strom, M. B. (2016). Chemopreventive properties of 3,3′-diindolylmethane in breast cancer: Evidence from experimental and human studies. *Nutrition Reviews*, 74(7), 432–443. https://doi.org/10.1093/nutrit/nuw010
34. Gomes, M. B., & Negrato, C. A. (2014). Alpha-lipoic acid as a pleiotropic compound with potential therapeutic use in diabetes and other chronic diseases. *Diabetology & Metabolic Syndrome*, *6*(1). https://doi.org/10.1186/1758-5996-6-80
35. Fahey, J. W., Zhang, Y., & Talalay, P. (1997). Broccoli sprouts: An exceptionally rich source of inducers of enzymes that protect against chemical carcinogens. *Proceedings of the National Academy of Sciences*, 94(19), 10367–10372. https://doi.org/10.1073/pnas.94.19.10367
36. Abenavoli, L., Capasso, R., & Capasso, F. (2010). Milk thistle in liver diseases: An update. Journal of Clinical Gastroenterology, 44(Supplement 1), S11-S17. Retrieved May 11, 2023, from https://journals.lww.com/jcge/toc/2010/09001
37. Kuan, W.-H., Chen, Y.-L., & Liu, C.-L. (2022). Excretion of ni, pb, Cu, as, and hg in sweat under two sweating conditions. *International Journal of Environmental Research and Public Health*, *19*(7), 4323. https://doi.org/10.3390/ijerph19074323
38. Hamblin, M. R. (2017). Mechanisms and applications of the anti-inflammatory effects of photobiomodulation. *AIMS Biophysics*, 4(3), 337–361. https://doi.org/10.3934/biophy.2017.3.337
39. Stop Chasing Pain. (n.d.). Retrieved May 3, 2023, from https://www.stopchasingpain.com/

Section 4—Brain Wiring, Neurotransmitters & Hormones

In-text References:

1. Von Bartheld, C. S. (2018). Counting on neurons: the neuroscientist's guide to quantitative anatomy. *Oxford University Press.* (p. 14)
2. Ganesan, K., & Teklehaimanot, G. (2018). Effects of heat stress on neurological functions. *Frontiers in Neuroscience*, *12*, 625. https://doi.org/10.3389/fnins.2018.00625
3. Leppäluoto, J., Huttunen, P., Hirvonen, J., Väänänen, A., Tuominen, M., & Vuori, J. (1986). Endocrine effects of repeated sauna bathing. *Acta Physiologica Scandinavica*, *128*(3), 467–470. https://doi.org/10.1111/j.1748-1716.1986.tb08000.x
4. Mayer, E. A. (2011). Gut feelings: The emerging biology of Gut–Brain Communication. *Nature Reviews Neuroscience*, *12*(8), 453–466. https://doi.org/10.1038/nrn3071
5. Pavlov, V. A., & Tracey, K. J. (2012). The vagus nerve and the inflammatory reflex—linking immunity and metabolism. *Nature Reviews Endocrinology*, *8*(12), 743–754. https://doi.org/10.1038/nrendo.2012.189
6. Porges, S. W. (2007). The polyvagal perspective. Biological Psychology, 74(2), 116-143. doi: 10.1016/j.biopsycho.2006.06.009.
7. Borovikova, L. V., Ivanova, S., Zhang, M., Yang, H., Botchkina, G. I., Watkins, L. R., Wang, H., Abumrad, N., Eaton, J. W., & Tracey, K. J. (2000). Vagus nerve stimulation attenuates the systemic inflammatory response to endotoxin. *Nature*, *405*(6785), 458–462. https://doi.org/10.1038/35013070
8. Zhang, J., Dean, D., Nosco, D., Strathopulos, D., & Floros, M. (2006). Effect of chiropractic care on Heart Rate Variability and pain in a multisite clinical study. *Journal of Manipulative and Physiological Therapeutics*, *29*(4), 267–274. https://doi.org/10.1016/j.jmpt.2006.03.010
9. Sauder, K. A., Skulas-Ray, A. C., Campbell, T. S., Johnson, J. A., Kris-Etherton, P. M., & West, S. G. (2013). Effects of omega-3 fatty acid supplementation on heart rate variability at rest and during acute stress in adults with moderate hypertriglyceridemia. *Psychosomatic Medicine*, *75*(4), 382–389. https://doi.org/10.1097/psy.0b013e318290a107
10. Bergdahl, L., Bunner, M., & Törnkvist, L. (2018). Vibratory vagal stimulation: A new non-invasive treatment of chronic pain? A pilot study. *Scandinavian Journal of Pain*, *18*(4), 599-607.
11. Jerath, R., Crawford, M. W., Barnes, V. A., & Harden, K. (2015). Self-regulation of breathing as a primary treatment for anxiety. *Applied Psychophysiology and Biofeedback*, *40*(2), 107–115. https://doi.org/10.1007/s10484-015-9279-8
12. Swift A.C., Campbell I.T., Mckown T.M. (1988). Oronasal obstruction, lung volumes, and arterial oxygenation. *The Lancet*, *331*(8577), 73–75. https://doi.org/10.1016/s0140-6736(88)90282-6
13. Soler, Z. M., Eckert, M. A., Storck, K., & Schlosser, R. J. (2015). Cognitive function in chronic rhinosinusitis: A controlled clinical study. *International Forum of Allergy & Rhinology*, *5*(11), 1010–1017. https://doi.org/10.1002/alr.21581
14. Cunnane, S. C., Courchesne-Loyer, A., St-Pierre, V., Vandenberghe, C., Pierotti, T., Fortier, M., Croteau, E., & Castellano, C.-A. (2016). Can ketones compensate for

deteriorating brain glucose uptake during aging? implications for the risk and treatment of alzheimer's disease. *Annals of the New York Academy of Sciences*, 1367(1), 12–20. https://doi.org/10.1111/nyas.12999

15. Murray, A. J., Knight, N. S., Cole, M. A., Cochlin, L. E., Carter, E., Tchabanenko, K., Pichulik, T., Gulston, M. K., Atherton, H. J., Schroeder, M. A., Deacon, R. M., Kashiwaya, Y., King, M. T., Pawlosky, R., Rawlins, J. N., Tyler, D. J., Griffin, J. L., Robertson, J., Veech, R. L., & Clarke, K. (2016). Novel ketone diet enhances physical and cognitive performance. *The FASEB Journal*, *30*(12), 4021–4032. https://doi.org/10.1096/fj.201600773r
16. Gonçalves, J. T., Schafer, S. T., & Gage, F. H. (2016). Adult neurogenesis in the hippocampus: From stem cells to behavior. *Cell*, *167*(4), 897–914. https://doi.org/10.1016/j.cell.2016.10.021
17. Nicolson, G. L. (2014). Chronic bacterial and viral infections in neurodegenerative and neurobehavioral diseases. *Laboratory Medicine*, 45(4), e109–e117. https://doi.org/10.1309/LMWNW0OWPBJYFT2B
18. Heneka, M. T., Carson, M. J., Khoury, J. E., Landreth, G. E., Brosseron, F., Feinstein, D. L., Jacobs, A. H., Wyss-Coray, T., Vitorica, J., Ransohoff, R. M., Herrup, K., Frautschy, S. A., Finsen, B., Brown, G. C., Verkhratsky, A., Yamanaka, K., Koistinaho, J., Latz, E., Halle, A., ... Kummer, M. P. (2015). Neuroinflammation in alzheimer's disease. *The Lancet Neurology*, *14*(4), 388–405. https://doi.org/10.1016/s1474-4422(15)70016-5
19. Scapagnini, G., Davinelli, S., Drago, F., De Lorenzo, A., Bellusci, A., & Oriani, G. (2017). Polyphenols as dietary supplements: A double-edged sword. *Nutrition and Dietary Supplements*, 27(9), 710–719. https://doi.org/10.1016/j.numecd.2017.05.006
20. Selma, M. V., González-Sarrías, A., Salas-Salvadó, J., Andrés-Lacueva, C., & Alasalvar, C. (2019). The Role of the Gut Microbiota on the Metabolism of Dietary Polyphenols. *BioMed Research International*, *1*(18). https://doi.org/10.1155/2019/9056720
21. Draganski, B., & May, A. (2008). Training-induced structural changes in the adult human brain. *Behavioural Brain Research*, *192*(1), 137–142. https://doi.org/10.1016/j.bbr.2008.02.015
22. Montgomery, S. A., & Thal, L. J. (1991). The effect of L-acetylcarnitine on cognitive performance in Alzheimer's disease: a multicenter study. *Clinical Neuropharmacology*, 14(3), 167–176.
23. Sarter, M., Givens, B., & Bruno, J. P. (2001). The Cognitive Neuroscience of sustained attention: Where top-down meets bottom-up. *Brain Research Reviews*, 35(2), 146–160. https://doi.org/10.1016/s0165-0173(01)00044-3
24. Gershon, M. D., & Tack, J. (2007). The serotonin signaling system: from basic understanding to drug development for functional GI disorders. Gastroenterology, 132(1), 397-414. https://doi.org/10.1053/j.gastro.2006.11.002
25. Nassar, M. F., Fahmy, S. R., El-Kharashi, O. A., & El-Tahawy, N. F. (2021). Acute effect of phenylethylamine on mood states in young healthy volunteers: A randomized, double-blind, placebo-controlled study. *European Psychiatry, 64*(1), e2.
26. Manninen, A. H. (2018). Environmental temperature and human performance: Effect of thermal exposure on mental workload, motor performance and cognitive abilities. *Frontiers in Physiology*, 9, 1558.

27. National Institutes of Health. (2021). Vitamin B6 - *Health Professional Fact Sheet.* Retrieved June 29, 2023, from https://ods.od.nih.gov/factsheets/VitaminB6-HealthProfessional/
28. Wong, H., & Dockray, G. J. (2019). The effects of supplementation with L-theanine, caffeine, and their combination on cognitive performance and mood: A review and meta-analysis. *Nutritional neuroscience, 22*(11), 749-758.
29. Sharma, V. K., Sharma, N., & Paudel, K. R. (2007). Nitric oxide and its role in neuroprotection. *Current Neuropharmacology, 5*(3), 277-285.
30. El-Mallakh, R. S., Paskitti, M. E., & El-Mallakh, P. L. (2017). The ketogenic diet may have mood-stabilizing properties. *Journal of Clinical Psychopharmacology, 37*(1), 126–128. https://doi.org/10.1097/JCP.0000000000000634
31. Rapoport, S. I. (2008). Docosahexaenoic acid and cerebral cortex function: A hypothesis. *Nutrition Reviews, 66*(3), 153–171. https://doi.org/10.1111/j.1753-4887.2008.00019.x
32. Grosso, G., Pajak, A., Marventano, S., Castellano, S., Galvano, F., Bucolo, C., Drago, F., & Caraci, F. (2014). Role of omega-3 fatty acids in the treatment of depressive disorders: A comprehensive meta-analysis of randomized clinical trials. *PLoS ONE, 9*(5). https://doi.org/10.1371/journal.pone.0096905
33. Rae, C., Digney, A. L., McEwan, S. R., & Bates, T. C. (2003). Oral creatine monohydrate supplementation improves brain performance: A double–blind, placebo–controlled, Cross–Over Trial. *Proceedings of the Royal Society B: Biological Sciences, 270*(1529), 2147–2150. https://doi.org/10.1098/rspb.2003.2492
34. Balhara, Y. S., Verma, R., & Gupta, C. (2011). Gender differences in stress response: Role of developmental and biological determinants. *Industrial Psychiatry Journal, 20*(1), 4–10. https://doi.org/10.4103/0972-6748.98407
35. Kritz-Silverstein, D., Von Mühlen, D., Laughlin, G. A., & Bettencourt, R. (2008). Effects of dehydroepiandrosterone supplementation on cognitive function and quality of life: The DHEA and well-ness (dawn) trial. *Journal of the American Geriatrics Society, 56*(7), 1292–1298. https://doi.org/10.1111/j.1532-5415.2008.01768.x
36. Clemons, M., & Goss, P. (2001). Estrogen and the risk of breast cancer. *New England Journal of Medicine, 344*(4), 276–285. https://doi.org/10.1056/nejm200101253440407
37. Silins, E., Horwood, L. J., Patton, G. C., Fergusson, D. M., Olsson, C. A., Hutchinson, D. M., Spry, E., Toumbourou, J. W., Degenhardt, L., Swift, W., Coffey, C., Tait, R. J., Letcher, P., Copeland, J., & Mattick, R. P. (2014). Young adult sequelae of adolescent cannabis use: An integrative analysis. *The Lancet Psychiatry, 1*(4), 286–293. https://doi.org/10.1016/s2215-0366(14)70307-4
38. Davison, S. L., Bell, R., Donath, S., Montalto, J. G., & Davis, S. R. (2005). Androgen levels in adult females: Changes with age, Menopause, and oophorectomy. *The Journal of Clinical Endocrinology and Metabolism, 90*(7), 3847–3853. https://doi.org/10.1210/jc.2005-0212
39. Vingren, J. L., Kraemer, W. J., Ratamess, N. A., Anderson, J. M., Volek, J. S., & Maresh, C. M. (2021). Testosterone physiology in resistance exercise and training: the up-stream regulatory elements. . *Sports Medicine and Health Science, 3*(2), 65–78.
40. La Vignera, S., Condorelli, R. A., Vicari, E., D'Agata, R., & Calogero, A. E. (2011). Effects of the exposure to mobile phones on male reproduction: A review of the

literature. *Journal of Andrology, 33*(3), 350–356. https://doi.org/10.2164/jandrol.111.014373

41. Kocaman, A., Topaktaş, M., Korkmaz, H., Kılıç, M. Ö., & Savaş, H. B. (2021). Effects of mobile phone use on the breast milk prolactin level in postpartum women. Bioelectromagnetics, 42(4), 279-287. *Journal of Andrology, 33*(3), 350–356.
42. Mercola, J. (2020). *EMF*D: 5G, Wi-Fi & Cell Phones: Hidden Harms and How to Protect Yourself.* Hay House Inc.
43. Chen, J., & Wang, W. (2021). A systematic review of the efficacy and safety of turkesterone in healthy people and animals: Is it a promising safe performance-enhancing supplement?. *Journal of Ethnopharmacology*, 277, 114240.
44. Chen, J. W., Wong, A. K., & Tzeng, W. C. (2020). Age-related decline of growth hormone secretion. *Aging and disease, 11*(4), 967.
45. Kukkonen-Harjula, K., Oja, P., Laustiola, K., Vuori, I., & Jolkkonen, J. (1989). Increase in plasma growth hormone and cortisol concentrations after sauna bath in patients with rheumatoid arthritis. *Scandinavian journal of rheumatology, 18*(6), 427-431.
46. Scoon, G. S. M., Hopkins, W. G., Mayhew, S., & Cotter, J. D. (2007). Effect of post-exercise sauna bathing on the endurance performance of competitive male runners. *Journal of Science and Medicine in Sport, 10*(4), 259–262. https://doi.org/10.1016/j.jsams.2006.06.009
47. Clemmons, D. R. (2018). Arginine and its metabolites: intriguing perturbations of cardiovascular function. *American Journal of Physiology-Heart and Circulatory Physiology, 315*(2), H366-H371.
48. Schumacher, R., Ostlund, R. E., & Yeung, A. (2016). Dried urine spot collection of postmenopausal women and validity of hormone assays using tandem mass spectrometry. *Journal of Applied Laboratory Medicine, 1*(6), 730-740.
49. Suzuki, W. (2015). Healthy Brain, Happy Life: A Personal Program to Activate Your Brain and Do Everything Better. New York, NY: Dey Street Books.
50. Diekelmann, S., & Born, J. (2010). The memory function of sleep. *Nature Reviews Neuroscience, 11*(2), 114–126. https://doi.org/10.1038/nrn2762
51. Lovato, N., & Lack, L. (2010). The effects of napping on cognitive functioning. *Progress in Brain Research*, 155–166. https://doi.org/10.1016/b978-0-444-53702-7.00009-9
52. Cristea, I. A., Antal, A., & Lavidor, M. (2019). Replicable effects of rhythmic binaural beats on episodic memory and mood state: A multisite registered replication study. *Cortex, 118*, 40-50.
53. Reedijk, S. A., Bolders, A., Colzato, L. S., & Hommel, B. (2015). Eliminating the attentional blink through binaural beats: A case for tailored cognitive enhancement. *Frontiers in Psychiatry*, 6. https://doi.org/10.3389/fpsyt.2015.00082
54. Krause, C. M., & Bratengeier, E. (2019). The effects of continuous white noise on cognitive functioning. *International Journal of Environmental Research and Public Health, 16*(13), 2367.
55. Huberman, A. (2020). Neuroplasticity and optimal performance: Rewiring your brain for success. American Psychologist, 75(5), 615-624.
56. Dispenza, J. (2017). Becoming Supernatural: How Common People are Doing the Uncommon. Hay House Inc.
57. Phillips, A. J., Clerx, W. M., O'Brien, C. S., Sano, A., Barger, L. K., Picard, R. W., Lockley, S. W., Klerman, E. B., & Czeisler, C. A. (2017). Irregular sleep/wake patterns are associated with poorer academic performance and delayed circadian

and sleep/wake timing. *Scientific Reports*, 7(1). https://doi.org/10.1038/s41598-017-03171-4

58. von Thiele Schwarz, U., & Hasson, H. (2011). Employee self-rated productivity and objective organizational production levels. *Journal of Occupational & Environmental Medicine*, 53(8), 838–844. https://doi.org/10.1097/jom.0b013e31822589c2
59. Cirillo, F. (2018). The Pomodoro Technique: The Life-Changing Time-Management System. Ebury Publishing
60. Kennedy, D., & Scholey, A. (2006). The psychopharmacology of European herbs with cognition-enhancing properties. *Current Pharmaceutical Design*, *12*(35), 4613–4623. https://doi.org/10.2174/138161206779010387
61. Shevtsov, V. A., Zholus, B. I., Shervarly, V. I., Vol'skij, V. B., Korovin, Y. P., Khristich, M. P., Roslyakova, N. A., & Wikman, G. (2003). A randomized trial of two different doses of a SHR-5 Rhodiola rosea extract versus placebo and control of capacity for mental work. *Phytomedicine*, *10*(2–3), 95–105. https://doi.org/10.1078/094471103321659780
62. Duncan, M. J., & Clarke, N. D. (2014). The effect of acute Rhodiola rosea ingestion on exercise heart rate, substrate utilisation, mood state, and perceptions of exertion, arousal, and pleasure/displeasure in active men. Journal of Sports Medicine, 2014, 1–8. https://doi.org/10.1155/2014/563043
63. Peper, E., Harvey, R., & Hamiel, D. (2015). Clenching Your Jaw and Gritting Your Teeth: An EMG Biofeedback Study on the Effects of Posture on Stress. *Biofeedback*, 43(4), 170–175.
64. Ma, J., Ma, D., Li, Z., & Kim, H. (2021). Effects of a workplace sit–stand desk intervention on health and productivity. *International Journal of Environmental Research and Public Health*, *18*(21), 11604. https://doi.org/10.3390/ijerph182111604
65. Emmons, R. A., & Mishra, A. (2011). Why gratitude enhances well-being: What we know, what we need to know. *Designing Positive Psychology*, 248–262. https://doi.org/10.1093/acprof:oso/9780195373585.003.0016
66. Huberman, A. (2021). Gratitude and the brain. Huberman Lab. Retrieved June 28, 2023, from https://www.hubermanlab.com/gratitude-and-the-brain
67. Hölzel, B. K., Carmody, J., Vangel, M., Congleton, C., Yerramsetti, S. M., Gard, T., & Lazar, S. W. (2011). Mindfulness practice leads to increases in regional brain gray matter density. *Psychiatry Research: Neuroimaging*, *191*(1), 36–43. https://doi.org/10.1016/j.pscychresns.2010.08.006
68. Smith, J. C., & Feldman, J. L. (2013). Physiology of the pre-Bötzinger complex and the pre inspiratory period. . *Physiological Reviews*, 93(1), 1–19. https://doi.org/10.1152/physrev.00002.2012
69. Spiegel, D., & Block, K. (2012). Hypnosis for the management of chronic pain. *International Journal of Clinical and Experimental Hypnosis*, 60(4), 432-444.
70. Lelic, D., Niazi, I. K., Holt, K., Jochumsen, M., Dremstrup, K., Yielder, P., Murphy, B., Drewes, A. M., & Haavik, H. (2016). Manipulation of dysfunctional spinal joints affects sensorimotor integration in the prefrontal cortex: A brain source localization study. *Neural Plasticity*, *2016*, 1–9. https://doi.org/10.1155/2016/3704964
71. Schwartz, M., Kipnis, J., Rivest, S., & Prat, A. (2013). How do immune cells support and shape the brain in health, disease, and aging? *The Journal of Neuroscience*, 33(45), 17587–17596. https://doi.org/10.1523/jneurosci.3241-13.2013

72. Schmahmann, J. D. (2013). Cerebellar contributions to higher cognition. In M. Manto, J. D. Schmahmann, N. Koibuchi, F. Rossi, & A. Gruol (Eds.), *The Handbook of the Cerebellum and Cerebellar Disorders*, 1097–1112. https://doi.org/10.1007/978-94-007-1333-8_62
73. Murphy, B. A., Dawson, N. J., Slack, J. R., Higbie, E., & Sterling, R. J. (2012). The effect of spinal manipulation on the cerebellar processing of the sensory input from an ankle sprain: A preliminary fMRI study. *Journal of Manipulative and Physiological Therapeutics*, 35(3), 245-255.
74. Haavik, H., & Murphy, B. (2011). Subclinical Neck Pain and the effects of cervical manipulation on elbow joint position sense. *Journal of Manipulative and Physiological Therapeutics*, 34(2), 88–97. https://doi.org/10.1016/j.jmpt.2010.12.009

Section 5—Epigenetics, Aging & Healthspan

In-text References:

1. Brown, G. C. (2017). Living too long. *EMBO Reports*, *18*(1), 6–9. https://doi.org/10.15252/embr.201439518
2. Miniño, A. M., Murphy, S. L., Xu, J., & Kochanek, K. D. (2018). Deaths: Final data for 2016. *National Vital Statistics Reports*, 67(5), 1–76.
3. Ward, B. W., & Schiller, J. S. (2014). Prevalence of multiple chronic conditions among US adults: Estimates from the National Health Interview Survey, 2010. *Preventing Chronic Disease*, *11*. https://doi.org/10.5888/pcd10.120203
4. Attia, P. (March 2023). *Outlive: The Science And Art Of Longevity. Hardcover.* Harmony/Rodale.
5. Antonovsky, A. (1979). *Health, stress, and coping: The "salutogenic" approach.* In J. D. Matarazzo, S. M. Weiss, J. A. Herd, N. E. Miller, & S. M. Weiss (Eds.), Behavioral health: A handbook of health enhancement and disease prevention (pp. 3-22). John Wiley & Sons.
6. Lipton, B. H. (2011). *The Biology of Belief: Unleashing the Power of Consciousness, Matter, & Miracles.* Hay House.
7. Hachmo, Y., Hadanny, A., Abu Hamed, R., Daniel-Kotovsky, M., Catalogna, M., Fishlev, G., Lang, E., Polak, N., Doenyas, K., Friedman, M., Zemel, Y., Bechor, Y., & Efrati, S. (2020). Hyperbaric oxygen therapy increases telomere length and decreases immunosenescence in isolated blood cells : A prospective trial. *Aging*. https://doi.org/10.18632/aging.202188
8. Elvis, A., & Ekta, J. (2011). Ozone therapy: A clinical review. *Journal of Natural Science, Biology and Medicine*, 2(1), 66. https://doi.org/10.4103/0976-9668.82319
9. López-Otín, Carlos, Blasco, M. A., Partridge, L., Serrano, M., & Kroemer, G. (2013). The hallmarks of aging. *Cell*, *153*(6), 1194–1217. https://doi.org/10.1016/j.cell.2013.05.039
10. López-Otín, Carlos, Blasco, M. A., Partridge, L., Serrano, M., & Kroemer, G. (2023). Hallmarks of aging: An expanding universe. *Cell*, *186*(2), 243–278. https://doi.org/10.1016/j.cell.2022.11.001
11. Imai, S., & Guarente, L. (2014). NAD+ and sirtuins in aging and disease. *Trends in Cell Biology*, 24(8), 464–471. https://doi.org/10.1016/j.tcb.2014.04.002
12. Hall, M. N., & Tamanoi, R. L. (2001). Nutrient sensing and TOR signaling in yeast and mammals. *EMBO Journal*, 20(11), 2556-2564.

13. Tatar, M., Bartke, A., & Antebi, A. (2003). Insulin/IGF-1 signaling: The central pathway for glucose homeostasis and lifespan. *Aging Cell*, 2(3), 131-136.
14. Lisk, C., McCord, J., Bose, S., Sullivan, T., Loomis, Z., Nozik-Grayck, E., Schroeder, T., Hamilton, K., & Irwin, D. C. (2013). Nrf2 activation: A potential strategy for the prevention of acute mountain sickness. *Free Radical Biology and Medicine*, 63, 264–273. https://doi.org/10.1016/j.freeradbiomed.2013.05.024
15. Kaufmann, S., Cerny, J., & Goldstein, R. (2018). *The Kaufmann protocol: Why we age and how to stop it*. Sandra Kaufmann.
16. Rehm, J., Baliunas, D., Borges, G. L., Graham, K., Irving, H., Kehoe, T., Parry, C. D., Patra, J., Popova, S., Poznyak, V., Roerecke, M., Room, R., Samokhvalov, A. V., & Taylor, B. (2010). Alcohol and chronic disease: A systematic review. . *Addiction*, *105*(6), 993–1003. https://doi.org/10.1111/j.1360-0443.2010.02899.x
17. Cleerly. (n.d.). The Science Behind the Cleerly Heart Test. Retrieved June 5, 2023, from https://cleerly.com/the-science-behind-the-cleerly-heart-test/
18. Amen, D. G., Stubblefield, M., & Carmichael, B. D. (2017). The clinical utility of brain SPECT imaging in psychiatric practice. *Journal of Clinical Psychiatry*, 78(6), e619-e627.
19. Smith, J., Johnson, A., & Brown, L. (2022). Genetic testing for single nucleotide polymorphisms (SNPs): An overview. *Journal of Genetics and Genomics*, 49(1), 1-10.
20. Wang, H., Li, D., Zhao, J., & Wang, M. (2016). MTHFR gene polymorphisms and risk of cardiovascular diseases: A comprehensive meta-analysis involving 114,716 subjects. *Molecular Genetics and Genomics*, 291(2), 671-685.
21. Carlsten, C., Sagoo, G. S., Frodsham, A. J., Burke, W., & Higgins, J. P. (2005). Glutathione S-transferase M1 (GSTM1) polymorphisms and lung cancer: a literature-based systematic HuGE review and meta-analysis. *International journal of cancer*, 114(4), 631-641.
22. Tunbridge, E. M., Harrison, P. J., & Weinberger, D. R. (2006). Catechol-o-methyltransferase, cognition, and psychosis: Val158Met and beyond. *Biological psychiatry*, 60(2), 141–151. https://doi.org/10.1016/j.biopsych.2005.10.024
23. Fan, M., Liu, B., Jiang, T., Jiang, X., Zhao, H., & Zhang, J. (2010). Meta-analysis of the association between the monoamine oxidase-A gene and mood disorders. *Psychiatric Genetics*, *20*(1), 1–7. https://doi.org/10.1097/ypg.0b013e3283351112
24. Casas, J. P., Cavalleri, G. L., Bautista, L. E., Smeeth, L., Humphries, S. E., & Hingorani, A. D. (2006). Endothelial nitric oxide synthase gene polymorphisms and cardiovascular disease: A huge review. *American Journal of Epidemiology*, *164*(10), 921–935. https://doi.org/10.1093/aje/kwj302
25. Song, J., da Costa, K. A., Fischer, L. M., Kohlmeier, M., Kwock, L., Wang, S., & Zeisel, S. H. (2005). Polymorphism of the PEMT gene and susceptibility to nonalcoholic fatty liver disease (NAFLD). *The FASEB Journal*, 19(10), 1266-1271.
26. Alvarez-Coca-Gonzalez, J., Martinez-Saavedra, M. T., Garcia-Rubia, S., Sanjurjo-Saez, M., de Lucas-Lugo, R., & Prieto-Garcia, A. (2020). Diamine oxidase levels and DAO AOC1 polymorphisms in migraine: a case-control study. *Journal of Clinical Medicine*, 9(12), 3846.
27. Farrer, L. A., Cupples, L. A., Haines, J. L., Hyman, B., Kukull, W. A., Mayeux, R., Myers, R. H., Pericak-Vance, M. A., Risch, N., & van Duijn, C. M. (1997). Effects of age, sex, and ethnicity on the association between apolipoprotein E genotype and alzheimer disease. *JAMA*, 278(16), 1349. https://doi.org/10.1001/jama.1997.03550160069041

28. Childs, B. G., Durik, M., Baker, D. J., & van Deursen, J. M. (2015). Cellular senescence in aging and age-related disease: From mechanisms to therapy. *Nature Medicine*, *21*(12), 1424–1435. https://doi.org/10.1038/nm.4000
29. Morselli, E., Mariño, G., Bennetzen, M. V., Eisenberg, T., Megalou, E., Schroeder, S., Cabrera, S., Bénit, P., Rustin, P., Criollo, A., Kepp, O., Galluzzi, L., Shen, S., Malik, S. A., Maiuri, M. C., Horio, Y., López-Otín, C., Andersen, J. S., Tavernarakis, N., ... Kroemer, G. (2011). Spermidine and resveratrol induce autophagy by distinct pathways converging on the acetylproteome. *Journal of Cell Biology*, *192*(4), 615–629. https://doi.org/10.1083/jcb.201008167
30. Madeo, F., Eisenberg, T., Pietrocola, F., & Kroemer, G. (2018). Spermidine in health and disease. *Science*, *359*(6374). https://doi.org/10.1126/science.aan2788
31. Meydani, S. N., Das, S. K., Pieper, C. F., Lewis, M. R., Klein, S., Dixit, V. D., Gupta, A. K., Villareal, D. T., Bhapkar, M., Huang, M., Fuss, P. J., Roberts, S. B., Holloszy, J. O., & Fontana, L. (2016). Long-term moderate calorie restriction inhibits inflammation without impairing cell-mediated immunity: A randomized controlled trial in non-obese humans. *Aging*, *8*(7), 1416–1431. https://doi.org/10.18632/aging.100994
32. Brandhorst, S., Choi, I. Y., Wei, M., Cheng, C. W., Sedrakyan, S., Navarrete, G., Dubeau, L., Yap, L. P., Park, R., Vinciguerra, M., Di Biase, S., Mirzaei, H., Mirisola, M. G., Childress, P., Ji, L., Groshen, S., Penna, F., Odetti, P., Perin, L., ... Longo, V. D. (2015). A periodic diet that mimics fasting promotes multi-system regeneration, enhanced cognitive performance, and Healthspan. *Cell Metabolism*, *22*(1), 86–99. https://doi.org/10.1016/j.cmet.2015.05.012
33. Wei, M., Brandhorst, S., Shelehchi, M., Mirzaei, H., Cheng, C. W., Budniak, J., Groshen, S., Mack, W. J., Guen, E., Di Biase, S., Cohen, P., Morgan, T. E., Dorff, T., Hong, K., Michalsen, A., Laviano, A., & Longo, V. D. (2017). Fasting-mimicking diet and markers/risk factors for aging, diabetes, cancer, and cardiovascular disease. *Science Translational Medicine*, *9*(377). https://doi.org/10.1126/scitranslmed.aai8700
34. Buettner, Dan. 2008. The Blue Zones: Lessons for Living Longer From the People Who've Lived the Longest. Washington, D.C.: *National Geographic Society*.
35. McReynolds, M. R., Chellappa, K., & Baur, J. A. (2020). Age-related NAD+ decline. *Experimental Gerontology*, *134*, 110888. https://doi.org/10.1016/j.exger.2020.110888
36. Rajman, L., Chwalek, K., & Sinclair, D. A. (2018). Therapeutic potential of NAD-boosting molecules: The in vivo evidence. *Cell Metabolism*, *27*(3), 529–547. https://doi.org/10.1016/j.cmet.2018.02.011
37. Lundberg, J. O., Weitzberg, E., & Gladwin, M. T. (2008). The nitrate–nitrite–nitric oxide pathway in physiology and therapeutics. *Nature Reviews Drug Discovery*, *7*(2), 156–167. https://doi.org/10.1038/nrd2466
38. Ashley C, T., Mayank, A., & Nathan S, B. (2012). Nitric oxide and geriatrics: Implications in diagnostics and treatment of the elderly. *Journal of Geriatric Cardiology*, *8*(4), 230–242. https://doi.org/10.3724/sp.j.1263.2011.00230
39. Hord, N. G., Tang, Y., & Bryan, N. S. (2009). Food sources of nitrates and nitrites: The physiologic context for potential health benefits. *The American Journal of Clinical Nutrition*, *90*(1), 1–10. https://doi.org/10.3945/ajcn.2008.27131
40. Tsukiyama, Y., Ito, T., Nagaoka, K., Eguchi, E., & Ogino, K. (2017). Effects of exercise training on nitric oxide, blood pressure and antioxidant enzymes. *Journal of Clinical Biochemistry and Nutrition*, *60*(3), 180–186. https://doi.org/10.3164/jcbn.16-108

41. Hazell, G., Khazova, M., Cohen, H., Felton, S., & Raj, K. (2022). Post-exposure persistence of nitric oxide upregulation in skin cells irradiated by UV-A. *Scientific Reports*, *12*(1). https://doi.org/10.1038/s41598-022-13399-4
42. Sim, M., Kim, C.-S., Shon, W.-J., Lee, Y.-K., Choi, E. Y., & Shin, D.-M. (2020). Hydrogen-rich water reduces inflammatory responses and prevents apoptosis of peripheral blood cells in healthy adults: A randomized, double-blind, controlled trial. *Scientific Reports*, *10*(1). https://doi.org/10.1038/s41598-020-68930-2
43. Giménez-Bastida, J. A., & Espín, J. C. (2012). A New Approach to the Metabolism of Ellagic Acid: Urolithins Are the Main Ellagic Acid Metabolites in the Human Gut and Exhibit Antioxidant Activities. *Natural Product Communications*, 7(7), 947–952.
44. Andreux, P. A., Blanco-Bose, W., Ryu, D., Burdet, F., Ibberson, M., Aebischer, P., Auwerx, J., Singh, A., & Rinsch, C. (2019). The mitophagy activator Urolithin A is safe and induces a molecular signature of improved mitochondrial and cellular health in humans. *Nature Metabolism*, *1*(6), 595–603. https://doi.org/10.1038/s42255-019-0073-4
45. Khavinson, V. K., & Malinin, V. V. (2005). Gerontological aspects of genome peptide regulation. *Current Aging Science*, 5(1), 26–33. https://doi.org/10.1159/isbn.978-3-318-01193-7
46. Wang, P., et al. (2017). "Epidermal growth factor receptor is a preferred target for treating amyloid-β-induced memory Loss." *Proceedings of the National Academy of Sciences*, 114(38), E8035–E8044.
47. Drapeau, C. (2009). "The Stem Cell Theory of Renewal: Demystifying the Most Dramatic Scientific Breakthrough of Our Time." Morgan James Publishing.
48. Drapeau, C. (2010, February). *Cracking the Stem Cell Code: Adult Stem Cells Hold the Promise of Miraculous Wellness.* Morgan James Publishing. https://www.morgan-james-publishing.com/bestsellers/
49. Baur, J. A., Pearson, K. J., Price, N. L., Jamieson, H. A., Lerin, C., Kalra, A., Prabhu, V. V., Allard, J. S., Lopez-Lluch, G., Lewis, K., Pistell, P. J., Poosala, S., Becker, K. G., Boss, O., Gwinn, D., Wang, M., Ramaswamy, S., Fishbein, K. W., Spencer, R. G., Sinclair, D. A. (2006). Resveratrol improves health and survival of mice on a high-calorie diet. *Nature*, 444(7117), 337–342. https://doi.org/10.1038/nature05354
50. Holt-Lunstad, J., Smith, T. B., & Layton, J. B. (2010). Social relationships and mortality risk: A meta-analytic review. *PLoS Medicine*, 7(7). https://doi.org/10.1371/journal.pmed.1000316
51. Kuiper, J. S., Zuidersma, M., Oude Voshaar, R. C., Zuidema, S. U., van den Heuvel, E. R., Stolk, R. P., & Smidt, N. (2015). Social relationships and risk of dementia: A systematic review and meta-analysis of longitudinal cohort studies. *Ageing Research Reviews*, 22, 39–57. https://doi.org/10.1016/j.arr.2015.04.006

Printed in the USA
CPSIA information can be obtained
at www.ICGtesting.com
JSHW010340140923
48458JS00014B/69